Pathology Facts

Richard C. Harruff, M.D., Ph.D.

Associate Medical Examiner
King County Medical Examiner Division
Division of Public Health
Seattle, Washington

formerly
Associate Professor of Pathology
Indiana University School of Medicine
Indianapolis, Indiana

Contributing Author
Ruth L. Viste, M.D.

Pathologist
Calumet Public Hospital
Laurium, Michigan

J.B. Lippincott Company
Philadelphia

Acquisitions Editor: Richard Winters
Sponsoring Editor: Jody Schott
Production Editor: Virginia Barishek
Indexer: M.L. Coughlin
Production: Berliner, Inc.
Printer/Binder: R.R. Donnelley & Sons Company / Crawfordsville

6 5 4 3

Library of Congress Cataloging-in-Publication Data

Harruff, Richard Charles, 1949-
    Pathology facts / Richard C. Harruff, contributing author [for]
Infectious diseases, Ruth Viste.
        p.   cm.
    Includes bibliographical references.
    ISBN 0-397-51258-9
    1. Pathology—Outlines, syllabi, etc. I. Viste, Ruth.
II. Title.
    [DNLM 1. Pathology—handbooks. QZ 39 H323p 1994]
RB32.H37 1994
616.07—dc20
DNLM/DLC
for Library of Congress   93-7717
                                                                    CIP

Preface

This book is designed as an educational tool for the student of pathology to assist in mastering the large amount of knowledge required for a basic understanding of human diseases. It presents the major topics of general pathology, infectious diseases, and systemic pathology in a concise and highly organized manner. The book is not intended to serve as a textbook but rather as a resource that assists the student in developing and organizing a personal knowledge base of pathology.

Because this book is not a standard textbook, it is necessary to describe its organization. There are three sections: General Pathology, Infectious Diseases, and Systemic Pathology. In the first section, each of the major concepts regarding general pathology are summarized in accordance with four categories, as follows: brief description of the concept, the causes and pathophysiologic mechanisms involved, morphologic features, and clinical correlations.

In the second and third sections, each page describes one disease process, with the information presented in a condensed format and organized under a consistent set of nineteen categories that cover epidemiology, etiology, pathogenesis, morphology, and clinical features. At the beginning of the chapters, the diseases are listed according to pathologic processes, and within the chapter they are arranged alphabetically.

In order to limit the size of this volume, it was necessary to be selective in the topics covered. In general, entries are limited to the most common diseases. Uncommon and rare diseases are included if they represent an especially distinctive aspect of etiology, pathogenesis, or morphology. Clinical information regarding each disease is included for purposes of showing the student the correspondence between pathology and clinical medicine. The few comments regarding treatment of disease are provided only as general guidelines; for specific therapy, standard textbooks of medicine need to be consulted.

Owing to its concise and highly ordered manner of presentation, this book should be a valuable resource for students of pathology, both during their formal course and later when they need to review. Students of pathology quickly learn that there is a vast amount of knowledge that they must acquire, and the most successful students are those that efficiently organize their personal knowledge base. The authors hope that this book will assist students to that goal.

Richard C. Harruff

Contents

General Pathology

Pathology Facts, by Richard C.
Harruff, J.B. Lippincott
Company, Philadelphia © 1994.

Chapter 1

Necrosis and
Cellular Adaptation

Necrosis

DESCRIPTION
Necrosis refers to a set of morphologic changes that accompany cell death within a living body. Coagulative necrosis is the basic and most common type of necrosis. In other types of necrosis, additional cellular changes occur that modify the processes of coagulative necrosis to produce distinctive morphologic patterns; these include: liquefactive necrosis, gangrenous necrosis, caseous necrosis, fat necrosis, and fibrinoid necrosis. Necrosis differs from autolysis, which is the process of cell death outside a living body.

CAUSES AND PATHOPHYSIOLOGIC MECHANISMS
Ischemia (loss of blood supply) is the most common cause of coagulative necrosis. Virus infections, physical injury (heat, cold, ionizing radiation), and toxins also cause coagulative necrosis. Liquefactive necrosis is a consequence of suppuration and abscesses; it is also the type of necrosis that occurs in the central nervous system. Gangrenous necrosis (gangrene) is the type of necrosis that affects an extremity or intestine. Caseous necrosis is typical of tuberculosis. Fat necrosis results from injury or inflammation of the pancreas or from trauma to adipose tissue. Fibrinoid necrosis occurs with immunological injuries of blood vessels.

Coagulative necrosis due to ischemia   With the absence of oxygen, oxidative phosphorylation ceases, ATP becomes depleted, and membrane functions fail. Calcium leaks out of mitochondria and cytosolic calcium rises. Phospholipases and proteases are activated by the calcium, and these enzymes digest membrane lipids and cytoskeletal components. The net result is loss of ion gradients, breakdown of cellular membranes, and denaturation of cellular proteins. Reperfusion of ischemic tissue compounds the damage by generating reactive oxygen-derived free radicals that react with membrane lipids.

Coagulative necrosis due to drugs, chemicals, viruses, and free radicals   Many chemicals and heavy metals are directly cytotoxic by their reaction with cellular lipids, proteins, or DNA. Other chemicals become cytotoxic after initial metabolism by the hepatic P-450 mixed function oxidase, which generates reactive intermediates, particularly free radicals. Viruses are cytopathic directly, due to the effects of the intracellular infection; and indirectly, due to the effects of the immune system. Ionizing radiation generates hydroxyl free radicals from cytosolic water. Free radicals damage cellular constituents by peroxidation of lipids, proteins, and DNA. Inflammatory reactions also generate oxygen-derived free radicals.

Liquefactive necrosis   Lytic enzymes released by PMNs digest and liquefy all cellular material in regions of intense acute inflammation (suppuration). Devitalized central nervous system tissue liquefies because of its composition and its high content of autolytic enzymes.

Gangrenous necrosis (gangrene)   This is a result of putrefactive bacteria acting on necrotic bowel or extremity; the bacteria metabolize blood to a green-black pigment and generate foul-smelling gases.

Caseous necrosis   Typical of tuberculosis; the waxy cell wall constituents of the mycobacteria are responsible for this variant of necrosis.

Fat necrosis   Lipases released from injured pancreas digest the surrounding fat to form free fatty acids and glycerol. A similar process occurs after crushing injuries of adipose tissue.

Fibrinoid necrosis   Fibrin and other plasma proteins are trapped within damaged vessel walls. The trapped proteins stain strongly eosinophilic, producing a distinctive morphologic change.

MORPHOLOGY
Coagulative necrosis   Grossly, a pale soft area in an organ or tissue; microscopically, cells are eosinophilic "ghost" figures lacking nuclei and cytoplasmic detail. Nuclei degenerate by pyknosis (contraction), karyorrhexis (fragmentation) or karyolysis (gradual fading of stain intensity).

Liquefactive necrosis Due to suppuration: dense accumulation of PMNs intermixed with cellular debris. In brain: discoloration and softening gradually disintegrating into a thick fluid.

Gangrenous necrosis Green-black discoloration and putrid odor; either wet or dry.

Caseous necrosis Grossly: resembles cottage cheese; microscopically: acellular, amorphous, granular eosinophilic debris.

Fat necrosis Grossly, whitish-yellow with a firm, dense texture and focal gritty calcifications; microscopically, digested fat and numerous foamy macrophages containing lipid

CLINICAL CORRELATIONS
Necrosis occurs in infarcts of any organ (e.g., myocardial infarct) as well as in infections, physical injury, immune reactions, and drug and chemical injury. The major consequence is the loss of function of an organ or tissue; inflammation is another consequence. After a cell becomes necrotic, enzymes leak from its cytoplasm and gain access to the blood; this provides the basis for detecting necrosis by laboratory tests. For example, elevations of creatine kinase, lactic dehydrogenase, and aspartate aminotransferase in serum are diagnostic of myocardial infarction.

Atrophy

DESCRIPTION
A reversible adaptive response to various injurious conditions that are insufficient to cause necrosis, characterized by decreased size and number of cells and reduction of mass and function of an organ or tissue.

CAUSES AND PATHOPHYSIOLOGIC MECHANISMS
Reduced functional demand (disuse, immobilization); gradual decrease in blood supply (chronic ischemia); starvation and malnutrition; denervation; loss of trophic hormones; chronic cell injury (toxins, pressure, chronic inflammation); aging. Cells deprived of oxygen or nutrients decrease in volume and lose their specialized functions. This also occurs in endocrine-responsive tissue with loss of trophic hormones and in skeletal muscle with loss of motor innervation. Chronic injury produces several effects: ischemia due to alterations of blood supply (e.g., fibrosis), deprivation of nutrients, pressure effects, and cellular toxins including free radicals. The effects of aging are multifactorial.

MORPHOLOGY
The affected organ or tissue is reduced in size and weight; the constituent parenchymal cells are decreased in size and number.

Chronic inflammation and chronic ischemia produce fibrosis. In skeletal muscle atrophy there is fatty replacement of muscle.

CLINICAL CORRELATIONS
Usually pathologic; occasionally physiologic (e.g., ovarian and endometrial atrophy following menopause). Pituitary lesions cause atrophy of gonads, thyroid, and adrenal cortex. Disuse, immobilization, strokes, and prolonged bed rest cause muscle and skeletal atrophy. Spinal cord and peripheral nerve lesions cause denervation atrophy of muscle. Fatty replacement of atrophic muscle in muscular dystrophy produces pseudohypertrophy. Atherosclerosis produces ischemic atrophy of muscle, kidney, and heart.

Hypertrophy

DESCRIPTION
A reversible adaptive response to exercise, functional demand, and hormonal stimulation, characterized by increased size of cells and mass of organ or tissue; may be either physiologic or pathologic.

CAUSES AND PATHOPHYSIOLOGIC MECHANISMS
Chemical signals mediate cellular enlargement by stimulating gene expression of synthetic enzymes. In tissues composed of cells capable of proliferation, hyperplasia occurs as well as hypertrophy. Skeletal and cardiac muscles are incapable of proliferation and enlarge by hypertrophy alone.

MORPHOLOGY
Cells are larger than normal, but their number remains constant. Skeletal and cardiac muscle fibers are increased in diameter.

CLINICAL CORRELATIONS
Exercise causes physiologic hypertrophy of skeletal muscle. Anabolic steroids are abused by athletes to stimulate skeletal muscle hypertrophy. Hypertension causes pathologic hypertrophy of cardiac muscle.

Hyperplasia

DESCRIPTION
A reversible adaptive response to functional demand, endocrine stimulation, and chronic inflammation or irritation, characterized by cellular proliferation that results in increased mass of organ or tissue; may be either physiologic or pathologic.

CAUSES AND PATHOPHYSIOLOGIC MECHANISMS

Occurs only in tissues where parenchymal cells are capable of mitotic division. Growth factors stimulate protein and DNA synthesis and cell division. Hyperplasia often occurs in combination with hypertrophy.

MORPHOLOGY

The number of cells is increased, and the tissue is hypercellular. During proliferation, mitotic figures are common; cells are small and appear crowded. The organ or tissue increases in size.

CLINICAL CORRELATIONS

Physiologic hyperplasia: Genital maturation during puberty; hyperplasia of breast lobules during pregnancy; hyperplasia of endometrium during the menstrual cycle. Granulocytic hyperplasia of the bone marrow is a response to bacterial infections; viral infections stimulate lymphocytic hyperplasia. Healing depends on hyperplasia for repair of injured tissue. *Pathologic hyperplasia:* abnormal endometrial hyperplasia occurs in anovulatory cycles and after menopause when there is excess estrogen without periodic cycling. Excess estrogen in males causes gynecomastia. Adrenocortical hyperplasia due to excess ACTH from a pituitary adenoma causes hypersecretion of cortisol and Cushing's syndrome. Parathyroid hyperplasia due to hypocalcemia causes bone resorption. Erythropoietin stimulates erythroid hyperplasia in response to hypoxia due to chronic lung disease or congenital heart disease. A skin callus represents epidermal hyperplasia produced by chronic irritation. *Differentiation of hyperplasia from neoplasia:* hyperplasia differs from neoplasia by being dependent on an extrinsic stimulus; in neoplasia there is cellular proliferation without an extrinsic stimulus.

Metaplasia

DESCRIPTION

A reversible adaptive response to persistent injury, in which one mature cell type is replaced by another.

CAUSES AND PATHOPHYSIOLOGIC MECHANISMS

Cells subjected to chronic infection or inflammation, exposure to toxins, and physical irritation acquire more resistant properties (e.g., keratin synthesis) and lose their specialized functions (e.g., secretory capabilities, presence of cilia). Metaplasia often occurs along with hyperplasia.

MORPHOLOGY

In squamous metaplasia, layers of cuboidal or flat epithelial cells lacking secretory vacuoles and cilia occupy sites normally covered by columnar cells. In goblet cell metaplasia occurring in bronchioles, mucus-secreting goblet cells are present where there should be none. Intestinal metaplasia is characterized by the presence of intestinal type mucosa in the stomach. In Barrett's esophagus, mucus-secreting columnar epithelium lines the distal third of the esophagus. Cystitis glandularis shows islands of glandular mucosa replacing regions of transitional epithelium in the urinary bladder.

CLINICAL CORRELATIONS
Squamous metaplasia is often present in Pap smears as a normal finding around the cervical os in sexually active women. It also occurs in the larynx and bronchi of smokers. Goblet cell metaplasia, another condition of smokers, plays a role in the pathogenesis of chronic obstructive lung disease. Intestinal metaplasia occurs with chronic gastritis. Barrett's esophagus is a result of chronic esophagitis. Cystitis glandularis is often present in chronic cystitis. Although metaplasia is not necessarily a precursor of cancer, neoplasms do develop at the same sites as metaplasia.

Dysplasia

DESCRIPTION
Disordered cellular growth and maturation that may be partly adaptive but is also a manifestation of genetic damage. Dysplasia may resolve after removal of the stimulus or persist and progress to a malignant neoplasm.

CAUSES AND PATHOPHYSIOLOGIC MECHANISMS
Stimuli producing hyperplasia and metaplasia, combined with exposure to a carcinogenic agent, may cause genetic damage and loss of control of cell growth, differentiation, and maturation. Dysplasia is a step in the transformation to neoplasia. It is often not reversible after the causative stimulus is removed. *Specific examples:* cervical dysplasia associated with human papilloma virus infection; actinic keratosis due to excessive long-term exposure to sunlight; bronchial dysplasia caused by aromatic hydrocarbons in cigarette smoke; oral mucosal dysplasia associated with smokeless tobacco; gastric mucosal dysplasia in chronic gastritis; epithelial dysplasia in ulcerative colitis.

MORPHOLOGY
In squamous dysplasia, there is disordered cellular maturation, with immature basal cells and mitoses present in upper levels of the epithelium. Other features are cellular pleomorphism, increased nuclear/cytoplasmic ratio, and nuclear hyperchromatism. Grossly, cervical dysplasia is not apparent. Actinic keratosis presents a scaly red lesion of sun-exposed skin. Dysplasia of oral mucosa or vulva may appear as white plaques (leukoplakia).

CLINICAL CORRELATIONS

Cervical dysplasia and carcinoma-in-situ are stages of cervical intraepithelial neoplasia, which may progress to invasive carcinoma. Squamous dysplasia also involves bronchus, skin, vulva and oral mucosa; in each site it is considered precancerous. Dysplasia also occurs in glandular epithelium (stomach, colon). Removal of dysplastic epithelium wherever it occurs successfully prevents cancer.

Pathology Facts, by Richard C.
Harruff, J.B. Lippincott
Company, Philadelphia © 1994.

Chapter 2

Hemodynamic Disorders

Edema and Congestion

DESCRIPTION
Edema is the accumulation of excessive fluid within the interstitial tissues or within body cavities. Congestion is the accumulation of excessive blood within the blood vessels of an organ or
tissue.

CAUSES AND PATHOPHYSIOLOGIC MECHANISMS
Localized congestion   Venous thrombosis, twisting of a mobile
vein, extrinsic compression. Cirrhosis produces congestion within
the portal venous system.

Generalized congestion   Right heart failure causes congestion in
the lower extremities and abdominal viscera; left heart failure
produces pulmonary congestion. Congestive heart failure occurs
when both sides of the heart fail.

Edema due to increased hydrostatic pressure   Increased pressure
due to congestion within capillaries forces fluid through the endothelial barrier into the interstitial tissues. Right heart failure
produces peripheral edema; left heart failure produces pulmonary edema. Gravitational forces further increase hydrostatic
pressure in the dependent portions of the body.

Edema due to reduced oncotic pressure   With hypoproteinemia
(hypoalbuminemia) the osmotic pressure of plasma is inadequate
to counterbalance normal hydrostatic pressure, and fluid leaks
from blood vessels into the interstitial space. Hypoproteinemia is
caused by excessive loss of protein in the urine (nephrotic syndrome), inadequate production of albumin by the liver, malnutrition, and certain protein-losing gastrointestinal diseases.

Lymphedema Lymphatic vessels normally return to the circulation the slight amount of fluid that leaks from blood vessels. Causes of lymphedema: obliteration of lymphatic vessels by inflammation, surgery, or radiation therapy; obstruction of lymphatics by neoplasm.

Cerebral edema Increased vascular permeability (vasogenic edema), cellular swelling (cytotoxic edema), and obstruction to the flow of cerebrospinal fluid (hydrocephalus).

Inflammatory edema Increased vascular permeability, resulting from endothelial damage, causes edema in inflammation.

MORPHOLOGY
Congestion Grossly, dark red (cyanotic) and bloody organs; microscopically, red cells distend blood vessels. "Nutmeg liver" refers to an enlarged liver with centrilobular congestion. "Heart-failure cells" (hemosiderin-laden macrophages in alveoli) characterize congested lung. Fibrotic nodules containing hemosiderin (Gamna-Gandy bodies) are features of congested spleen.

Peripheral edema In heart failure, dependent "pitting edema" appears at the ankles and feet in an ambulatory patient (pedal edema) or at the lower back in a bedridden patient (presacral edema). With hypoproteinemia, edema is not dependent but collects in loose tissues (periorbital edema). Anasarca refers to massive generalized edema. Elephantiasis describes extreme edema of the legs.

Pulmonary edema Frothy white or pink fluid exudes from bronchi and cut surfaces of lung; this same froth comes from the nose and mouth of a patient dying with pulmonary edema. Microscopically, there is acellular, hyaline, eosinophilic residue within alveoli.

Effusions The fluid is thin, clear, and straw-colored and has a low specific gravity and protein content (transudate).

CLINICAL CORRELATIONS
Heart failure This is a condition produced by many heart diseases: ischemic heart disease, hypertensive heart disease, valvular heart disease, myocarditis, and cardiomyopathy. Usually the left ventricle fails first, soon followed by right-sided failure. In congestive heart failure, pulmonary edema causes hypoxia and shortness of breath that is worse when lying flat (orthopnea); the liver is enlarged; and dependent edema (pedal or presacral) is evident. Pure right heart failure is a result of lung disease (cor pulmonale).

Hypoproteinemia Certain diseases involving the renal glomerular basement membrane cause the nephrotic syndrome, characterized by heavy proteinuria, hypoproteinemia, and generalized edema. Cirrhosis is another cause of hypoproteinemia. Kwashiorkor is the condition of generalized edema in malnutrition.

Lymphedema This is sometimes present in the skin overlying a breast cancer, producing "peau d'orange." After mastectomy, lymphedema of the arm develops because of surgical disruption of axillary lymphatics; subsequent radiation therapy to the area worsens this effect. Filariasis causes elephantiasis.

Effusions Pleural effusions occur in heart failure and with intrathoracic tumors or inflammation. Large effusions limit full expansion of the lungs. Pericardial effusion causes cardiac tamponade. Ascites is peritoneal effusion developing in cirrhosis. Compared with a transudative effusion due to hemodynamic forces, an exudative effusion due to inflammation has a higher protein concentration, greater specific gravity, and greater number of inflammatory cells.

Cerebral edema Cerebral edema is a consequence of trauma, intracranial hemorrhage, infarcts, infection, neoplasms, hypoxia, and chemical or toxic injury. Increased intracranial pressure produced by the edema causes herniations. With herniation through the foramen magnum, compression of vital respiratory centers of the medulla is fatal.

Infarction

DESCRIPTION
An infarct is a localized region of necrosis caused by reduction of arterial perfusion below a level required for cell viability.

CAUSES AND PATHOPHYSIOLOGIC MECHANISMS
Arterial obstruction due to atherosclerosis, arterial thrombosis, or embolism causes ischemia that results in necrosis when oxygen supply fails to meet oxygen requirements of the tissue. Venous obstruction due to thrombosis, torsion, or strangulation produces ischemia by causing stagnation of blood and reducing arterial inflow.

Critical factors for infarction Major factors are the extent of vascular occlusion, the rate at which it develops, and the length of time it persists. Occlusion that is partial, develops gradually, or is relieved within several minutes may cause only reversible ischemia. Infarcts are more likely in organs with end-arteries (heart, kidney, spleen). Organs with a dual blood supply (lung, liver) or well-developed anastomoses (intestine) are less likely to develop infarcts. The heart has rudimentary anastomoses, and protective collateral blood flow develops if coronary stenosis progresses gradually. The cells most sensitive to ischemia are cerebral cortical neurons. Myocardial cells are also vulnerable; their vulnerability depends on the myocardial workload.

MORPHOLOGY

Gross features   Infarcts are either red (hemorrhagic) or pale (anemic). *Kidney and spleen infarcts* are wedge-shaped lesions with central pallor and peripheral redness; the base is toward the capsule, away from the blood supply. A *myocardial infarct* is a pale zone surrounded by a red border within the left ventricular wall. *Pulmonary infarcts* are wedge-shaped and hemorrhagic, due to the dual blood supply. *Intestinal infarcts* are initially red and swollen, then later turn black and gangrenous. A *cerebral infarct* is initially soft, swollen and discolored; it subsequently undergoes liquefactive necrosis. A *healed infarct* appears as a depressed and contracted region composed of fibrous scar tissue. Healed infarcts of brain are cystic cavities (cystic encephalomalacia).

Microscopic features   Coagulation necrosis occurs. Numerous red cells are present in red infarcts; pale infarcts show no hemorrhage except in the red border with normal tissue. With time, there is acute inflammation followed by healing, which starts at the periphery of the infarct and progresses inward. In a septic infarct, there is suppuration that produces an abscess.

CLINICAL CORRELATIONS

Myocardial infarcts are a consequence of coronary atherosclerosis; thrombosis may be superimposed. Bed rest effectively reduces the workload and oxygen demand of the myocardium and limits the size of an infarct. Myocardial infarcts cause sudden heart failure and death or weaken the heart to produce chronic congestive heart failure. *Cerebral infarcts* are the most frequent type of stroke. Atherosclerosis, followed by embolism, are the most common causes. Strokes result in rapid functional neurologic impairment, depending on the size of the infarct and the region involved. Pulmonary embolism causes *pulmonary infarction*. Because of the dual blood supply of the lung, arterial occlusion does not necessarily cause an infarct. With large pulmonary emboli, the patient dies before an infarct develops. Atherosclerosis, embolism, strangulated hernias, and volvulus cause *intestinal infarcts*. Gangrene develops rapidly and gram-negative bacteria enter the blood to cause septic shock and death. *Infarcts of the lower extremity* cause gangrene and require amputation. This is particularly common in diabetics. *Liver infarcts* are uncommon. *Infarcts of kidney and spleen* are most often embolic and clinically of minor significance, unless the embolus originates from infective endocarditis and causes an abscess. Septic emboli are common causes for abscesses of brain and lung.

Thrombosis and Embolism

DESCRIPTION
A thrombus is a solid mass of clotted blood within an intact blood vessel or chamber of the heart. An embolus is a mass of solid, liquid, or gas that moves within a blood vessel to lodge at a site distant from its place of origin. Most emboli are thromboemboli.

CAUSES AND PATHOPHYSIOLOGIC MECHANISMS
Major factors in thrombosis and thromboembolism Thrombosis results from pathologic activation of the hemostatic mechanisms involving platelets, coagulation factors, and blood vessel walls. Endothelial injury, alteration in blood flow (stasis and turbulence), and hypercoagulability of the blood promote thrombosis and thromboembolism.

Consequences of a thrombus Dissolution due to the fibrinolytic system; organization and recanalization or incorporation into the vessel wall; embolization. The whole thrombus may detach to form a large embolus or fragments may break off to generate small emboli.

Pulmonary embolism and systemic (arterial) embolism Pulmonary emboli originate from thrombi in deep leg veins that detach and migrate through the vena cava and right heart to lodge in pulmonary arteries. Systemic emboli originate from a mural thrombus in the heart or aorta or from aortic or mitral valve vegetations of endocarditis; they lodge in the distal systemic arteries to produce infarcts.

Other types of embolism Traumatic injuries, especially those with fractured bones, cause fat embolism by mechanical disruption of bone marrow fat and by alterations in plasma lipids. Bubbles of air or gas in the blood are other forms of embolism. Any foreign body can cause an embolus if it gains access to the circulation.

MORPHOLOGY
An arterial thrombus shows alternating red and white laminations (lines of Zahn). Venous thrombi are more uniformly red; the lines are indistinct. Microscopically, there are platelet aggregates and a fibrin meshwork containing entrapped red cells and leukocytes. Organization starts at the periphery of the thrombus, adjacent to the vessel wall. Arterial and venous thrombi are usually occlusive. A mural thrombus is a nonocclusive mass of blood clot, with prominent yellow and red laminations, attached to the luminal surface of the heart or aorta.

Pulmonary emboli The largest ones form a "saddle embolus" across the bifurcation of the main pulmonary artery. Smaller thromboemboli lodge within distal pulmonary arteries; these are usually multiple and produce pulmonary hemorrhages or infarcts.

Arterial emboli These are generally small and are most easily recognized by the infarcts they produce. A septic embolus from infective endocarditis produces an abscess.

Thrombus versus postmortem clot A blood clot formed after death shows only two layers: an upper pale layer resembling chicken fat and a lower red layer resembling currant jelly. There are no lines of Zahn.

Fat emboli These are not visualized by routine histologic methods and require frozen sections stained with fat stains (Oil Red O).

CLINICAL CORRELATIONS

Conditions predisposing to thrombosis Atherosclerosis is the most important contributor to arterial thrombosis. Conditions predisposing to venous thrombosis include heart failure, extensive tissue damage (trauma, surgery, burns), bed rest and immobilization, cancer, hematologic diseases, pregnancy, oral contraceptives, hyperlipidemia, nephrotic syndrome, age, obesity, and smoking. Mural thrombosis complicates myocardial infarction, atrial fibrillation, and atherosclerosis of the abdominal aorta. Thrombus constitutes the vegetations on cardiac valves in infective endocarditis, nonbacterial thrombotic endocarditis, and Libman-Sacks endocarditis of SLE. Thrombosis is one complication of prosthetic cardiac valves.

Infarcts secondary to arterial thrombosis and systemic embolism Myocardial infarct, cerebral infarct (stroke), intestinal infarct, and gangrene of leg are consequences of arterial thrombosis. Arterial embolism from mural thrombi and from valve vegetations cause infarcts in brain, kidney, spleen, intestine, and extremities. Prophylactic anticoagulation with warfarin reduces the risk of thrombosis and embolism in patients with chronic atrial fibrillation and abnormal or prosthetic cardiac valves.

Pulmonary embolism This is the most common cause of sudden death in hospitalized patients. Thrombi in deep leg veins are the source of most pulmonary emboli; thrombosis of superficial veins is not a factor. Massive pulmonary embolism (saddle embolus) causes sudden death; smaller emboli cause pulmonary infarcts. The predisposing conditions are the same as for venous thrombosis. High-risk patients require preventative measures, such as exercise, early ambulation, and prophylactic anticoagulation. Pulmonary embolism occurs suddenly, without warning; nuclear ventilation-perfusion scans and pulmonary arteriography are methods to confirm the diagnosis.

Treatment of thrombosis Anticoagulation with heparin prevents further thrombosis and allows the plasmin fibrinolytic system to dissolve formed thrombi. Pharmacologic fibrinolysis with streptokinase, urokinase, and tissue plasminogen activator is effective for arterial thrombosis and pulmonary embolism.

Fat embolism syndrome This occurs a few days after trauma, particularly with multiple fractures, and carries a high mortality. Shortness of breath, hypoxia, and showers of petechiae are presenting signs; fat globules in the urine confirm the diagnosis.

Air and gas embolism A defect in a large neck vein, from trauma or surgery, can allow air to enter the circulation and embolize to the right heart; a defective infusion pump can also cause air embolism. Fatalities occur with 100–150 ml of air. Nitrogen gas embolism causes decompression sickness, a hazard of underwater diving with pressurized air.

Shock

DESCRIPTION
Shock consists of a set of hemodynamic changes that diminish blood flow below a level that provides adequate oxygen for the metabolic needs of organs and tissues.

CAUSES AND PATHOPHYSIOLOGIC MECHANISMS
Major categories of shock: hypovolemic, cardiogenic, and septic. Hemorrhage, dehydration, vomiting, diarrhea, and fluid loss from burns cause hypovolemic shock. Myocardial infarction is the usual cause of cardiogenic shock. Septicemia complicating infections by gram-negative bacteria and, less often, gram-positive bacteria cause septic shock. Neurogenic shock is a minor category of shock that results from injury to the central nervous system. Anaphylactic shock occurs with severe allergic reactions.

Hypovolemic shock Intravascular blood or fluid loss greater than 10–15% of the total blood volume produces shock. In early *compensated shock,* there is increased heart rate, cardiac contractility, and vasoconstriction of arteries and arterioles acting to maintain blood pressure and tissue perfusion. Vasoconstriction maintains blood pressure by increasing arterial resistance and reducing blood flow to all tissues, except heart and brain. Prolonged vasoconstriction produces tissue hypoxia, leading to *decompensated shock* as vasodilatation supervenes. Blood pressure falls and all organs are poorly perfused, including heart and brain. Without rapid correction of the hemodynamic deterioration, *irreversible shock* develops and the patient dies.

Cardiogenic shock With primary pump failure, cardiac function is insufficient to maintain tissue perfusion. Initial compensatory vasoconstriction acts to maintain the blood pressure but stresses the weakened myocardium. Decompensated and irreversible shock develop rapidly.

Septic shock Endotoxin from gram-negative bacteria in the blood causes generalized vasodilatation and altered vascular permeability, resulting in intractable hypotension and fluid loss into the interstitium. Perfusion pressure falls and tissue hypoxia develops. Compensatory mechanisms are ineffective.

Chemical mediators Catecholamines (epinephrine and norepinephrine), antidiuretic hormone, renin-angiotensin system, and aldosterone are active in compensated shock. Hypoxemia and lactic acidosis contribute to the vasodilatation of decompensated shock. Hypoxia injures endothelial cells, which increases vascular permeability and leads to activation of platelets and leukocytes. Platelets release vasoactive amines, histamine, and serotonin. Arachidonic acid metabolites (prostaglandins and leukotrienes) mediate local vascular changes and activate leukocytes. Products of activated leukocytes cause endothelial damage. Lipopolysaccharide endotoxin activates the complement, coagulation, and kinin systems; stimulates release of tumor necrosis factor and interleukins from macrophages; and damages cell membranes. Additional mediators include endorphins and myocardial depressant factor. As shock progresses, essentially all vasoactive and inflammatory mechanisms are active, but in an uncontrolled and chaotic fashion.

Organ damage in shock Hypoxia injures both parenchymal and endothelial cells. Reduced perfusion of kidneys, largely due to vasoconstriction, causes acute tubular necrosis. The pulmonary microvasculature is damaged by products of activated leukocytes and by activation of the coagulation system, which causes diffuse alveolar damage and adult respiratory distress syndrome (ARDS).

MORPHOLOGY

The *heart* is dilated and flabby; subendocardial hemorrhages may be present; contraction band necrosis is seen microscopically. *Lungs* are heavy, airless, congested, and edematous; bronchopneumonia may be present. Microscopically, there are hyaline membranes that later organize to produce alveolar fibrosis. *Liver* shows centrilobular congestion; fatty change and centrilobular necrosis may be apparent microscopically. *Kidneys* are edematous and show cortical pallor; histologically, there is tubular cell necrosis and tubular regeneration. Within the *gastrointestinal tract,* segments of mucosal hemorrhage are common; gastric or duodenal ulcers may be present. The *pancreas* is often soft and hemorrhagic. The *brain* may show changes of hypoxic encephalopathy, consisting of hypereosinophilia of cerebral cortical neurons and cerebellar Purkinje cells; watershed zone infarcts may also be present. The *adrenal glands* sometimes show bilateral hemorrhage and necrosis, especially in sepsis (Waterhouse-Friderichsen syndrome).

CLINICAL SIGNIFICANCE

Hypovolemic shock   Shock is the most difficult problem in the management of trauma patients. Despite initial success in resuscitation and repair of wounds, ARDS and acute renal failure are likely to develop. ARDS has a high mortality rate. Acute renal failure can usually be managed by dialysis until renal function returns. Sepsis, disseminated intravascular coagulation, gastrointestinal hemorrhage, and multisystem organ failure too often complicate trauma cases; these situations are usually irreversible. Fluid loss from the gastrointestinal tract, due to vomiting and diarrhea, may also produce hypovolemic shock. Infants and young children are especially vulnerable, and there is a high mortality in infant diarrhea.

Septic shock   Also called endotoxin shock and gram-negative sepsis, this may develop suddenly during infections with gram-negative organisms, such as urinary tract infection and bacterial peritonitis. It may also complicate shock from other causes when endotoxin leaks into the blood through the intestinal mucosa damaged by hypoxia. The toxic shock syndrome is an example of septic shock produced by products of gram-positive organisms.

Signs of shock   The rapid but weak pulse, and cool, pale, and moist skin are manifestations of the compensatory sympathetic mechanisms that occur in early hypovolemic and cardiogenic shock. In septic shock, the skin is warm and flushed, and there is a bounding pulse with wide pulse pressure; these are due to increased cardiac output, vasodilatation, and systemic effects of infection. Management of any case of shock requires constant monitoring of multiple hemodynamic parameters. The final prognosis depends on speedy control or reversal of the initiating conditions.

Pathology Facts, by Richard C.
Harruff, J.B. Lippincott
Company, Philadelphia © 1994.

Inflammation and Healing

Acute Inflammation

DESCRIPTION

The initial response of tissue to injury, particularly bacterial infections and necrosis, involving vascular and cellular responses.

CAUSES AND PATHOPHYSIOLOGIC MECHANISMS

Vascular phase Transient vasoconstriction, followed by vasodilatation and increased vascular permeability occurs in the microvasculature. Protein-rich fluid leaks through the endothelium into the interstitial tissue to produce an exudate (inflammatory edema). These changes are reversible with mild injury. With more severe or persistent injury, endothelial damage is permanent.

Cellular phase Leukocytes accumulate at the site of injury by first marginating within blood vessels and then emigrating into the extravascular space where they migrate toward the injured site by chemotaxis. Leukocytes attach to and engulf particulate material (bacteria, antigen-antibody complexes, necrotic cellular debris) by phagocytosis. The engulfed material becomes a phagosome that combines with lysosomal granules to form a phagolysosome. Lysosomal granules contain potent hydrolytic enzymes and generate reactive oxygen-derived metabolites that digest the engulfed material and kill bacteria.

Cellular mediators of acute inflammation PMNs are the predominant leukocyte in the cellular phase. Basophils, tissue mast cells, and platelets are important in the vascular phase. Macrophages appear in the later cellular phase and represent a transition between acute and chronic inflammation. Phagocytes include PMNs and macrophages.

Chemical mediators of the vascular response   Agents that increase vascular permeability include histamine and serotonin, platelet activating factor, bradykinin, certain components of complement, and arachidonic acid metabolites. Hageman factor (clotting factor XII) activates the coagulation system, the plasmin fibrinolytic system, the kinin system, and complement. Antigen-antibody reactions also activate complement. Prostaglandins and leukotrienes mediate a divergent set of responses; prostacyclin (PGI_2) is a potent vasoconstrictor secreted by endothelial cells whereas thromboxane (TxA_2) is a powerful vasoconstrictor released from platelets. Arachidonic acid is derived from cell membranes by action of phospholipase; synthesis of leukotrienes follows the lipoxygenase pathway of arachidonic acid metabolism, and prostaglandin synthesis follows the cyclo-oxygenase route.

Chemical mediators of the cellular phase   Chemotactic factors include complement component C5a, leukotriene LTB_4, and bacterial peptides; these factors bind to cell surface receptors and activate leukocytes by stimulating synthesis of cyclic nucleotides (cAMP and cGMP). Subsequent intracellular responses include an increase in intracellular calcium; activation of protein kinases and phospholipases; and assembly of actin-myosin and other cytoskeletal proteins for locomotion. Phospholipase A releases arachidonic acid from membranes; subsequent metabolism produces prostaglandins and leukotrienes. Membrane adhesion proteins are expressed on the surface of activated leukocytes that bind to endothelial cells. Following adhesion, leukocytes migrate through the vessel wall and move in the direction of increasing concentrations of chemotactic agents.

Opsonization   Opsonins consist of antibodies and complement components that facilitate phagocytosis by coating the surface of particulate material. PMNs and macrophages bind to opsonins via membrane receptors for the Fc portion of immunoglobulin and for complement component C3b.

Degradation and killing   There are three types of PMN granules that contain hydrolytic enzymes capable of digesting cellular and extracellular proteins, lipids, and carbohydrates. Granules also contain myeloperoxidase, which generates reactive oxygen metabolites. Phagocytosis activates synthesis of superoxide anion, which reacts to form hydroxyl free radical and hydrogen peroxide, both of which are bacteriostatic. Myeloperoxidase catalyzes formation of hypochlorite from chloride and hydrogen peroxide; hypochlorite is a potent oxidant and the most important reactive oxygen metabolite.

Damage of normal tissue by acute inflammation   Activated PMNs and macrophages release into the extracellular space proteolytic enzymes and reactive oxygen metabolites that are toxic and cause necrosis of normal cells. Mechanisms that limit the damage include antiproteases, such as serum alpha-1-antitrypsin. Superoxide dismutase, glutathione peroxidase, and catalase neutralize reactive oxygen metabolites.

MORPHOLOGY
Patterns of acute inflammation   Acute inflammatory exudates consist of fluid, PMNs, and protein. *Serous exudate* is nearly all fluid. *Purulent exudate,* or suppuration, is a thick yellow-green fluid (pus) containing degenerating PMNs and other cell debris. An *abscess* is localized suppuration with liquefactive necrosis of the underlying tissue. *Fibrinous exudate* is a flaky gray coating on the surface of organs that is microscopically acellular and eosinophilic. Fibrinopurulent exudate shows admixture of abundant fibrin with PMNs.

Complications of acute inflammation   Resolution of inflammation restores the tissue to normal; otherwise one of the following complications occurs: suppuration, organization, or progression to chronic inflammation. Organization is similar to scarring and complicates fibrinous exudates and inflammation where there is significant tissue necrosis.

CLINICAL CORRELATIONS
Local signs of acute inflammation   Redness (rubor), warmth (calor), swelling (tumor), pain (dolor), and loss of function.

Examples of acute inflammation   In acute meningitis, pneumonia, acute peritonitis, and acute pyelonephritis, there is purulent exudate in response to bacterial infection. Tissue necrosis elicits acute inflammation in myocardial infarcts, burns, and traumatic wounds. The fluid-filled blisters of second-degree burns are an example of serous inflammation. An ulcer of skin or mucosa shows purulent exudate at its base. Fibrinous pleuritis and pericarditis organize to form adhesions; occasionally, constrictive pericarditis occurs. Abscesses complicate pneumonia when there is excessive suppuration. Organizing pneumonia occurs when there is excess fibrin that PMNs cannot digest and clear from alveoli.

Systemic effects of acute inflammation   These include fever, tachycardia, and a hypermetabolic state. Acute phase proteins are elevated in the blood (C-reactive protein, serum amyloid A, complement, and coagulation factors). The white blood cell count is elevated (leukocytosis), specifically the neutrophil count (neutrophilia or granulocytosis). Increased immature PMNs (left shift) may indicate a serious bacterial infection.

Chronic Inflammation

DESCRIPTION
The tissue response to injury where there is accumulation of mononuclear inflammatory cells (lymphocytes, plasma cells, and macrophages) and production of fibrous connective tissue (fibrosis).

CAUSES AND PATHOPHYSIOLOGIC MECHANISMS
Persistent injury, repeated episodes of acute inflammation, infection by intracellular organisms (viruses, TB), cell-mediated immune responses, and foreign body reactions. Healing involves processes similar to chronic inflammation.

Cellular mediators Primarily macrophages and lymphocytes, attracted to the site of injury by specific antigens and chemotactic factors. T-lymphocytes mediate cellular immune reactions and serve regulatory functions. B-lymphocytes, including plasma cells, secrete antibodies. Monocytes originate in the bone marrow and become macrophages after entering tissue in response to chemotactic stimuli.

Functions of macrophages Microbial degradation and killing by means of granules containing proteases and enzymes that generate reactive oxygen metabolites; activation of T-cells by processing and presenting antigen; secretion of cytokines and growth factors that attract additional inflammatory cells and stimulate proliferation of fibroblasts and blood vessels; synthesis of complement and coagulation proteins.

Eosinophils Active in chronic inflammatory reactions directed against parasites and in allergic reactions. They respond to eosinophil chemotactic factor secreted by mast cells, and their large granules contain a major basic protein toxic to parasites.

Cytokines (lymphokines and monokines) These include proteins secreted by activated T-cells and macrophages: macrophage migration inhibition factor, macrophage chemotactic factors, interferon-gamma, tumor necrosis factor, and several types of interleukins.

Fibrosis This is the reactive formation of connective tissue, predominantly fibroblasts and small blood vessels, that progressively obliterates and replaces normal tissue. Growth factors secreted by macrophages cause proliferation of fibroblasts and endothelial cells.

MORPHOLOGY
Mononuclear cell infiltrates (lymphocytes, plasma cells, macrophages) and fibrosis are microscopic features of chronic inflammation. Perivascular cuffing by lymphocytes is a feature of viral

infections. Multinucleated giant cells are a feature of granuloma-tous inflammation. Fibroblasts and small blood vessels, along with collagen fibers synthesized by fibroblasts, constitute fibrosis. Grossly, fibrotic tissue is light gray with a dense, firm texture that contracts the normal tissue.

CLINICAL CORRELATIONS
Chronic inflammation develops at a site of injury that persists longer than several days. The associated fibrosis causes progres-sive tissue damage and loss of function.

Examples of chronic inflammation   Chronic interstitial pneumo-nias, chronic hepatitis, chronic pyelonephritis; autoimmune dis-eases. Rheumatoid arthritis causes progressive destruction of joints due to fibrosis of the periarticular tissues. Progressive sys-temic sclerosis causes fibrosis and contraction of the skin, esopha-gus, and other tissues. Chronic infections display either a purely chronic inflammatory pattern or a combination of acute and chronic inflammation, as in fungal infections. Viral infections elic-it a lymphocytic response from their onset. Chronic inflammation produces the dense fibrotic margin of an abscess.

Systemic effects of chronic inflammation   Low-grade fever, malaise, weight loss, anemia, and fatigue; leukocytosis; lympho-cytosis is characteristic of viral infection. The erythrocyte sedi-mentation rate (ESR) is a sensitive indicator of inflammatory ac-tivity that corresponds to elevation of acute phase proteins.

Granulomatous Inflammation

DESCRIPTION
A subtype of chronic inflammation characterized morphological-ly by granulomas.

CAUSES AND PATHOPHYSIOLOGIC MECHANISMS
Insoluble particulate material, micro-organisms that resist intra-cellular degradation, and the high molecular weight fatty acids of mycobacteria produce granulomas. *Granulomatous infections:* my-cobacterial diseases (tuberculosis, leprosy); fungal diseases (histo-plasmosis, blastomycosis, coccidioidomycosis); parasitic diseases (schistosomiasis); also syphilis and cat-scratch disease. Sterile for-eign bodies provoke a granulomatous response. Silicosis and berylliosis are granulomatous lung diseases produced by occupa-tional exposure to dusts. Sarcoidosis is a granulomatous disease of unknown etiology. *Mediators of delayed hypersensitivity:* lym-phokines, secreted by sensitized T-cells, recruit, immobilize, and transform macrophages. Macrophages transform into epithelioid cells. Multinucleated giant cells are formed as adjacent epithe-lioid cells fuse their cytoplasm into a syncytium. Other processes

of chronic inflammation produce fibrosis and obliteration of normal tissue.

MORPHOLOGY
Granulomas are nodules of epithelioid cells, usually 2 mm or less in diameter, although several granulomas may coalesce into much larger lesions. The distinctive epithelioid cell is a modified macrophage with abundant eosinophilic cytoplasm. Lymphocytes, plasma cells, and fibroblasts surround the nodule of epithelioid cells. Eosinophils may be present, depending on the etiology. A few PMNs may be present; a large number is characteristic of certain fungal infections. Multinucleated giant cells are usually present. Langhan's giant cells are typical of tuberculosis; their nuclei are distributed about the periphery of the cytoplasm. The nuclei of foreign body giant cells are arranged within in the central part of the cytoplasm.

Granulomas in tuberculosis   Caseation necrosis is present as a cheesy, white, disintegrating substance in the midst of multiple confluent granulomas. Cavitation occurs when the caseous material discharges into a bronchus. Microscopically, a caseous granuloma shows amorphous, granular eosinophilic debris surrounded by epithelioid cells, Langhan's giant cells, lymphocytes, and fibroblasts. Progressive fibrosis produces a firm margin of the granuloma that may calcify in older lesions.

Etiology of granulomatous inflammation   This may be obvious microscopically; for example, large fragments of foreign material or eggs of a parasite. Polarized light may reveal small crystals of inorganic material (e.g., silica) within macrophages and giant cells. Special stains for infective organisms facilitate visualization and identification of the agent. Acid-fast stains (e.g., Ziehl-Neelsen) detect mycobacteria; silver and PAS stains are useful for fungi.

CLINICAL CORRELATIONS
Recognition of granulomatous inflammation narrows the range of diagnostic possibilities. Tuberculosis and other infectious diseases are excluded first by tissue examination, microbiologic cultures, and skin tests for TB. Environmental and occupational exposure to dusts can produce the debilitating chronic lung disease, silicosis. Suture material and talc from surgeon's gloves produce granulomatous foreign body reaction that may cause intestinal adhesions. Sarcoidosis is a disease of unknown etiology associated with non-necrotizing granulomas; its diagnosis requires exclusion of all other causes.

Healing

DESCRIPTION
The repair of damaged tissue by two coordinated processes, regeneration and scarring. In regeneration, there is proliferation of parenchymal cells to replace those lost by injury. In scarring, there is formation of fibrous connective tissue.

CAUSES AND PATHOPHYSIOLOGIC MECHANISMS
Disruption or necrosis of tissue by physical wounds, infections, infarcts, and surgical incisions. The relative contributions of regeneration and scarring depend on the proliferative capacity of the injured tissue and the extent of damage to its mesenchymal framework. The amount of scarring is a function of the tissue injured, the nature of the injury, and the quality of surgical and medical care. Fibrosis in chronic inflammation involves processes similar to scarring.

Regeneration   *Permanent cells* cannot undergo mitosis, and regeneration does not occur; examples are neurons and cardiac and skeletal muscle cells. *Stable cells,* including parenchymal cells of organs and most mesenchymal cells, are mitotically inactive but can undergo rapid cell division when stimulated. *Labile cells* continuously divide and mature from stem cells; these include epithelial cells of skin and mucosa, bone marrow hematopoietic cells, and lymphoid cells. Tissues composed of labile and stable cells have the best potential for healing by regeneration. Successful regeneration requires an intact stromal framework to re-establish normal structure. Significant necrosis or disruption of the mesenchymal stroma precludes effective regeneration, and healing occurs predominantly by scarring.

Scarring   Scarring involves granulation tissue, composed of proliferating fibroblasts and small blood vessels, that forms during the later phases of acute inflammation when PMNs and macrophages are still active. Granulation tissue grows into the necrotic defect that has been "cleaned out" by the acute inflammatory reaction. Myofibroblasts contract the defect, and fibroblasts synthesize collagen. With time, the defect progressively contracts, blood vessels become less numerous, and collagen matures to strengthen the scar.

Collagen and extracellular matrix components   Collagen is the major constituent of the extracellular matrix and basement membranes; glycoproteins, elastic fibers, and proteoglycans are other components. There are at least 11 different types of collagen. Type I is the most abundant collagen in normal tissues and in mature scars, where it provides the major tensile strength. Type III collagen is present in immature scars. Fibroblasts synthesize collagen as a triple helix; a critical posttranslational modification is hydroxylation of proline to hydroxyproline, a reaction dependent on ascorbic acid (vitamin C). Fibroblasts secrete soluble procollagen into the extracellular space where proteases cleave peptides from each end to produce insoluble collagen fibrils. Cross-linking of the fibrils by a process involving hydroxylation of lysine provides the full tensile strength of mature collagen. Mature collagen is stable under normal conditions but can be digested by collagenases from PMNs, macrophages, fibroblasts, and others cells.

Laminin and fibronectin   These are two glycoproteins that mediate cellular interactions with the extracellular matrix. Along with Type IV collagen and proteoglycans, laminin is a major component of basement membranes surrounding cells. Laminin simultaneously binds to specific cell surface receptors, Type IV collagen, and proteoglycans, thereby anchoring cells into the basement membrane. Fibronectin binds to several different extracellular macromolecules (fibrin, collagen, proteoglycans) and to cell surfaces via the membrane integrin receptors. Fibronectin is a chemotactic agent for macrophages and fibroblasts and an opsonin for phagocytosis of fibrin, collagen, and other extracellular components. Fibronectin and laminin together provide signals that regulate cell growth and differentiation of parenchymal cells, fibroblasts, and endothelial cells.

Growth factors   Chemical signals that stimulate parenchymal cells, fibroblasts, and endothelial cells to undergo mitosis and proliferation include platelet-derived growth factor, epidermal growth factor, fibroblast growth factors, transforming growth factors and the cytokines, interleukin-1 and tumor necrosis factor. Macrophages secrete many of these. Fibroblast growth factor stimulates angiogenesis, critical for the formation of granulation tissue.

MORPHOLOGY
Healing and inflammation are both present in proportions that depend on the type of injury, the tissue injured, and the time after injury. Regeneration and scarring appear simultaneously.

Granulation tissue and scarring   Following initial infiltration by PMNs that digest fibrin and necrotic debris, macrophages are prominent. After the third day, small blood vessels are apparent at the periphery of the lesion. Later, numerous blood vessels and plump fibroblasts invade the lesion. Sparse, pale-staining collagen fibers are present around the fourth day. The fibers become more abundant and stain more eosinophilic thereafter. Fibroblasts continue to increase during the second week, while leukocytes and blood vessels diminish. In the following weeks, cellularity and number of blood vessels decrease. Dense collagen with a few fibroblasts and blood vessels constitutes the final scar obtained after several months. Grossly, within an organ or tissue, a mature scar appears as a dense, firm, white to gray, irregular region that contracts the surrounding parenchyma.

Regeneration   Epithelial cells proliferate at the edges of a wound and then migrate into the region of repair or across the surface of the wound. Epidermis and mucosal epithelium are likely to regenerate effectively to cover a surface defect. Within organs, the framework is often destroyed, and regeneration is either ineffective or causes distortion of the tissue. In cirrhosis, scarring and regeneration occur together but are uncoordinated and result in a nodular, distorted liver.

CLINICAL CORRELATIONS
Skin wounds   Healing by first intention occurs when sutures approximate the skin edges of a surgical incision. With well-approximated wounds, there is little granulation tissue, and the final scar is minimal. Healing occurs by second intention when nonsurgical wounds fill in with abundant granulation tissue, producing large irregular scars.

Complications of healing   Contracture, or cicatrization, occurs when scar contraction produces deformity or functional impairment. A keloid results from excessive scar formation.

Local and systemic factors influencing healing   *Local:* infection, blood supply, extent of necrosis, presence of foreign bodies, protection from further trauma or movement. *Systemic:* general nutritional status (especially protein and vitamin C), cardiovascular disease, hematological disorders (neutropenia), systemic infections, diabetes mellitus, corticosteroid therapy.

Healing in specific organs   Myocardial infarcts heal exclusively by scarring, and the heart is permanently weakened. In the central nervous system, a stroke causes permanent disability, and healing occurs by gliosis rather than by collagenous scar formation. In other organs, effective regeneration depends on the nature of injury. Necrosis of only parenchymal cells, with retention of the existing stroma, may permit regeneration and restoration of normal anatomy. However, necrosis that involves the mesenchymal framework favors scar formation.

Pathology Facts, by Richard C.
Harruff, J.B. Lippincott
Company, Philadelphia © 1994.

Chapter 4

Immunopathology

Hypersensitivity Diseases

DESCRIPTION
Four types of disease processes mediated by immune mechanisms, in which antibodies and cellular responses cause tissue damage.

Type I hypersensitivity (immediate type or anaphylaxis) Mediated by antibodies of the IgE class. Antigen (allergen) reacting with IgE attached to the surface of mast cells by the Fc receptor causes mast cell degranulation. Histamine is released, which causes bronchospasm, vascular congestion, edema, and increased mucus secretion. Other mediators released from mast cells are chemotactic factors, especially eosinophil chemotactic factor; prostaglandins and leukotrienes, which enhance and prolong the responses initiated by histamine; and platelet activating factor, which stimulates release of vasoactive amines and other substances.

Type II hypersensitivity (cytolytic/cytotoxic type) Several mechanisms are involved. Most typically, IgM or IgG antibodies react with cell surface antigens and activate complement, which mediates either cell lysis or opsonization that leads to phagocytosis. In antibody-dependent cell-mediated cytotoxicity, phagocytes and cytotoxic lymphocytes react directly, via their Fc receptors, with target cells coated with antibody; complement is not required for cell lysis. Antibodies that react with extracellular components produce a local acute inflammatory reaction in which PMNs and other mediators cause tissue injury and cell necrosis. Antibodies that react with cell membrane receptors interfere with receptor function or cause inappropriate stimulation.

Type III hypersensitivity (immune complex disease) Immune complexes are antigen-antibody complexes that circulate in the bloodstream or form in the tissues. Antigens are either exogenous or endogenous, and antibodies belong to classes IgG, IgM, or IgA. Circulating immune complexes deposit in tissue around blood vessels, where they activate complement to cause acute inflammation and tissue injury. Sites of deposition depend on the size and charge of the immune complexes as well as the characteristics of the blood vessels; renal glomerular capillaries are frequently involved. Models of immune complex disease are serum sickness and the Arthus reaction.

Type IV hypersensitivity (cell-mediated immunity) *Delayed hypersensitivity:* macrophages sensitize T-cells by presenting fragments of antigen on their surface in combination with HLA Class II molecules. Upon subsequent antigen exposure, the sensitized T-lymphocytes secrete lymphokines that recruit and activate macrophages and other lymphocytes. Persistent antigenic stimulation leads to granuloma formation. In addition to macrophages, antigen-presenting cells include Langerhans cells in skin, which mediate contact dermatitis, and dendritic cells in lymphoid tissue. HLA Class II molecules. *T-cell–mediated cytotoxicity:* sensitized cytotoxic (CD8+) T-cells react directly, via the T-cell receptor, with target cells bearing surface antigen in association with Class I HLA molecules to cause cell lysis. Helper (CD4+) T-cells participate by secreting lymphokines that stimulate proliferation of cytotoxic T-cells. Cells with altered or foreign Class I HLA antigens are targets for T-cell–mediated cytotoxicity; these include cells infected with viruses, neoplastic cells, and transplanted cells. Natural killer cells cause cell lysis directly, mediated by a special receptor or by the Fc receptor, as described for antibody-dependent cell-mediated cytotoxicity.

MORPHOLOGY

Anaphylaxis: interstitial edema and infiltrates of eosinophils are major features. In bronchial asthma, thick mucus and swollen mucosa obstruct bronchi; cords of mucus are present in sputum as Curschmann's spirals. Microscopically, there is hyperplasia of mucous glands and bronchial smooth muscle. Infiltrates of eosinophils are present in bronchial walls, and bronchial basement membranes are thickened. *Cytolytic/cytotoxic hypersensitivity:* these are a diverse assortment of diseases that are described separately in Systemic Pathology. *Immune complex diseases:* blood vessels and renal glomeruli are most often affected, consistent with the common sites of complex deposition. Acute necrotizing vasculitis, with fibrinoid necrosis, and acute proliferative glomerulonephritis are typical lesions. *Cell-mediated immunity:* granulomatous inflammation is the characteristic histologic feature of delayed hypersensitivity. The lesions of contact dermatitis are also produced by delayed hypersensitivity reactions. Mononuclear inflammatory infiltrates, particularly cuffs of lymphocytes around blood vessels, are present in T-cell–mediated cytotoxicity, e.g., in viral infections.

CLINICAL CORRELATIONS
Anaphylaxis   This represents a variety of allergic conditions. *Systemic anaphylaxis* is a serious condition that occurs suddenly in an allergic individual exposed to an antigen (e.g., penicillin injection). Laryngeal edema, bronchoconstriction, generalized urticaria, and shock develop and often result in death. *Localized anaphylaxis* includes urticaria, allergic rhinitis (hay fever), bronchial asthma, and atopic dermatitis.

Cytolytic/cytotoxic hypersensitivity   Cytolytic reactions include incompatible transfusion reactions, autoimmune hemolytic anemia, and erythroblastosis fetalis (Rh hemolytic disease of the newborn). Antibody reactions occurring in extracellular tissues cause Goodpasture's disease, bullous skin diseases (pemphigus and pemphigoid), and rheumatic heart disease. Antibody reactions that involve cell surface receptors cause myasthenia gravis, Grave's disease, and Hashimoto's thyroiditis.

Immune complex diseases   Polyarteritis nodosa is a typical vasculitis caused by immune complexes; the antigen is often hepatitis B surface antigen. Antigens from streptococcal pharyngitis, complexed with antistreptococcal antibodies, cause acute post-streptococcal glomerulonephritis. In the autoimmune disease, systemic lupus erythematosus, anti-DNA autoantibodies combine with endogenous DNA to form immune complexes that cause systemic disease and glomerulonephritis.

Cell-mediated immunity   Delayed hypersensitivity is an important cause of tissue damage in granulomatous diseases, such as tuberculosis, fungal infections, and sarcoidosis. Similar reactions mediate contact dermatitis, e.g., the poison ivy reaction. T-cell–mediated cytotoxicity is active in the responses to viral infections, in tumor immunology and in transplant rejection.

Transplant Rejection and Graft-Versus-Host Disease

DESCRIPTION
In allograft (transplant) rejection, immune mechanisms of the host attack and injure the foreign tissue. In graft-versus-host disease, immunocompetent cells in grafted bone marrow attack the immunosuppressed host's tissue.

CAUSES AND PATHOPHYSIOLOGIC MECHANISMS

Both antibody and cell-mediated immune mechanisms are involved in allograft rejection. After sensitization by foreign HLA Class I and II antigens, cytotoxic T-cells attack the grafted tissue directly, and helper T-cells secrete lymphokines that provoke a delayed hypersensitivity response. Antibodies to the graft are either preformed or formed after the graft is in place. Both T-cell and B-cell responses attack the vasculature of the graft and thereby produce ischemia. Preformed antibodies immediately attack graft blood vessels to cause hyperacute rejection. Acute rejection involves humoral rejection, cellular rejection, or both. In chronic rejection, there are progressive changes in the blood vessels, possibly due to repeated episodes of cellular rejection.

MORPHOLOGY

Rejected renal transplants exemplify the morphology of rejection. In hyperacute rejection, the kidneys are pale, mottled, swollen, and focally infarcted. Microscopically, there is necrotizing vasculitis with fibrin thrombi in blood vessels and glomeruli. In acute cellular rejection, there are mononuclear infiltrates in the interstitium surrounding damaged tubules. In acute humoral rejection, vasculitis and infarcts are present. In chronic rejection, there is narrowing of arteries and arterioles by intimal thickening, and the parenchyma shows chronic ischemic damage. In other rejected organs, infiltration by mononuclear cells, particularly in and around vascular structures, is a common feature.

CLINICAL CORRELATIONS

HLA Matching   Identical twins are perfectly HLA matched, and their grafts survive well. Close HLA matching is possible for nonidentical twin and familial grafts, but graft survival depends on immunosuppressive therapy. Graft rejection is usually most serious in cadaveric transplants from nonrelated donors where HLA matching is only partial. Graft versus host disease is a complication of bone marrow transplantation, and the likelihood of occurrence depends on HLA matching.

Immunosuppressive therapy   This is usually necessary for all transplants except those from an identical twin. Agents include azathioprine, corticosteroids, cyclosporine, and antilymphocyte globulin. Cyclosporine is effective by its action against CD4+ (helper) T-cells. Complications of immunosuppressive therapy include opportunistic infections and increased risk of developing a lymphoid neoplasm.

Diagnosis of rejection   Graft rejection causes rapid loss or gradual decline in function of the transplanted organ. In kidney transplants, hyperacute rejection causes renal failure within the first few hours or days; acute rejection, in the first few weeks or months or sometimes much later; chronic rejection causes progressive renal failure over a period of many months or years. Biopsies of the graft monitor immunosuppressive therapy, confirm rejection in cases of organ failure, and assess the type of rejection.

Graft-versus-host (GVH) disease   This occurs in bone marrow transplant recipients, who are treated aggressively for leukemia, metastatic breast cancer, or aplastic anemia. Principal sites of involvement are skin, liver, and intestine. The incidence of GVH disease is reduced by treating the marrow with anti–T-cell antibodies prior to transplantation.

Autoimmune Diseases

DESCRIPTION
A category of diseases in which the etiology involves immune mechanisms directed against self antigens. Some diseases in this category are systemic; others involve a single organ.

CAUSES AND PATHOPHYSIOLOGIC MECHANISMS
Hypotheses to explain autoimmune diseases   Escape of a normally sequestered antigen; production of antibodies against micro-organisms that cross-react with normal tissue components; modification of cell surface antigens; depression of T-suppressor cell activity; inappropriate T-helper cell activity; and polyclonal B-cell stimulation. There is a genetic susceptibility; certain HLA types show increased risk, most notably ankylosing spondylitis with HLA-B27.

Hypersensitivity reactions that mediate autoimmune diseases
Cytolytic/cytotoxic reactions produce autoimmune hemolytic anemia, Graves' disease, Hashimoto's thyroiditis, myasthenia gravis, Type I diabetes mellitus, and Goodpasture's syndrome. Immune complex hypersensitivity causes much of the tissue damage in systemic autoimmune diseases, such as systemic lupus erythematosus (SLE), rheumatoid arthritis, and progressive systemic sclerosis.

Antinuclear antibodies   Many autoimmune diseases are associated with characteristic autoantibodies. SLE: anti-DNA and anti-Sm antigen; Sjogren's syndrome: anti-ribonucleoprotein (SS-A and SS-B); progressive systemic sclerosis: anti-centromere and anti-Scl-70 (DNA topoisomerase); polymyositis-dermatomyositis: anti-Jo (transfer RNA synthetase); mixed connective tissue disease: anti-ribonucleoprotein without anti-DNA.

MORPHOLOGY
Systemic lupus erythematosus   SLE involves skin, serosa, joints, kidneys, heart, blood vessels, blood cells, and central nervous system. The classic skin lesion is a "butterfly rash" over the face.

Fibrinous inflammation affects serosa, causing pericarditis and pleuritis; organization produces fibrous adhesions. Chronic synovitis affects joints. In Libman-Sacks endocarditis, there are fibrinous vegetations on the heart valves. Immune complex vasculitis and glomerulonephritis are common. There are four types of lupus glomerulonephritis: mesangial, focal proliferative, diffuse proliferative, and membranous. The "LE cell" is a phagocyte containing a disrupted cell's nucleus; this is a laboratory test demonstrating opsonization of nuclear material.

Sjogren's syndrome   There is chronic inflammation of salivary and lacrimal glands that usually progresses to fibrosis and atrophy of the glands. Occasionally, the lymphocytic infiltration is massive and causes enlargement of the glands (Miculicz's syndrome). In some cases, immunoblastic lymphoma develops.

Progressive systemic sclerosis (scleroderma)   In PSS there is fibrosis of connective tissue in skin and other tissues. The dermis is densely collagenized, and the epidermis is atrophic. In advanced cases, the dermis resembles scar tissue. The wall of the esophagus is also fibrotic. Fibrosis of lung leads to "honeycomb" lung. In the kidney there is intimal proliferation of arterioles and arteries, with "onion-skin" thickening of their walls and narrowing of their lumen; fibrinoid necrosis is sometimes present. These vascular changes are similar to those in malignant hypertension.

CLINICAL CORRELATIONS

Systemic lupus erythematosus typically affects young adult women, with acute attacks and remissions recurring over several years. Joints, kidney, and skin are involved most frequently. Hematologic disorders (hemolytic anemia, anemia of chronic disease, leukopenia, thrombocytopenia) are common. Renal failure occurs in most patients and is the usual cause of death. Central nervous system involvement is sometimes serious, but the mechanism is unclear. Immunosuppressive therapy allows prolonged survival. *Sjogren's syndrome* presents with keratoconjunctivitis sicca (dry eyes) and xerostomia (dry mouth) due to destruction of salivary and lacrimal glands. Other autoimmune diseases, particularly rheumatoid arthritis, are often associated. Respiratory tract involvement causes bronchitis and pneumonitis. The fibrosis in *progressive systemic sclerosis* contracts the skin, drawing it tight on the fingers and face, resulting in sclerodactyly and a mask-like grimace. In rapidly progressive cases with visceral involvement, there are gastrointestinal obstruction, respiratory failure, and malignant hypertension. The CREST syndrome refers to less severe cases with calcinosis cutis, Raynaud's phenomenon, esophageal dysmotility, sclerodactyly, and telangiectasia.

Immunodeficiency Diseases

DESCRIPTION

Congenital or acquired failure of one or more functions of the immune system, predisposing the affected patient to infections that a normal human easily resists.

CAUSES AND PATHOPHYSIOLOGIC MECHANISMS

Primary (congenital) immunodeficiency   These are due to failure of organ development necessary for lymphocyte maturation, a specific enzyme deficiency, or an undefined failure of normal lymphocyte maturation. In *DiGeorge syndrome,* there is intrauterine failure of the third and fourth pharyngeal pouches to develop thymus and parathyroid glands; the absence of thymus results in T-cell deficiency. In *X-linked agammaglobulinemia of Bruton,* pre–B-cells fail to mature, and B-cell deficiency develops. Normal maturation of IgA-secreting B-cells is defective in *selective IgA deficiency;* this is an inherited or acquired defect. *Severe combined immunodeficiency* results in both T-cell and B-cell deficiencies; about half of these are autosomal recessive and lack the enzyme, adenosine deaminase. Without this enzyme, there is accumulation of deoxyadenosine and other metabolites, which are toxic to lymphocytes and kill the common stem cell precursor for both T-cells and B-cells.

Secondary (acquired) immunodeficiency due to nonspecific causes   Multiple, diverse and nonspecific defects in the immune defenses occur in: viral and other infections, malnutrition, alcoholism, aging, autoimmune diseases, diabetes mellitus, cancer, chronic diseases, steroid therapy, cancer chemotherapeutic agents, and radiation.

Acquired immunodeficiency syndrome (AIDS)   The RNA retrovirus, HIV, causes AIDS by infecting T-helper cells and macrophages. The virus binds to membrane CD4 molecules on target cells via its gp120 glycoprotein and becomes internalized. Viral RNA serves as a template for viral reverse transcriptase to synthesize DNA, which is incorporated into the infected cell's genome. After a latent period, the infected cell's genome is activated to synthesize HIV viral particles. The virus selectively destroys CD4+ cells and produces a number of defects in the immune system, particularly those related to T-helper function. This results in faulty antibody responses, defective T-cell–mediated cytotoxicity, and poor macrophage function.

Consequences of immunodeficiency   Predisposition to opportunistic infections produces the clinical manifestations. Selective B-cell deficiencies predispose to bacterial infections; T-cell deficiencies predispose to viral and fungal infections. Combined deficiencies, including AIDS, are particularly severe because they predispose to all kinds of infection.

MORPHOLOGY

In *DiGeorge syndrome,* thymus and parathyroid glands are absent; defects of the lower face, heart, and great vessels may be present. In *X-linked agammaglobulinemia of Bruton,* pre–B-cells are present in blood, but mature B-cells, plasma cells, and germinal centers are absent from lymphoid tissue. In *selective IgA deficiency* there is absence of IgA-secreting plasma cells from gastrointestinal and respiratory mucosa. In *severe combined immunodeficiency,* lymphocytes are absent from thymus, spleen, gastrointestinal tract, and lymph nodes. During early stages of *HIV infection,* there is atypical follicular hyperplasia producing generalized lymphadenopathy. Generalized lymphocyte depletion occurs in the terminal stages of AIDS. *Opportunistic infections* produce the major morphologic changes. The inflammatory response is diminished or atypical; in severe immunodeficiency, the cellular inflammatory reaction may be nearly absent. *Kaposi's sarcoma* in AIDS produces multiple lesions on the skin and mucosa; these are flat or slightly elevated, blue to red-brown spots, usually less than 2–3 cm in diameter.

CLINICAL CORRELATIONS

Infants with *DiGeorge syndrome* develop tetany due to hypocalcemia and are likely to die from overwhelming viral infection at an early age. Those with *X-linked agammaglobulinemia of Bruton* develop recurrent bacterial infections of the respiratory tract and skin; antibiotics and immunoglobulin therapy allow prolonged survival. Some patients with *selective IgA deficiency* show no clinical disease while others have recurrent sinus infections and gastroenteritis. Infants with *severe combined immunodeficiency* usually die at an early age; genetic replacement of adenosine deaminase holds promise for the future.

Transmission of HIV infection Sexual contact; parenteral inoculation; and mother to infant during the perinatal period. High risk groups: homosexual or bisexual males; intravenous drug abusers; hemophiliacs and recipients of blood or blood products who received these products before uniform testing for HIV; and heterosexual contacts of the foregoing risk groups. Occupational exposure to health care workers, usually via accidental needle punctures, has resulted in a few cases; transmission to patients from infected health care workers is rare and controversial.

Spectrum of HIV-associated disease Asymptomatic carrier state, acute HIV syndrome, persistent generalized lymphadenopathy, and AIDS. Persistent generalized lymphadenopathy, as a group, is usually accompanied by fever, weight loss, and other constitutional symptoms; CD4+ cells may or may not be depressed; and there is no identifiable opportunistic infection. Diagnosis of AIDS requires evidence of HIV infection, plus one or more opportunistic infections or one of a specified set of malignant neoplasms. In 1992, CDC further defined AIDS to include any patient with HIV infection who has less than $200 \times 10^6/L$ CD4$^+$ lymphocytes.

Opportunistic infections and malignancies in AIDS Pneumocystis carinii pneumonia; cytomegalovirus infection (pneumonia or disseminated); cryptosporidiosis or isosporidiosis enteritis with chronic diarrhea; candidiasis; oral hairy leukoplakia; disseminated mycobacterial infections *(M. avium-intracellulare, M. tuberculosis)*. Malignant neoplasms include Kaposi's sarcoma and malignant B-cell lymphoma.

Malignant lymphoma and autoimmune diseases Patients with primary and secondary immunodeficiencies are at increased risk for developing malignant lymphoma. Patients with survivable primary immunodeficiencies develop autoimmune diseases, such as rheumatoid arthritis and SLE.

Pathology Facts, by Richard C.
Harruff, J.B. Lippincott
Company, Philadelphia © 1994.

Chapter 5

Neoplasia

See also Dysplasia 8

Neoplasia

DESCRIPTION

A neoplasm, or tumor, is an abnormal growth of cells that is uncontrolled and uncoordinated with the surrounding tissue. The
classification of a neoplasm indicates its cell or tissue of origin
and whether it is benign or malignant. Neoplasms are of either
epithelial or mesenchymal origin. The suffix "carcinoma" indicates a malignant tumor of epithelial origin. "Sarcoma" indicates
a malignant tumor of mesenchymal origin. The suffix "oma" indicates a benign neoplasm of either origin. "Cancer" is a general
term referring to any malignant neoplasm. Modifiers attached to
the name of a tumor describe distinctive growth patterns and its
primary anatomic site of origin. Neoplasms of bone marrow end
with "emia", and neoplasms of embryonic precursor cells end
with "blastoma". A hamartoma is an overgrowth of normal tissue
that is not neoplastic. A choristoma is an ectopic mass of non-neoplastic tissue.

Examples of naming conventions Squamous papilloma of
tongue, squamous cell carcinoma of lung, pituitary adenoma, villous adenoma of colon, adenocarcinoma of stomach, cystadenocarcinoma of ovary, osteoma of humerus, osteosarcoma of tibia,
lipoma of breast, liposarcoma of thigh, leiomyoma of uterus,
leiomyosarcoma of ileum, rhabdomyoma of heart, rhabdomyosarcoma of vagina, acute lymphoblastic leukemia, neuroblastoma of adrenal medulla. *Exceptions:* hepatoma, melanoma,
lymphoma, seminoma.

Incidence Cancer is the second most common cause of death, accounting for about 20% of all deaths. The death rate is higher in
men, and the incidence of most cancers increases with age. The
most common fatal cancers in men are, in descending order according to site: lung, colon and rectum, prostate, and pancreas; in
women: lung, breast, colon and rectum, and uterus or ovary.

Cancers showing trends related to time, race, cultural habits, and geography Carcinomas of lung, uterine cervix, skin, colon, stomach, breast, liver, nasopharynx, urinary bladder, and penis; Burkitt's lymphoma and T-cell leukemia.

Cancers in childhood Cancer is the most common natural cause of death in children. Childhood tumors include acute leukemias, brain tumors, neuroblastoma, retinoblastoma, Wilm's tumor (nephroblastoma), rhabdomyosarcoma, osteosarcoma, teratoma.

CAUSES AND PATHOPHYSIOLOGIC MECHANISMS
Carcinogens There are chemical, viral, and physical carcinogens. Chemical carcinogens: polycyclic aromatic hydrocarbons, aromatic amines (beta-naphthylamine) and azo dyes, vinyl chloride, nitrosamines, aflatoxin, heavy metals, alkylating agents. Oncogenic DNA viruses: hepatitis B virus, Epstein-Barr virus, human papilloma virus; oncogenic RNA virus: human T-cell leukemia virus (HTLV). Physical carcinogens: ultraviolet light, ionizing radiation, asbestos.

Preneoplastic, precancerous, and inherited conditions *Inherited:* retinoblastoma, multiple polyposis, multiple endocrine neoplasia syndromes, neurofibromatosis, tuberous sclerosis, von Hippel-Lindau syndrome, xeroderma pigmentosa, X-linked lymphoproliferative syndrome; *Acquired:* cirrhosis, atrophic gastritis, endometrial hyperplasia, solar keratosis, squamous dysplasia of cervix, oral leukoplakia, ulcerative colitis.

Chemical carcinogenesis Carcinogenesis is a multistep process that involves damage to DNA; carcinogens are also mutagens. The first stage of chemical carcinogenesis is *initiation;* an initiator is a chemical that reacts with DNA. Except for alkylating agents, metabolism by hepatic P-450 mixed function oxidase is required before most chemical carcinogen initiators react with and permanently alter DNA. The second stage of chemical carcinogenesis is *promotion.* A promoter does not damage DNA directly but does stimulate certain cellular events, such as mitosis, which causes the DNA alteration of the initiation stage to become "fixed" and carried into succeeding generations of the altered cell. Promoters may also be initiators. Examples of promoters include phorbol esters, hormones (e.g., estrogen), food additives (saccharin), and drugs. The third stage of chemical carcinogenesis is *tumor progression,* where the altered cells develop into a neoplasm capable of autonomous growth.

Radiation *Ultraviolet radiation* produces DNA damage by the formation of pyrimidine dimers that cause transcription errors and mutations. A series of enzymes normally repairs a damaged segment by excision-repair. In xeroderma pigmentosa there is a high rate of skin cancers related to UV radiation of sunlight because of a genetic deficiency of an excision-repair enzyme, most commonly an endonuclease. *Ionizing radiation* (x-rays, gamma-rays) produces reactive free radicals within cells that react with and thus damage DNA.

Oncogenic viruses   Oncogenic viruses transform normal cells into neoplastic cells by inserting part of the viral genome into the host genome. DNA viruses insert segments of their DNA directly; oncogenic RNA retroviruses first transcribe their code into new DNA by reverse transcriptase. The inserted DNA segments causing neoplastic transformation represent viral oncogenes.

Oncogenes and antioncogenes   *Oncogenes* exist as cellular genes that normally code for a variety of proteins involved in regulation of cell growth. The normally expressed genes are proto-oncogenes; when activated and expressed inappropriately they represent cellular oncogenes. Transforming agents activate proto-oncogenes by insertional mutagenesis or by transduction. Chemical carcinogens and radiation activate oncogenes by producing point mutations, translocations, and gene amplification. *Anti-cancer genes* (anti-oncogenes) normally inhibit cell proliferation. Inactivation of an anti-oncogene by mutation or viral interaction results in unregulated cell growth. The retinoblastoma gene represents an inactivated anti-oncogene present in inherited cases of retinoblastoma; the same or similar inactivated anti-oncogenes are present in other human cancers.

Clonality, growth kinetics, and tumor progression   Most neoplasms are monoclonal, indicating that they originate from a single transformed cell. Tumor growth is due to imbalance between cell proliferation and cell death; not all tumors enlarge because their cells proliferate faster than normal. Tumor cells show loss of differentiation to a greater or lesser extent; some express oncofetal antigens. Loss of terminal differentiation may produce immortalized cells and cause tumor growth, not because the cells are growing fast but because they fail to mature and die. *Angiogenesis* refers to the proliferation of non-neoplastic vascular connective tissue that forms in response to an invading or enlarging tumor. The connective tissue supplies a supporting stroma for the neoplastic cells and the newly formed blood vessels supply their nutritional needs. A rapidly growing tumor is likely to outgrow its blood supply and become centrally necrotic. Cancers often stimulate abundant collagen formation (desmoplasia).

Evasion of immune surveillance   This allows a tumor to survive. Tumor cells may evade the immune defenses by: absence of tumor-specific or altered HLA antigens; release of antigens into the circulation that block antibodies and inhibit cellular responses; stimulation of suppressor T-cells; and nonspecific immune suppression. Immunodeficiency syndromes predispose to tumors, usually malignant lymphomas.

Invasion and metastasis   As a malignant tumor progresses, subsets of cells emerge possessing properties that promote invasion and metastasis, such as collagenase activity and laminin receptors. These properties enable cells to migrate through tissue without the normal inhibitions imposed by the extracellular matrix. Metastasis involves a mechanism by which cancer cells attach to endothelial surfaces.

MORPHOLOGY
Key morphologic features regarding any neoplasm   Site of origin, cell type of origin, degree of differentiation, growth pattern, size, and extent of spread by local invasion or metastasis.

Criteria of malignancy   Features indicating malignancy: loss of histologic differentiation (or presence of anaplasia), hypercellularity, nuclear hyperchromatism, increased nuclear/cytoplasmic ratio, pleomorphism, abundant and abnormal mitotic figures, rapid growth rate and large size, necrosis, hard "scirrhous" texture; most importantly—invasive growth pattern and metastasis.

Differentiation and anaplasia   Differentiation is a measure of a tumor's resemblance to normal tissue. Anaplasia is absence of differentiation. In poorly and undifferentiated tumors, assessing cell of origin requires special techniques to reveal evidence of cellular differentiation, such as histochemical stains, electron microscopy, and immunoperoxidase techniques.

Patterns of invasion and metastasis   Benign tumors grow by expansion. Cancers spread by local invasion and metastasis. Metastasis is the spread of a tumor to a secondary site distant and separated from its primary site; metastasis is an absolute indicator of malignancy. Metastasis occurs by the lymphatic or hematogenous route. With *lymphatic metastasis,* the tumor first spreads to local and regional lymph nodes draining the primary site. The local lymph nodes are able to temporarily arrest the spread of the cancer cells; eventually this barrier fails and the cancer disseminates via the blood. With *hematogenous metastasis,* secondary tumor nodules develop in liver, lung, brain, bone marrow, and sometimes spleen and soft tissue. Metastatic tumors are often deceptively round and well circumscribed; however, their multiplicity, central umbilication (depression due to necrosis), and microscopic appearance are features that distinguish them from benign tumors.

Chromosomal abnormalities in cancers Translocations are the most common chromosomal abnormality, especially in leukemias and lymphomas. Translocations can activate the expression of a proto-oncogene. The Philadelphia chromosome, present in chronic myelogenous leukemia, represents a translocation between chromosomes 9 and 22. Deletions are other karyotypic abnormalities; a chromosomal deletion may inactivate an anti-oncogene. In retinoblastoma, there is deletion of a segment from chromosome 13.

CLINICAL CORRELATIONS
Local effects of a tumor Compression or invasion of an organ, obstruction, hemorrhage, ulceration, fistula formation, infection. *Examples:* obstruction of a proximal bronchus by bronchogenic carcinoma causes dysfunction of the entire lung and pneumonia; obstruction of ureters by cervical carcinoma produces renal failure and pyelonephritis; obstruction of pleural lymphatics by metastases causes pleural effusions; colon carcinomas cause intestinal obstruction; esophageal carcinoma can invade the trachea to produce tracheoesophageal fistula and subsequent pneumonia or lung abscess; an aortoesophageal fistula from an esophageal carcinoma produces exsanguinating gastrointestinal hemorrhage; obstruction of the common bile duct by a pancreatic carcinoma produces obstructive jaundice..

Systemic effects Advanced cancers produce cachexia, (wasting) by multiple mechanisms. The cytokine, tumor necrosis factor (cachectin), is partly responsible. Paraneoplastic syndromes are produced by mechanisms other than direct tumor invasion; ectopic hormones mediate many of these. *Examples:* hypercalcemia in cases of lung cancer that secrete a peptide with parathyroid hormone activity; Cushing's syndrome caused by ectopic secretion of ACTH; polycythemia due to secretion of erythropoietin by renal cell carcinoma; neuromuscular disorders, such as Eaton-Lambert syndrome; polymyositis-dermatomyositis; acanthosis nigricans; and hypertrophic pulmonary osteoarthropathy.

Anemia and coagulation disorders Anemia is usually present in a cancer patient; granulocyte and platelet abnormalities are also common. Inappropriate activation of coagulation factors (hypercoagulable blood) produces migratory thrombophlebitis (Trousseau's syndrome), disseminated intravascular coagulation, and nonbacterial thrombotic endocarditis.

Clinical diagnosis Patients may present with symptoms referable to a tumor; less often, an unsuspected tumor is found during routine medical examination. Screening methods, such as Pap smears and mammography, can detect cancers at an early stage when therapy is easiest and most effective. Diagnosis starts with history and physical examination; habits such as cigarette smoking are important. X-rays, CT scans, and MRI scans localize the tumor and assess its size and extent of spread. Nuclear bone scans detect bone metastases that are not apparent with routine x-rays. Diagnosis requires histologic confirmation; obtaining a biopsy may require a surgical procedure. Fiberoptic bronchoscopy and gastrointestinal endoscopy can visualize a tumor and permit biopsy without major operation. Needle biopsy of liver and fine needle aspiration cytology are other approaches to secure a tissue diagnosis.

Laboratory diagnosis   Routine histology is the standard method. Frozen section histology renders an accurate diagnosis within a few minutes. Cytologic methods are valuable for screening and early detection of cancer; the cervical Pap smear is an example of exfoliative cytology. Fine needle aspiration cytology is used to diagnose both superficial and deep lesions. Other tissue studies include assay of hormone receptors in breast cancers, immunohistochemistry, electron microscopy, and flow cytometry.

Tumor markers   Examples: carcinoembryonic antigen for colorectal and other carcinomas; alpha-fetoprotein for hepatocellular carcinoma and yolk sac tumor; acid phosphatase and prostate-specific antigen for prostate cancer; human chorionic gonadotropin for choriocarcinoma; catecholamine metabolites for pheochromocytoma and neuroblastoma; monoclonal immunoglobulin for multiple myeloma. Tumor markers are most useful for classifying a particular tumor, evaluating the adequacy of its treatment, and detecting recurrence of the tumor after resection.

Staging and grading   The *stage* of a tumor is a clinical estimation of size, extent of local invasion, regional lymph node metastasis, and distant metastasis. The TNM classification is a uniform system for expressing the stage. The *grade* of a tumor is a histologic assessment by the pathologist of the degree of differentiation. The stage of a tumor is almost always more important than its grade for selecting appropriate therapy and estimating prognosis.

Treatment   Modalities include surgery, chemotherapy, and radiation therapy. The objective of therapy is either cure or palliation. Surgery offers the best chance for cure in solid tumors. An advanced tumor may be "inoperable" for technical reasons or if the procedure would not materially add to quantity or quality of survival. Chemotherapy is potentially curative in certain cases of acute lymphoblastic leukemia and Hodgkin's disease. For most solid tumors, chemotherapy is an adjunct to surgery or a palliative measure. Bone marrow suppression is an expected complication of chemotherapy. Radiation therapy is either adjunctive to surgery or palliative. Complications of radiation that limit its effectiveness include radiation necrosis and radiation fibrosis of normal tissues.

Pathology Facts, by Richard C.
Harruff, J.B. Lippincott
Company, Philadelphia © 1994.

Chapter 6

Environmental and Nutritional Pathology

Physical Injuries

DESCRIPTION
Injuries produced by external mechanical, thermal, and electrical forces.

CAUSES AND PATHOPHYSIOLOGIC MECHANISMS
Mechanical injuries   Sharp force, blunt force, gunshot wounds. High-velocity gunshot wounds are more destructive than ordinary gunshot wounds because of the $E = 1/2MV^2$ relationship.

Hypothermia   *Generalized:* heat loss exceeds heat production; peripheral vasoconstriction acts to preserve core heat; shivering generates muscular heat; metabolic processes slow, producing cerebral dysfunction and cardiac arrhythmias; blood viscosity increases. *Localized:* freezing of tissues crystallizes cell water; membranes rupture on rewarming; vasoconstriction and damage to endothelium produce ischemia; increased vascular permeability produces edema.

Hyperthermia   *Generalized:* heat production exceeds heat loss; CNS and cardiac dysfunction occur in heat stroke. *Localized:* temperature and duration of heating are factors in production of partial or full-thickness cutaneous burns. Necrosis of large areas of skin leads to severe clinical complications.

Electrical injury   Extent of injury depends on voltage, amperage and resistance, related by Ohm's law $(V = IR)$; skin offers the greatest resistance, which is decreased when wet; the amount of amperage through the heart or brain stem determines the likelihood of electrocution death; less than 100 mA is potentially lethal; alternating current is more dangerous than direct current in producing ventricular fibrillation.

MORPHOLOGY
Blunt force injuries   *Contusions* (bruises) are initially red, purple, or blue and later turn green, brown, and yellow before fading away. Microscopically, there is bleeding from small blood vessels. After about 48 hours, hemosiderin is present in macrophages. In *abrasions*, varying depths of epidermis are scraped off. In *lacerations*, the skin is torn; the edges are irregular and there is tissue bridging in the depths of the wound. Internal organs may also show contusions and lacerations; bones are fractured.

Sharp force injury   Incised wounds have sharp edges and show no bridging. Incisions, cuts, and slashes are longer than deep; stab wounds are deeper than long.

Gunshot wounds   *Entrance wounds:* round or oval, marginal abrasion; exit wounds: often irregular, lacerated, no marginal abrasion. *Contact wounds:* soot and gunpowder residue in the wound and at the margin of the wound; intermediate range wounds: stippling around the wound; distant range wounds: no gunpowder residue deposits around or in the wound. *Shotgun wounds:* large, often irregular entrance wounds at close range; individual pellet wounds at distant range; exit wounds are uncommon. *High-velocity rifle wounds:* exit wound much larger than entrance wound; extensive visceral damage.

Thermal and electrical burns   *First-degree burns:* erythema of skin, no necrosis; *second degree:* necrosis of epidermis, blister formation, serous exudate; *third degree:* necrosis of epidermis and dermis. Epidermal regeneration following second-degree burns progresses from preserved rete ridges and appendages; epidermal regeneration does not occur following third-degree burns, and healing occurs by scarring. Electrical burns may be similar to thermal burns and occur at points of electrical contact and/or grounding. More characteristic electrical burns are silvery-white, raised and hard. Microscopically, there is nuclear streaming of the epidermal cells. High-voltage electrical burns show extensive charring and incineration.

CLINICAL CORRELATIONS
Physical injuries are a major part of clinical medicine. Debridement and repair of tissue injuries require surgical expertise; intensive medical care is needed to treat the common complications

of trauma: shock, sepsis, adult respiratory distress syndrome (ARDS), acute renal failure, and disseminated intravascular coagulation (DIC). Prognosis in thermal injuries depends on total body surface area (TBSA) burned, which is estimated by the rule of 9's. Extensive skin burns cause copious fluid and protein loss leading to hypovolemic shock. Infections by Pseudomonas and Candida occur on the denuded, devitalized skin surface; secondary sepsis causes many deaths. In house fires, inhalation of hot gases injures the airway and results in pulmonary edema, ARDS, atelectasis, and pneumonia; CO poisoning is also likely. Treatment involves fluid and electrolyte therapy, respiratory care, infection control, debridement, and skin grafting. Excessive scarring produces contractures.

Chemical Injuries

DESCRIPTION
Harmful effects produced by environmental exposure to a variety of man-made and naturally occurring chemicals.

CAUSES AND PATHOPHYSIOLOGIC MECHANISMS
Solvents and vapors   Carbon tetrachloride: hepatotoxicity due to free radical generation; *chloroform, fluorocarbons:* CNS depression (anesthesia), cardiac arrhythmias; *ethylene glycol:* acute renal tubular necrosis; *methanol:* metabolic acidosis, CNS and retinal damage due to formaldehyde and formic acid metabolites; *benzene:* aplastic anemia, acute myeloblastic leukemia.

Pesticides   Chlorinated hydrocarbons (DDT, dieldrin): CNS and liver toxicity; *organophosphates* (malathion, parathion): nervous system toxicity due to acetylcholinesterase inhibition.

Herbicides and polychlorinated biphenyls   Dioxin (TCDD, contaminant of 2,4,5-T): blocks epidermal growth factor, causes chloracne, hepatotoxicity; dioxin, PCBs, and hexachlorophene are much more toxic to certain laboratory animals than to humans, due to different metabolic pathways.

Mushroom poisoning   Amanitin from *Amanita phalloides* inhibits RNA polymerase and causes necrosis of liver and other tissues; *muscarin* from *Amanita muscaria* causes parasympathomimetic effects (bradycardia, hypotension).

Asphyxiant gases   Carbon monoxide: hypoxia due to formation of carboxyhemoglobin; *cyanide:* inhibition of cellular cytochrome oxidase.

Heavy metals   Lead: denaturation of cellular enzymes by binding to disulfide groups; disrupts heme synthesis by inhibition of delta-aminolevulinic acid dehydratase and ferrochetalase. *Mercury:* denatures proteins, inhibits enzymes; inorganic mercury is toxic to renal tubules, organic mercury is neurotoxic. *Arsenic:* cytoplasmic poison, produces gastroenteritis and neurotoxicity.

MORPHOLOGY
Chronic lead poisoning produces rather specific lesions: lead line at epiphysis of child's long bones, gingival discoloration, basophilic stippling of red cells, nuclear inclusions in renal tubule cells, cerebral edema (lead encephalopathy). Several toxins cause liver lesions: carbon tetrachloride and amanitin produce hepatic necrosis; aflatoxin causes hepatocellular carcinoma. Acute tubular necrosis is characteristic of elemental mercury poisoning; cerebral and cerebellar degeneration occurs with organic mercury. Ethylene glycol poisoning produces oxalate crystals in renal tubules. Chlorinated aromatic hydrocarbons (dioxin) cause chloracne. Carbon monoxide and cyanide produce a cherry-red discoloration of skin, mucosa, and tissues.

CLINICAL CORRELATIONS
Injuries are often related to occupational exposures or industrial and agricultural accidents; the clinical presentation usually correlates with the level of exposure and known toxicity of the agent. *Organophospate poisoning* causes excessive secretions, dilatation of pupils, motor paralysis, and occasionally permanent neuropathy. *Chlorinated hydrocarbons* cause CNS hyperexcitability and convulsions. Dioxin and PCBs produce chloracne but evidence of additional toxicity is disputed. *Carbon monoxide poisoning* occurs in house fires and is a common suicide method. Importantly, CO poisoning is a subtle cause of neurologic symptoms and occasionally produces multiple fatalities due to faulty home appliances. *Methanol* and *ethylene glycol* poisoning occasionally occurs in chronic alcoholics desperate for a cheap drunk or consuming adulterated beverage. *Lead poisoning* often occurs in children who eat lead paint chips in old homes. Irritability and intellectual impairment occur with low doses; convulsions and death with high doses. Adults are exposed to lead through occupation and develop peripheral neuropathy (wrist or foot drop). Other effects of lead poisoning are abdominal pain, anemia, and renal tubular dysfunction (Fanconi's syndrome). Therapy requires chelators to remove the lead from body stores where it is tightly complexed in the inorganic matrix of bones.

Adverse Drug Reactions

DESCRIPTION
Harmful effects produced by drugs that are prescribed by a physician.

CAUSES AND PATHOPHYSIOLOGIC MECHANISMS

Dose-related effects (predictable drug injury) Toxicity of drug or metabolite due to overdose; variations in pharmaceutical preparation; genetic variations in drug metabolism; pre-existing liver disease, renal failure, heart failure, thyroid disease; drug interactions; bone marrow and immune system suppression by antineoplastic drugs.

Non–dose-related effects (unpredictable drug injury) Immunologic reactions: immediate hypersensitivity or anaphylaxis, cytotoxic reactions, immune complex reactions, delayed hypersensitivity. Idiosyncratic reactions are due to individual susceptibility related to nonimmunologic and poorly understood factors.

MORPHOLOGY

Heart *Cardiomyopathy:* adriamycin; *myocardial infarct:* oral contraceptives.

Lung *Alveolitis and interstitial fibrosis:* nitrofurantoin, busulfan, bleomycin; *asthma:* aspirin, propranolol; *pneumonia:* steroids, immunosuppressive therapy.

Gastrointestinal tract *Gingival hyperplasia:* dilantin; *gastritis* and *peptic ulcer:* steroids, aspirin, and other nonsteroid anti-inflammatory agents; *pseudomembranous colitis:* broad-spectrum antibiotics, especially clindamycin.

Liver *Fatty change:* tetracycline, aspirin in children with viral illness (Reye's syndrome); *cholestatic jaundice:* phenothiazines, sex steroids; *hepatitis:* halothane, isoniazid; *massive necrosis:* halothane, acetaminophen; *adenoma:* oral contraceptives.

Kidneys *Acute interstitial nephritis:* methicillin, other antibiotics; *acute tubular necrosis:* gentamicin, amphotericin B; *chronic interstitial nephritis* and *papillary necrosis:* phenacetin, acetaminophen, aspirin.

Endocrine system *Adrenocortical atrophy:* steroids.

Skeletal system *Osteoporosis:* steroids.

Central nervous system *Intracranial hemorrhage:* warfarin, heparin; *cerebral infarct:* oral contraceptives.

Blood and bone marrow *Autoimmune hemolytic anemia:* penicillins, cephalosporins, quinidine, methyldopa; *G6PD hemolytic anemia:* antimalarial drugs, sulfonamides, nitrofurantoin; *megaloblastic anemia:* methotrexate, dilantin; *aplastic anemia:* chloramphenicol, antineoplastic agents; *neutropenia:* chloramphenicol, chlorpromazine, sulfonamides; *thrombocytopenia:* quinidine.

Skin *Urticaria:* penicillins, sulfonamides, x-ray contrast media; *fixed drug eruptions:* sulfonamides; *erythema nodosum:* sulfonamides, oral contraceptives; *toxic epidermal necrolysis, Stevens-Johnson syndrome, erythema multiforme:* penicillin, sulfonamides, phenylbutazone, phenytoin.

Fetal injury *Phocomelia:* thalidomide; *vaginal adenosis* and *vaginal carcinoma:* diethylstilbestrol; *yellow discoloration of teeth:* tetracycline: *multiple congenital abnormalities:* antineoplastic agents, phenytoin, *sodium warfarin.*

CLINICAL CORRELATIONS
Up to 5% of hospitalized patients experience an adverse drug reaction; 2–12% may be fatal reactions. The risk is increased in elderly patients taking multiple drugs. Skin rashes, fever, and jaundice are common signs. Monitoring of blood cell counts, liver enzymes, electrolytes, BUN, and creatinine is indicated for certain drug therapies. Digoxin and other cardiotropic drugs cause arrhythmias that require ECG monitoring. Halothane-induced hepatic necrosis and anaphylactic reaction to penicillin are among the most common fatal reactions.

Radiation Injuries

DESCRIPTION
The range of cellular and tissue injuries produced by machine-generated x-rays and by gamma-rays from radioisotope disintegration. Alpha- and beta-particles are other forms of ionizing radiation that are much less important because of their limited penetrability.

CAUSES AND PATHOPHYSIOLOGIC MECHANISMS
Measurement of radiation Roentgen (R): emitted radiation; gray (Gy): absorbed radiation; 1 rad = 1 centigray; curie (ci): isotopic disintegration; half-life: time for one-half of an isotope to disintegrate; linear energy transfer (LET): rate at which radiation transfers energy to the tissue along the path it traverses; relative biologic effectiveness (RBE): relative measure of different types of radiation in producing a similar biologic effect; roentgen equivalent man (rem): another unit comparing effects of different types of radiation.

Production of cellular injury Most damage occurs by indirect action; photons collide with water molecules to produce free radicals that then react with cellular macromolecules; the most important target is nuclear DNA. The presence of oxygen increases the formation of free radicals and enhances the damage (the oxygen effect). Many lesions of DNA can be repaired; others are irreparable and lead to cell death or mutations due to genetic damage. The effects of the DNA damage are expressed when the cell is unable to divide normally (reproductive failure). *Tissue sensitivity* to radiation thus depends on cellular proliferation; the earliest effects are most pronounced in tissues with a high mitotic rate. Late effects of radiation injury depend partly on similar damage to parenchymal cells that proliferate slowly. More important in producing chronic radiation injury is damage to endothelial cells, which leads to occlusion of small blood vessels and consequent ischemia and fibrosis. Other long-term effects are cellular mutations that may be carcinogenic.

Sensitivity of cells to radiation *High radiosensitivity:* lymphocytes, bone marrow hematopoietic cells, epithelial cells of the gastrointestinal tract, pneumocytes, spermatogonia, germ cells of ovary and granulosa cells of follicle. *Low radiosensitivity:* mature bone and cartilage, skeletal muscle.

MORPHOLOGY
Early changes *Gastrointestinal tract:* epithelial cells fail to regenerate at the normal rate and after about three days the mucosa is edematous, hyperemic, and ulcerated. *Lungs:* alveolar lining cells show degenerative changes; alveoli are filled with protein-rich edema fluid. *Liver:* fibrin thrombi in central veins, leading to hepatic veno-occlusive disease. *Urinary bladder:* loss of urothelial cells, edema of wall. *Skin:* erythema, edema, desquamation, alopecia. *Gonads:* loss of germ cells, collapse of seminiferous tubules, loss of ovarian follicles. *Lymphoid tissue:* necrosis and disappearance of lymphocytes. *Bone marrow:* necrosis of hematopoietic elements, aplastic marrow. *Brain:* cerebral edema.

Late or delayed changes Within most tissues, the changes are similar; blood vessels and connective tissue are most affected. Walls of small arteries and arterioles are thickened with hyalinized collagen; endothelial cells proliferate and are vacuolated; vessel lumens are narrowed or obliterated. Connective tissue is increased and densely collagenized; parenchymal cells are degenerated and atrophic; large abnormal fibroblasts with hyperchromatic and sometimes bizarre nuclei are present. The vascular changes correlate with delayed radiation necrosis of brain and transverse myelitis of spinal cord. Radiation nephritis is characterized by vascular damage, interstitial fibrosis, and tubular atrophy. The connective tissue changes produce pulmonary fibrosis, hepatic fibrosis, fibrous strictures of GI tract, fibrosis and contraction of urinary bladder, and fibrosis and atrophy of gonads. Cataracts develop in the lens of the eye. In chronic radiation dermatitis, there are epidermal atrophy, hyperkeratosis, and hyperpigmentation; squamous cell carcinoma develops after several years.

CLINICAL CORRELATIONS

Localized radiation   Localized radiation therapy for tumors accounts for most instances of radiation injury. Normal tissue is shielded to minimize peripheral damage, which often limits the amount of radiation that can be safely administered. Fractionation of the total dose allows higher doses to be delivered because normal cells are better able than neoplastic cells to repair the damage in the interval between fractions. Nausea, vomiting, and diarrhea are common complications of radiation therapy.

Whole body radiation   Occurs with nuclear reactor accidents, nuclear explosions, and is administered prior to bone marrow transplantation. Low doses are more toxic when directed at the whole body, compared with localized radiation. Acute radiation sickness syndromes depend on the dose absorbed. Hematopoietic syndrome (2–5 Gy): mild GI symptoms; thrombocytopenia and granulocytopenia, leading to bleeding and fatal infections. Gastrointestinal syndrome (5–10 Gy): nausea, vomiting, profuse diarrhea; hypovolemic shock, sepsis; hematopoietic syndrome in survivors. Cerebral syndrome (20–50 Gy or more): convulsions, coma; cerebral edema and rapid death.

Cancers produced by radiation in various exposed groups   Squamous cell carcinoma of skin: early radiologists; lung cancers: uranium miners exposed to radon; leukemia of all types except chronic lymphocytic leukemia: atomic bomb survivors, early radiologists, patients irradiated for ankylosing spondylitis; thyroid cancers: atomic bomb survivors, children who received thymic radiation, Marshall Islanders; angiosarcoma of liver: patients who received Thorotrast (thorium dioxide); osteosarcoma: radium dial painters; breast cancer: atomic bomb survivors.

Congenital anomalies after intrauterine exposure   Microcephaly, growth and mental retardation, hydrocephalus, spina bifida, blindness, cleft palate, club foot.

Diseases Due to Smoking, Alcoholism, and Drug Abuse

DESCRIPTION
Diseases directly caused by major habits.

CAUSES AND PATHOPHYSIOLOGIC MECHANISMS
Cigarette smoking   Carcinogenic (polycyclic aromatic hydrocarbons); damages respiratory cilia; physically irritates airways; risk factor for atherosclerosis; promotes hypertension; elevates blood lipids; affects the female reproductive cycle; produces adverse fetal effects.

Ethyl alcohol   Acute effects: central nervous system depressant. Chronic effects: toxic to liver, pancreas, gastrointestinal tract, heart, brain, bone marrow, immune system, and fetus; promotes nutritional deficiencies. Cellular metabolic effects: increases NADH/NAD ratio, generates acetaldehyde, destabilizes cell membranes.

Drug abuse   Major categories of abused drugs: opiates, stimulants, depressants, psychoactive agents, inhalants. Adverse effects: overdose, dependence/addiction, local and systemic infections, injury of renal glomeruli and lung.

MORPHOLOGY
Smoking   Bronchogenic carcinoma; chronic obstructive pulmonary disease (emphysema and chronic bronchitis); carcinoma of larynx and oral cavity; increased incidence of carcinoma of esophagus, pancreas, kidney, and bladder; peptic ulcer disease; low-birth-weight infants; placental disorders (abruption, previa), premature rupture of membranes.

Alcoholism   Fatty liver, alcoholic hepatitis, cirrhosis and the complications thereof; gastritis, peptic ulcers; acute and chronic pancreatitis; alcoholic cardiomyopathy; gynecomastia, testicular atrophy; necrosis of mamillary bodies, cerebellar degeneration, central pontine myelinolysis.

Drug abuse   Linear scars on forearms (tracks); hepatitis; AIDS; talc granulomas in lung; infective endocarditis; abscesses at injection sites; marked pulmonary edema in overdose deaths.

CLINICAL CORRELATIONS
Smoking is responsible for enormous health problems and accounts for 350,000 deaths per year, particularly due to its effects on the respiratory and cardiovascular systems. After quitting for 15 years, ex-smokers' mortality rates return to normal. In *alcoholism,* acute intoxication contributes greatly to traumatic injuries and all types of violent death. Effects are dose related; one drink in a 150-lb person elevates the blood alcohol concentration by 20 mg/dL; potentially fatal respiratory depression occurs at 400 mg/dL. Cirrhosis is a major cause of death in chronic alcoholics due to its complications (liver failure, bleeding esophageal varices). With *drug abuse,* heroin and cocaine are the drugs most commonly injected. Alcohol is frequently abused in combination with drugs. Respiratory depression is a common mechanism of overdose deaths with opiates and depressants; seizures and cardiac arrhythmias are produced by stimulants. Cocaine causes seizures and cardiac complications. Viral hepatitis B and C and AIDS are major problems of intravenous drug abuse.

Diseases of Nutritional Deficiency

DESCRIPTION
The various diseases caused by deficiency of one or several nutrients. The deficiency may be primary (the nutrient is lacking in the diet) or secondary to another condition.

CAUSES AND PATHOPHYSIOLOGIC MECHANISMS
Protein–calorie malnutrition   Inadequate intake of protein, carbohydrate, and lipid. Kwashiorkor results from protein deficiency; marasmus occurs when all caloric sources are inadequate.

Malabsorption   Due to small intestinal disease (Crohn's disease, celiac disease, disaccharidase deficiency), pancreatic disease (cystic fibrosis, chronic pancreatitis), or biliary disease. Absorption of fat-soluble vitamins A, D, E, and K are affected to the greatest extent. Vitamin B_{12} malabsorption occurs in pernicious anemia due to absence of intrinsic factor, caused by destruction of gastric parietal cells. Vitamin B_{12} malabsorption also occurs with Crohn's disease affecting the ileum. Folate deficiency may also result from small intestinal malabsorption.

Chronic alcoholism   Interferes with proper nutrition due to multiple factors including inadequate intake. Deficiencies of B vitamins are most common; malabsorption of fat-soluble vitamins occurs with alcoholic chronic pancreatitis.

Chronic blood loss   Peptic ulcers and cancers of the gastrointestinal tract produce iron deficiency.

Liver disease   Cirrhosis and hepatitis result in deficient production of vitamin K-dependent coagulation factors (II, VII, IX, X).

Increased demand   Folate deficiency may develop in cases of severe chronic hemolytic anemia. *Infants, children, and women:* Neonates are deficient in vitamin K. Infants may receive inadequate nutrition after weaning. During growth of children and during pregnancy, nutritional demands are high and deficiencies are likely to appear. Menstruating females are predisposed to iron deficiency.

Dietary factors   Vegetarian diets may be deficient in protein, vitamin B_{12}, and iron. Overcooking destroys vitamin C and folate. "Tea and toast" diet of apathetic elderly leads to vitamin C deficiency. Certain infant formulas have been produced without pyridoxine; any infant formula prepared too diluted delivers insufficient nutrients. A maize diet leads to pellagra because the niacin is tightly bound and unavailable; a millet diet contains excess leucine, which blocks conversion of tryptophan to niacin and predisposes to pellagra.

Parasites Hookworm infestation produces iron-deficiency anemia due to chronic blood loss. *Diphyllobothrium latum* (fish tapeworm) produces vitamin B_{12} deficiency.

Drug-induced deficiencies Warfarin: vitamin K; isoniazid: vitamin B_6; methotrexate: folate; cholestyramine: fat-soluble vitamins.

Iatrogenic causes Hemodialysis; total parenteral nutrition; small bowel resection; partial gastrectomy.

MORPHOLOGY
Protein-calorie malnutrition Kwashiorkor is characterized by fatty liver and generalized edema; in marasmus, there is emaciation and stunting of growth. Intestinal mucosal atrophy is common, which may complicate absorption of nutrients when food becomes available. Mental development may be retarded.

Vitamin A deficiency Xerophthalmia, keratomalacia; squamous metaplasia of glandular epithelium; susceptibility to measles pneumonia.

Vitamin B_1 (thiamine) deficiency Dry beriberi: polyneuropathy with demyelination; wet beriberi: high-output heart failure with right heart dilatation and generalized edema; Wernicke-Korsakoff syndrome: focal brain lesions with necrosis in the thalamus, hypothalamus (especially mamillary bodies), paraventricular and periaqueductal regions.

Vitamin B_2 (niacin, nicotinic acid) deficiency Pellagra: rough scaly dermatitis often involving hands; diarrhea due to intestinal mucosal atrophy and ulceration; dementia due to degeneration of CNS neurons; demyelination of spinal cord tracts; glossitis.

Vitamin B_3 (riboflavin) deficiency Ariboflavinosis: cheilosis (cracking at corners of mouth); glossitis; seborrheic dermatitis; interstitial keratitis.

Vitamin B_6 (pyridoxine) deficiency Deficiency is uncommon. Dermatologic conditions similar to deficiencies of other B vitamins; peripheral neuropathy in alcoholics and with isoniazid therapy for TB; convulsions in infants eating deficient formula; anemia and convulsions in pyridoxine-dependency syndromes.

Vitamin B_{12} (cyanocobalamin) deficiency Megaloblastic (macrocytic) anemia: megaloblastic erythroid precursors in bone marrow; chronic atrophic gastritis in pernicious anemia; subacute combined degeneration of spinal cord.

Vitamin C (ascorbic acid) deficiency Scurvy: deficient synthesis of collagen; defective production of osteoid in growing bones with cartilaginous overgrowth at epiphysis; subperiosteal and intra-articular hemorrhage; ecchymoses and purpura of skin and gingiva; periodontal disease; loosened teeth; poor wound healing due to inadequate scar tissue.

Vitamin D deficiency   Rickets in children: excessive osteoid and cartilage at epiphysis, producing rachitic rosary; frontal bossing of skull; pigeon breast deformity of chest; bowing of legs. Osteomalacia in adults, predisposing to fractures, especially of hip and vertebra.

Vitamin E deficiency   Degeneration of posterior columns of the spinal cord.

Vitamin K deficiency   Hypoprothrombinemia: ecchymosis and purpura of skin and mucosa; soft tissue hematomas; gastrointestinal and intracerebral hemorrhages; hemorrhagic disease of the newborn.

Folic acid deficiency   Megaloblastic (macrocytic) anemia: megaloblastic erythroid precursors in bone marrow; similar to vitamin B_{12} deficiency but without the neurologic degeneration.

Iodine deficiency   Thyroid goiter.

Iron deficiency   Hypochromic microcytic anemia; absence of iron stores in bone marrow; glossitis; koilonychia; Plummer-Vinson syndrome.

Zinc deficiency   Acrodermatitis enteropathica; growth retardation; male hypogonadism; exacerbation of vitamin A deficiency; congenital defects in offspring of deficient mother.

Copper deficiency   Anemia, neutropenia, osteoporosis, depigmentation of hair; worse in children.

Selenium deficiency   Congestive cardiomyopathy.

CLINICAL CORRELATIONS
In the US, deficiency states are usually secondary to other conditions. Chronic alcoholism and malabsorption due to intestinal, pancreatic, or biliary disease account for most cases. Small intestinal malabsorption is most likely to produce deficiencies of fat-soluble vitamins; cystic fibrosis is another common cause of fat malabsorption. Iron deficiency is quite common, especially in menstruating and postpartum females and in children; iron deficiency in an adult male or postmenopausal female is a sign of chronic blood loss from cancer, ulcers or other serious disease. Elderly people living alone and eating poorly are a vulnerable group; vitamin C deficiency may become evident when an older

person does not heal properly after surgery. Vitamin D deficiency may occur in this same group, due to inadequate dietary intake combined with absence of sunlight exposure; the resulting osteomalacia contributes to hip and other fractures. Drug-induced vitamin K deficiency is common in patients with congestive heart failure, atrial fibrillation, and prosthetic heart valves, who are treated prophylactically with warfarin. Folic acid supplements can reverse the macrocytic anemia of pernicious anemia without affecting the neurologic degeneration; thus, vitamin B_{12} deficiency must be excluded before folic acid is given to treat anemia.

Pathology Facts, by Richard C.
Harruff, J.B. Lippincott
Company, Philadelphia © 1994.

Chapter 7

Congenital Malformations and Genetic Diseases

Congenital Malformations

DESCRIPTION
Structural defects that are present at birth caused by errors of morphogenesis.

CAUSES AND PATHOPHYSIOLOGIC MECHANISMS
Known causes: chromosomal abnormalities, inherited diseases, and environmental factors. The cause of most malformations is unknown.

Environmental factors   Maternal infections that cross the placenta: toxoplasmosis, rubella, cytomegalovirus, herpes simplex type I or II, syphilis (TORCH complex). Maternal drugs: alcohol, thalidomide, androgens, folate antagonists, alkylating agents, anticonvulsants (phenytoin), warfarin, retinoic acid. Maternal radiation. Maternal diabetes mellitus or other metabolic disease. During the first 8 weeks of gestation (during organogenesis), exposure to an environmental teratogen causes major malformations; after this period, similar exposures produce less severe malformations.

Patterns of malformations   Preimplantation: incomplete separation of blastomeres (siamese twins, sacrococcygeal teratoma). Postimplantation: agenesis, aplasia, hypoplasia; dysplasia; failures of involution, division, or fusion; atresia; ectopias, heterotopias. Multiple simultaneous malformations may constitute a syndrome.

MORPHOLOGY

Fetal alcohol syndrome   Microcephaly, growth and mental retardation, facial abnormalities (short palpebral fissure, epicanthic folds, maxillary hypoplasia), abnormalities of extremities, heart (atrial septal defect), and kidney.

Thalidomide-associated malformations   Amelia, phocomelia, defects of ears and heart.

TORCH infections   *Rubella syndrome:* triad of cataracts, heart defects, and deafness; also microcephaly, mental retardation, hepatosplenomegaly, growth retardation. *Toxoplasmosis:* chorioretinitis, cerebral calcifications; intracellular parasites and cysts. *Cytomegalovirus:* thrombocytopenia with purpura, hemolytic anemia with jaundice, hepatosplenomegaly, necrotic brain lesions; cellular enlargement with "bulls-eye" nuclear inclusions. *Herpes:* keratoconjunctivitis, skin vesicles, necrotic lesions in various organs, including brain; multinucleated cells, "ground-glass" nuclear inclusions. *Syphilis:* vasculitis, gummas, skin lesions; Hutchinson's teeth, mulberry molars; saddle nose, hard palate perforation; periostitis, saber shin; interstitial keratitis; optic nerve atrophy, 8th nerve deafness; pneumonia alba.

Common malformations   Hypospadias; clubfoot; congenital heart defects (ventricular septal defect, patent ductus arteriosus, atrial septal defect); cleft lip/cleft palate; congenital hip dislocation; neural tube defects (anencephaly, spina bifida, meningocele, myelomeningocele); fetal hydantoin syndrome; cystic disease of kidney; malformations associated with chromosomal abnormalities; malformations due to inherited diseases.

Deformations   Structural abnormalities that are produced by an adverse uterine environment, such as amniotic bands and oligohydramnios (Potter's syndrome).

CLINICAL CORRELATIONS

Known maternal infections and exposure to drugs, chemicals, and radiation account for less than 5% of congenital malformations; chromosomal abnormalities are responsible for about 5%; and hereditary diseases, 15%; most of the remainder have no known cause. The list of drugs that are known teratogens is relatively small; alcohol is the most common chemical teratogen. Recognition of particular syndromes and inherited diseases is important so that parents can receive genetic counseling. Cytogenetic studies detect chromosomal abnormalities. Rubella is the most important teratogenic maternal infection; during the first 16 weeks of pregnancy it can produce malformations, with the greatest risk and worst malformations during the first 8 weeks. All TORCH infections produce similar effects during early pregnancy; differentiation requires serologic studies and viral cultures. Neonatal herpes results from passage of the infant through an infected birth canal; cesarean section is performed to avoid this exposure. *Treponema pallidum* infects the fetus after 16 weeks to produce congenital syphilis; in worst cases, lesions are present at birth; in the tardive form, lesions appear after several years.

Cytogenetic Diseases

DESCRIPTION
Diseases due to an abnormal number of chromosomes or abnormal structure of one or more chromosomes.

CAUSES AND PATHOPHYSIOLOGIC MECHANISMS
Autosomal trisomies *Down's syndrome:* trisomy 21, most often due to meiotic nondisjunction, usually involving the maternal chromosomes; about 5% of cases are due to translocations of the long arm of chromosome 21 to another chromosome; 1% are mosaics, with part of the cells having normal karyotype and other cells trisomy 21. *Edwards' syndrome (trisomy 18), and Patau's syndrome (trisomy 13):* both due to meiotic nondisjunction.

Sex chromosome abnormalities *Klinefelter's syndrome (47,XXY):* meiotic nondisjunction of the X chromosome received from either parent; variants include mosaics and karyotypes with more than 2 X chromosomes. *Turner's syndrome:* half of cases have monosomy of the X chromosome (45,X), usually due to paternal meiotic nondisjunction. In the remainder, there is a structurally defective X chromosome, usually from the father, or a mosaic.

MORPHOLOGY
Down's syndrome Flat face, oblique palpebral fissures, narrow interpupillary distance, epicanthic folds; Brushfield spots on iris; enlarged tongue; low-set ears; transverse (simian) palmar crease; hypoplastic and incurved middle finger; short trunk, short neck; high rate of cardiac defects, especially septal defects; increased risk of acute leukemia, especially lymphoblastic leukemia.

Klinefelter's syndrome Tall male, eunichoid, long legs; gynecomastia; female hair distribution; testicular atrophy with interstitial fibrosis, atrophic tubules, and aspermatogenesis.

Turner's syndrome Short female; webbed neck, lymphedema, cystic hygroma; broad chest, widely spaced nipples with absent breast development; absent sexual maturation; coarctation of aorta and other heart defects; multiple melanocytic nevi; streak ovaries without ova or follicles.

CLINICAL CORRELATIONS
Down's syndrome occurs in 1 of 700–800 live births and is highly associated with maternal age, especially after age 40. It is a leading cause of mental retardation. Cardiac septal defects are common; there is increased susceptibility to respiratory infection; and the risk of acute leukemia is increased. Death in early life is due to cardiac disease or pneumonia. Those living past 40 years develop Alzheimer-type dementia; postmortem brain examination shows neuritic plaques and neurofibrillary tangles. *Klinefelter's syndrome* occurs in 1 of 850–1000 live births but is not apparent until sexual maturity. It is the most common cause of male infertility. Intelligence is subnormal. Testosterone is low; serum gonadotropins are elevated. *Turner's syndrome* occurs in 1 of 3000 live births; many more are seen as stillbirths. Apparent at birth because of the webbed neck and lymphedema. Later there is short stature, primary amenorrhea, failure of secondary sexual development, and infertility; intelligence is usually normal. Estrogens are low, serum gonadotropins are elevated.

Inherited Diseases

DESCRIPTION
Diseases that are transmitted from one generation to the next as gene mutations on the autosomes or sex chromosomes. Single gene mutations are transmitted according to mendelian principles; those involving several genes are more complex in their inheritance patterns.

CAUSES AND PATHOPHYSIOLOGIC MECHANISMS
Single gene disorders   Mutation produces a synthetically defective enzyme, receptor, transport, or structural protein or results in diminished production of normal protein. Enzyme defects may result in either absence of a critical metabolite or accumulation of a toxic intermediate. Defects in receptor or transport proteins cause metabolic failure or accumulation of metabolic products. Structural protein defects cause inadequate cell membranes or connective tissue. Mutations of regulatory genes result in neoplasms. Transmission may be autosomal dominant, autosomal recessive, or sex-linked. In a certain percentage, a new mutation produces the disease and there is no inheritance.

Multifactorial (polygenic) disorders   More than one mutation is involved, and expression depends on the number of mutant genes inherited. Extent of expression may be continuous, with all levels of expression possible, or discontinuous, when there is a threshold effect producing either expression or nonexpression. Environmental factors greatly modify expression of polygenic inherited diseases.

MORPHOLOGY

Autosomal dominant diseases   *Enzyme deficiency:* porphyria. *Receptor protein defects:* familial hypercholesterolemia, von Willebrand's disease. *Structural protein deficiencies:* Ehlers-Danlos syndrome, Marfan's syndrome, osteogenesis imperfecta, hereditary spherocytosis. *Neoplasms:* familial polyposis coli, von Recklinghausen's neurofibromatosis, tuberous sclerosis, von Hippel-Lindau syndrome. *Others:* achondroplasia, adult polycystic kidney disease, Huntington's disease, Osler-Weber-Rendu disease (hereditary hemorrhagic telangiectasia).

Autosomal recessive diseases   *Enzyme deficiency:* disorders of amino acid metabolism (albinism, alkaptonuria or ochronosis, phenylketonuria, tyrosinemia), galactosemia, lysosomal storage diseases (sphingolipidoses: Tay-Sachs, Niemann-Pick, Gaucher's; mucopolysaccharidoses: Hurler's; glycogenoses: McArdle's, Pompe's, von Gierke's), severe combined immunodeficiency. Enzyme inhibitor deficiency: alpha-1-antitrypsin deficiency. Transport protein deficiency: sickle cell anemia, thalassemia, cystic fibrosis, possibly Wilson's disease and hemochromatosis.

Sex-linked recessive diseases   *Enzyme deficiency:* chronic granulomatous disease, Fabry's disease, hemolytic anemia with glucose-6-phosphate dehydrogenase deficiency, Lesch-Nyhan syndrome. *Enzyme cofactor deficiency:* hemophilia. *Cytoskeletal/regulatory protein defect:* Duchenne muscular dystrophy. *Others:* Wiskott-Aldrich syndrome, X-linked agammaglobulinemia of Bruton, fragile-X syndrome.

Multifactorial genetic diseases   Atherosclerosis, cleft lip and/or palate, congenital dislocation of hip, congenital heart disease, diabetes mellitus, gout, hypertension, congenital pyloric stenosis, neural tube defects.

CLINICAL CORRELATIONS

Autosomal dominant diseases are expressed in every generation; males and females are affected; heterozygotes express the disease, depending on the gene's penetrance and expressivity, and transmit the disease to half of their children. *Autosomal recessive diseases* may not be expressed in every generation; males and females are affected; only homozygotes are affected; both parents of the affected are heterozygotes (carriers) and do not express the disease but do transmit the disease to one quarter and the carrier state to half of their children. *Sex-linked recessive diseases* may not be expressed in every generation; only males and rare homozygous females are affected (an occasional heterozygous female may partially express the disease due to unfavorable lyonization); only females are carriers and transmit the disease to half of their sons and the carrier state to half of their daughters; affected males transmit the carrier state to their daughters. *Multifactorial diseases* occur at a lower rate in affected families, compared with single gene diseases, but at a higher rate than in the general population. Approximately 2–7% of first-degree relatives express the disease. If one child is affected, the risk for the next child is 2–7%; if two children are affected, the risk for the next is 9%. More severe defects indicate a greater chance for the same defect to recur in succeeding pregnancies. *Diagnosis of single gene diseases* requires evaluation of the family history; negative family history indicates uncertain parentage or a new mutation. Methods for confirming the presence of a defective gene include: enzyme assays, electrophoresis, immunochemical methods, and DNA probe analysis using blood or tissue cells or cells obtained by amniocentesis for prenatal diagnosis.

Infectious
Diseases

Pathology Facts, by Richard C. Harruff, J.B. Lippincott Company, Philadelphia © 1994.

Chapter 8

Viral Infections

Cytomegalovirus Infection

DESCRIPTION   Infection with cytomegalovirus, a DNA virus of the Herpes group; infection may be congenital, peri- or postnatal, or disseminated in immunocompromised persons.

DISEASE ENTITIES; SYNONYMS AND ACRONYMS   Cytomegalic inclusion disease, CID; CMV infection.

INCIDENCE   Common; increases with age.

AGE   1% of newborns are infected; 50–80% of adults are seropositive.

ETIOLOGY, PATHOGENESIS, AND PREDISPOSING FACTORS   Cytomegalovirus may be transmitted through the placenta, perinatally, via mother's milk, sexually, through blood transfusions and transplanted organs.

SITES INVOLVED   In utero infections involve the brain and cause mental retardation. The infection may be disseminated involving the salivary glands, kidneys, liver, lung, pancreas, thyroid, adrenals, and GI tract.

GROSS LESIONS   Lesions include diffuse interstitial pneumonitis leading to respiratory distress syndrome; hepatitis, adrenalitis, intestinal ulcerations; calcifications around ventricles in neonatal CNS infections.

MICROSCOPIC LESIONS   Intranuclear or intracytoplasmic inclusions; enlargement of the infected cells; intranuclear inclusions are eosinophilic with a surrounding halo ("bulls-eye").

COMPLICATIONS   In utero infections can cause mental retardation and neurologic deficits. Transplant patients or immunocompromised patients may have fatal disseminated infections with respiratory failure.

SIGNS AND SYMPTOMS   In normal adults, the infection is usually asymptomatic; in immunosuppressed patients, there may be fever, splenomegaly, hepatitis, or pneumonitis.

CLINICAL DIAGNOSIS AND OTHER CLINICAL FEATURES   Signs of pulmonary, hepatic or multisystem involvement in immunocompromised patients, transplant patients, or neonates. Purpuric skin rash may develop in neonatal CID.

LABORATORY DIAGNOSIS   Isolation of virus in cultures of urine or mouth swabs; demonstration of characteristic viral inclusions in tissue biopsies; serum antibody titers may indicate prior infection that is reactivated.

PROGNOSIS   Poor for immunodeficient patients. Most infections in immunocompetent adults are asymptomatic.

THERAPY   Ganciclovir has been shown to be effective; acyclovir is ineffective.

OTHER INFORMATION   CMV may be transmitted to susceptible patients through blood transfusion; thus, using seronegative donors for CMV, seronegative transplant patients, or neonates is appropriate.

Dengue Fever

DESCRIPTION   An arthropod-borne viral infection that may be complicated by fever, hemorrhage, and shock (dengue shock syndrome). The skin rash is maculopapular and petechial.

DISEASE ENTITIES; SYNONYMS AND ACRONYMS   Breakbone, dandy, aden, polka, or solar fever; dengue shock syndrome; dengue hemorrhagic fever.

INCIDENCE   Common in tropical regions; may occur in epidemics; hemorrhagic fever in Southeast Asia.

AGE   Any age; shock syndrome is most common in children with repeated infections.

ETIOLOGY, PATHOGENESIS, AND PREDISPOSING FACTORS   Arbovirus transmitted to humans by Aedes aegypti mosquitoes, especially in rainy season; children with repeated infections by different serotypes of virus are predisposed to the shock syndrome.

SITES INVOLVED   Viremia; skin, joints, hematopoietic system and muscles; bleeding from body orifices and petechial hemorrhages in skin and mucous membranes with shock syndrome.

GROSS LESIONS   Petechial hemorrhages in skin, mucous membranes, and gastrointestinal tract.

MICROSCOPIC LESIONS   Blood film may show leukopenia and thrombocytopenia. Perivascular hemorrhage around capillaries is present in the petechial lesions.

COMPLICATIONS   Death in 3% of patients with shock syndrome even if patient receives good medical care. Uncomplicated dengue fever resolves completely.

SIGNS AND SYMPTOMS   Fever, maculopapular rash, painful joints and muscles, headache, "saddle-back" temperature curve. Shock syndrome: bleeding from body orifices and petechial hemorrhages.

CLINICAL DIAGNOSIS AND OTHER CLINICAL FEATURES   Recognition of above signs in a person who has been in an endemic area; hypotension; petechiae produced by the tourniquet test.

LABORATORY DIAGNOSIS   Serologic tests such as hemagglutination inhibition or complement fixation; thrombocytopenia in severe cases.

PROGNOSIS   Fairly good for shock syndrome if treated; uncomplicated cases recover completely.

THERAPY   Supportive medical care; avoid aspirin. No vaccine is yet available.

OTHER INFORMATION   Dengue fever is widespread and found in Asia, Africa, the Pacific islands, Mexico, South America, and the Caribbean. Twenty-four cases in US in 1990, all imported from endemic areas.

Encephalitis, Arthropod-Borne

DESCRIPTION   Meningoencephalitis caused by one of eight arboviruses including Western Equine, Eastern equine, Venezuelan equine, St. Louis, Japanese, West Nile, and California encephalitis viruses.

DISEASE ENTITIES; SYNONYMS AND ACRONYMS   WEE, EEE, VEE, SLE, JBE, CE.

INCIDENCE   Sporadic cases in mid-summer and autumn; viruses vary by geographic location; occasional epidemics.

AGE   Any age but some types are more common in the elderly or young.

ETIOLOGY, PATHOGENESIS, AND PREDISPOSING FACTORS   All have mosquitoes as their vector; reservoirs are birds and rodents primarily. Horses and humans have "dead-end" infections: mosquitoes do not transmit from them to other people or animals.

SITES INVOLVED   Central nervous system; inflammation and necrosis are most severe around blood vessels.

GROSS LESIONS   Varies from mild congestion of meninges to extensive encephalitis with multifocal cerebral cortical necrosis in severe cases; petechial hemorrhages are often present within brain substance.

MICROSCOPIC LESIONS   Mild infection: lymphocytic meningoencephalitis with perivascular cuffing (except EEE which has a PMN infiltrate); severe cases: focal cerebral cortical necrosis, vasculitis, and thrombosis.

COMPLICATIONS   Residual neurologic deficits which are more severe in the very young.

SIGNS AND SYMPTOMS   Fever, headache, and body aches progressing to neck rigidity and drowsiness; confusion, convulsions, coma, or death in most severe cases.

CLINICAL DIAGNOSIS AND OTHER CLINICAL FEATURES   Recognition of the above signs; CT, MRI, and brain scans to exclude mass lesions; cases are most frequent in late summer in second consecutive year of heavy rainfall.

LABORATORY DIAGNOSIS   Serology; hemagglutination inhibition and complement fixation testing.

PROGNOSIS   EEE mortality rate of >50%; WEE, 3%; SLE, 2–12%; California, <2%.

THERAPY   Supportive care.

OTHER INFORMATION   St. Louis virus can cause urban epidemics; California virus is a major cause of encephalitis in the Midwestern United States.

German Measles

DESCRIPTION   Infection with rubella virus, which causes a mild childhood illness with rash resembling measles; infection in a pregnant woman causes fetal damage (rubella syndrome).

DISEASE ENTITIES; SYNONYMS AND ACRONYMS   Rubella, 3-day measles; rubella syndrome.

INCIDENCE   Previously a common childhood illness but now uncommon due to widespread immunization.

AGE   Any age person without protective antibodies; usually children.

ETIOLOGY, PATHOGENESIS, AND PREDISPOSING FACTORS   Rubella virus, an RNA togavirus; transplacental fetal infection in pregnant nonimmune women who contract rubella may cause congenital malformations or intrauterine death.

SITES INVOLVED   Many infections are subclinical. The virus is shed from the nasopharynx and has a 12–21 day incubation. The lymph nodes behind the ears may be enlarged and a skin rash may appear.

GROSS LESIONS   Erythematous morbilliform skin rash; congenital malformations include cardiovascular defects, cataracts, deafness, mental retardation, and microcephaly.

MICROSCOPIC LESIONS   No specific microscopic lesions.

COMPLICATIONS   Intrauterine fetal infections cause serious congenital malformations of brain, heart, and eyes; otherwise the disease is clinically insignificant.

SIGNS AND SYMPTOMS   A low-grade fever accompanied by a skin rash that spares the palms and soles along with enlarged lymph nodes behind the ears or in the back of the head.

CLINICAL DIAGNOSIS AND OTHER CLINICAL FEATURES   Recognition of the above signs in a person who is not immune to the virus.

LABORATORY DIAGNOSIS   Serology demonstrates immune status, which is important to know in a newly pregnant woman.

PROGNOSIS   Good; except for intrauterine infections and very rare cases of meningoencephalitis.

THERAPY   Supportive care; prevention with attenuated live virus vaccine.

OTHER INFORMATION   Congenitally infected infants may shed virus for several months after birth. Joint pain and swelling may occur in adult infections.

Hepatitis C

DESCRIPTION   Infection with an as yet poorly defined virus that causes necrosis of the liver; the infection is likely to become chronic and progress to cirrhosis.

DISEASE ENTITIES; SYNONYMS AND ACRONYMS   Non-A and non-B hepatitis, NANB hepatitis, HCV.

INCIDENCE   20–40% of all acute viral hepatitis cases are due to HCV.

AGE   Any age.

ETIOLOGY, PATHOGENESIS, AND PREDISPOSING FACTORS   The virus may be transmitted through transfusion of cellular blood components or through drug abuse, occupational blood exposure, or household contact with an infected person.

SITES INVOLVED   Liver; hepatocytes.

GROSS LESIONS   Acute hepatitis: liver may be swollen or shrunken and yellow; chronic infection may progress to macronodular cirrhosis with fibrosis surrounding regenerating hepatic nodules.

MICROSCOPIC LESIONS   Acutely there is hepatocellular necrosis that may be massive, with associated inflammation; in chronic infections there is portal inflammation with piece-meal necrosis and progressive fibrosis.

COMPLICATIONS   Cirrhosis, liver failure, bleeding diathesis, hepatic encephalopathy.

SIGNS AND SYMPTOMS   Mild and asymptomatic infections are common; 25% have jaundice and other signs of hepatitis including fatigue, anorexia, and malaise.

CLINICAL DIAGNOSIS AND OTHER CLINICAL FEATURES   Recognition of the signs of hepatitis in a person having a history of transfusion, blood exposure, or intravenous drug use.

LABORATORY DIAGNOSIS   Elevation of serum liver enzymes indicating liver damage. Antibody testing is not useful to diagnose acute infections as seroconversion takes up to 6 months.

PROGNOSIS   Often poor; up to 40% of transfusion-associated cases develop chronic active hepatitis.

THERAPY   Supportive treatment of liver failure; interferon alfa-2b is FDA approved for chronic active cases.

OTHER INFORMATION   The current antibody test detects antibodies against a nonstructural viral protein; there is no confirmatory test yet available.

Herpes Simplex Infections

DESCRIPTION   Infection with either herpes simplex virus type 1 or 2. Primary infections occur in those not previously exposed; recurrent lesions are due to latent virus infection of sensory nerve ganglia.

DISEASE ENTITIES; SYNONYMS AND ACRONYMS   Herpes labialis, cold sores, fever blisters; herpes gingivostomatitis; herpes genitalis; herpetic whitlow.

INCIDENCE   Common and world-wide distribution.

AGE   Any age. Neonates can acquire the infection at birth from an infected mother.

ETIOLOGY, PATHOGENESIS, AND PREDISPOSING FACTORS   Herpes is an enveloped, double stranded DNA virus. Herpes simplex type 1 may be transmitted by direct contact or by fomites. Type 2 is spread by sexual contact.

SITES INVOLVED   Type 1: lips, face skin, oral mucosa; type 2: skin and mucosa of genital and anal region; dissemination with widespread skin, CNS, and visceral lesions in neonate and immunocompromised patients.

GROSS LESIONS   Red vesicular lesions in clusters, initially filled with clear fluid; ulceration and oozing; secondary bacterial infection with purulent exudate.

MICROSCOPIC LESIONS   Superficial vesicles with multinucleated epithelial cells containing intranuclear inclusions; lymphocytic inflammation.

COMPLICATIONS   Meningoencephalitis;   keratoconjunctivitis; aseptic meningitis; dissemination to CNS and viscera in immunocompromised patients and neonates.

SIGNS AND SYMPTOMS   Painful, vesicular skin lesions on the face or lips in type 1 infection, or on the genitalia in type 2 infections.

CLINICAL DIAGNOSIS AND OTHER CLINICAL FEATURES   Recognition of the skin lesions or related mucosal lesions (e.g., herpetic gingivostomatitis); differentiate pharyngeal infection from "strep throat" and genital infection from syphilis.

LABORATORY DIAGNOSIS   Tzanck preparation from skin lesion to visualize the intranuclear viral inclusions; meningoencephalitis may require brain biopsy of the temporal lobe; viral culture; immunofluorescence.

PROGNOSIS   Recurrent skin lesions are common; reactivation of the virus is often related to stress or trauma.

THERAPY   Acyclovir improves the course of the infection and decreases the duration of the lesions.

OTHER INFORMATION   Neonatal herpes infections are acquired as an ascending infection from the mother or during delivery due to passage through an infected birth canal.

Infectious Mononucleosis

DESCRIPTION Infection with Epstein-Barr virus (EBV), a herpesvirus that causes lymphoid proliferation in the blood, lymph nodes, and spleen.

DISEASE ENTITIES; SYNONYMS AND ACRONYMS Mono, glandular fever; IM; EBV.

INCIDENCE Common; most adults are seropositive for EBV; IM is a disease of youth.

AGE Most common in children, adolescents, and young adults.

ETIOLOGY, PATHOGENESIS, AND PREDISPOSING FACTORS Epstein-Barr virus; spread by oral-oral contact (kissing); EBV immortalizes B-cells to cause lymphocytosis; T-cells react to the infected B-cells and appear as atypical lymphocytes.

SITES INVOLVED Lymphoid system including lymph nodes, spleen, and peripheral blood; EBV is tropic for B-cells and for epithelial cells of the nasopharynx and uterine cervix.

GROSS LESIONS Enlargement of lymph nodes and spleen; spleen may be enlarged 2–3 times normal.

MICROSCOPIC LESIONS Lymphoid hyperplasia, diffuse and follicular; prominent germinal centers; Reed-Sternberg cells may be seen; hyperplasia of splenic red pulp; lymphocytosis in blood.

COMPLICATIONS Hepatitis; splenic rupture; tonsillar enlargement may compromise airway; rare meningoencephalitis.

SIGNS AND SYMPTOMS Fever, sore throat, and lymphadenopathy are the most common presenting signs; splenomegaly, headache, anorexia, and jaundice are less common.

CLINICAL DIAGNOSIS AND OTHER CLINICAL FEATURES Recognition of the presenting symptoms in children and adolescents; persistent left upper abdominal pain and tenderness may indicate splenic rupture.

LABORATORY DIAGNOSIS CBC: absolute lymphocytosis with atypical lymphocytes; positive Monospot or heterophile antibody test; abnormal liver enzymes in 95% but jaundice in only 4%.

PROGNOSIS Excellent.

THERAPY Rest and supportive care.

OTHER INFORMATION EBV has been implicated in the causation of African Burkitt's lymphoma and nasopharyngeal carcinoma in the Orient. Chronic infection with EBV may cause chronic fatigue syndrome.

Measles

DESCRIPTION An acute viral illness characterized by fever, sore throat, respiratory symptoms, and skin rash (exanthem) due to infection with measles virus.

DISEASE ENTITIES; SYNONYMS AND ACRONYMS Red measles; rubeola; black (hemorrhagic) measles.

INCIDENCE Decreased due to childhood immunization. May cause outbreaks in adolescents and college students.

AGE Previously a childhood illness, now seen in college-aged persons.

ETIOLOGY, PATHOGENESIS, AND PREDISPOSING FACTORS Measles virus, RNA paramyxovirus, respiratory droplet transmission; college students are susceptible due to loss of protective antibodies or suboptimal immunization standards during their childhood.

SITES INVOLVED Virus infects respiratory tract and spreads by viremia to involve lymphoid tissue; skin shows characteristic rash; Koplik's spots are present in oral mucosa; lungs occasionally develop pneumonia.

GROSS LESIONS An erythematous rash that becomes maculopapular, involving the face, neck, trunk, and limbs. Lymph nodes and spleen may be enlarged. Koplik's spots are red with central white speck.

MICROSCOPIC LESIONS Lymph nodes are hyperplastic with multinucleated Warthin-Finkeldey giant cells containing intranuclear and intracytoplasmic viral inclusions. Cells in Koplik's spots contain similar viral inclusions.

COMPLICATIONS Measles giant-cell pneumonia, hemorrhagic (black) measles, measles encephalitis, subacute sclerosing panencephalitis, juvenile diabetes mellitus; secondary bacterial pneumonia.

SIGNS AND SYMPTOMS Viral prodrome with development of typical morbilliform rash after 3–5 days; fever, nonproductive cough, and photophobia with conjunctivitis resolve as the rash develops.

CLINICAL DIAGNOSIS AND OTHER CLINICAL FEATURES Recognition of the clinical signs; Koplik's spots in the mouth are nearly diagnostic and may precede the skin rash by several days; malnourished children are at risk for developing pneumonia.

LABORATORY DIAGNOSIS Serologic demonstration of IgM class antibodies in the acute phase of the illness, or a significant increase in IgG antibody titers between acute and convalescent sera.

PROGNOSIS Good in children; increased risk of serious complications in immunosupressed or older people.

THERAPY Supportive care; prevention with live attenuated vaccine is highly effective.

OTHER INFORMATION Epidemics throughout history have occurred when indigenous populations were exposed to the virus by explorers. Malnutrition, especially vitamin A deficiency, causes high morbidity and mortality.

Mumps

DESCRIPTION Infection with mumps virus, a paramyxovirus, that affects the glandular tissues of the body.

DISEASE ENTITIES; SYNONYMS AND ACRONYMS Infectious parotitis.

INCIDENCE The frequency is low due to childhood vaccinations.

AGE Mumps was a common childhood illness but can affect any nonimmune person.

ETIOLOGY, PATHOGENESIS, AND PREDISPOSING FACTORS Mumps virus is an RNA paramyxovirus, transmitted by respiratory droplet inhalation or by direct nasopharyngeal or oral contact with secretions from an infected person.

SITES INVOLVED Initial infection of pharynx with incubation of 2–4 weeks; viremic spread to salivary glands, especially parotid glands; may also involve pancreas, ovaries, and testes.

GROSS LESIONS The salivary glands are swollen and inflamed; gonads may also be swollen.

MICROSCOPIC LESIONS Salivary glands are edematous and infiltrated with chronic inflammatory cells, including lymphocytes and plasma cells; microinfarcts may be present in the swollen testis.

COMPLICATIONS Epididymo-orchitis, pancreatitis, mastitis, oophoritis; infrequent meningitis, encephalitis, and myocarditis.

SIGNS AND SYMPTOMS Fever, malaise, headache, and other viral signs along with swelling and pain of the salivary glands, most notably the parotid glands.

CLINICAL DIAGNOSIS AND OTHER CLINICAL FEATURES Recognition of the above clinical signs; differential may include bacterial sialoadenitis, which causes acute unilateral swelling and tenderness with signs of acute inflammation.

LABORATORY DIAGNOSIS Demonstration of a significant rise in titer between acute and convalescent sera is diagnostic; elevation of serum amylase indicates pancreatitis.

PROGNOSIS Good.

THERAPY Supportive care.

OTHER INFORMATION Orchitis, if it occurs, is usually unilateral and thus seldom causes male sterility. Adults who are infected often have a longer course and convalescence.

Poliomyelitis

DESCRIPTION   Infection with poliovirus, an enterovirus that affects anterior horn cells of the spinal cord; disease manifestations include asymptomatic and minor infections, aseptic meningitis, and paralytic polio.

DISEASE ENTITIES; SYNONYMS AND ACRONYMS   Polio, infantile paralysis; bulbar poliomyelitis.

INCIDENCE   Endemic in underdeveloped regions; rare in US due to vaccinations; more common in summer and autumn.

AGE   Symptomatic disease more common in infants and children.

ETIOLOGY, PATHOGENESIS, AND PREDISPOSING FACTORS   Poliovirus is an enterovirus with tropism for motor neurons, transmitted by consumption of water with fecal contamination.

SITES INVOLVED   Virus replicates in mucosa of the pharynx and GI tract and then produces a viremia. The virus reaches the CNS through the blood and infects the anterior horn cells.

GROSS LESIONS   No distinctive acute gross lesions; atrophy of anterior spinal nerve roots months or years after infection.

MICROSCOPIC LESIONS   Swelling and necrosis of neurons; dispersion of the Nissl substance; neuronophagia by macrophages; progressive loss of motor neurons in anterior cord; early PMN infiltrate, later lymphocytic.

COMPLICATIONS   Paralysis, muscle atrophy; respiratory paralysis, death; late progression or recurrence.

SIGNS AND SYMPTOMS   Fever, malaise, headache, vomiting in minor infection; paralysis may follow or be the presenting symptom; paralysis is asymmetric and flaccid; spasm of unaffected muscles.

CLINICAL DIAGNOSIS AND OTHER CLINICAL FEATURES   Recognition of the above; infection produces no symptoms in 95% of cases; in others, there is gastroenteritis (minor infection), meningitis, or paralytic polio.

LABORATORY DIAGNOSIS   Viral cultures from throat in early stages and from stool in later stages; CSF cultures have poor yield; CSF examination: lymphocytosis, elevated protein, normal glucose.

PROGNOSIS   Mortality rate 5–10% for paralytic disease; residual deficits related to severity of presentation.

THERAPY   Supportive care with physical therapy.

OTHER INFORMATION   Infection of neurons in the brainstem (bulbar) causes paralysis of respiratory muscles; postpolio syndrome presents decades after infection with muscle weakness and fatigue.

Varicella-Zoster Infection

DESCRIPTION   Varicella (chickenpox) is an acute viral exanthem caused by varicella-zoster virus (VZV). Herpes zoster (shingles) is a reactivated latent infection caused by the same virus.

DISEASE ENTITIES; SYNONYMS AND ACRONYMS   Chickenpox; herpes zoster, shingles; VZV.

INCIDENCE   Initial infection is common during childhood; worldwide distribution.

AGE   Chickenpox, usually in children but can be any age; shingles, usually older adults.

ETIOLOGY, PATHOGENESIS, AND PREDISPOSING FACTORS   VZV is a member of the herpesvirus group; chickenpox: respiratory or direct transmission; shingles: history of previous chickenpox, advanced age, immunosuppression, underlying malignancy.

SITES INVOLVED   Skin, diffuse in chickenpox, dermatome distribution in shingles; virus persists latent in spinal ganglion; dissemination to all organs may occur in immunocompromised patients.

GROSS LESIONS   Chickenpox: vesicular skin lesions occurring in crops for 3–6 days; shingles: vesicular skin lesions confined to the distribution of infected nerve root.

MICROSCOPIC LESIONS   Vesicular skin lesions with herpes viral inclusions, which are intranuclear, acidophilic inclusions with a clear halo around them (Cowdry type A inclusions); syncytial giant cells are also seen.

COMPLICATIONS   Pneumonia, encephalitis, hepatitis, carditis, keratitis, orchitis; Reye's syndrome in children given aspirin; postherpetic neuralgia; dissemination with immunosuppression, lymphoma, or leukemia.

SIGNS AND SYMPTOMS   Fever, malaise, anorexia, and vesicular skin lesions appearing in crops all over skin (chickenpox) or along a dermatome distribution (shingles).

CLINICAL DIAGNOSIS AND OTHER CLINICAL FEATURES   Recognition of the skin lesions and systemic signs of infection; differential includes disseminated herpes simplex, bug bites, scabies, impetigo.

LABORATORY DIAGNOSIS   Isolation of organism from skin lesions; histologic examination of skin biopsy; diagnosis is made on clinical grounds in nearly all cases.

PROGNOSIS   Excellent in chickenpox; postherpetic pain syndrome may occur after shingles.

THERAPY   Acyclovir in immunocompromised patients.

OTHER INFORMATION   Adults with shingles are infectious to persons who have not had chickenpox. Adults with chickenpox may have a more severe infection and are at higher risk for developing pneumonia.

Viral Respiratory Infections

DESCRIPTION   Infection of the upper or lower respiratory system, causing diseases that include rhinitis, pharyngitis, laryngitis, tracheitis, bronchitis, bronchiolitis, and interstitial pneumonia.

DISEASE ENTITIES; SYNONYMS AND ACRONYMS   Common cold, URI; sore throat; croup; influenza; viral pneumonia, interstitial pneumonia.

INCIDENCE   Very common and may occur in epidemics or pandemics.

AGE   Any age may be infected; RSV is more common and severe in infants and children.

ETIOLOGY, PATHOGENESIS, AND PREDISPOSING FACTORS   Influenza virus, rhinovirus, coronavirus, adenovirus, parainfluenza virus, respiratory syncytial virus (RSV); spread by respiratory droplets or direct contact with secretions from an infected person.

SITES INVOLVED   Epithelium of upper and lower airways and nasal sinuses; alveolar septa of lung in pneumonia.

GROSS LESIONS   Edema and redness of mucous membranes with watery discharge; hyperemia of airway mucosa with edema. Lungs may be red, firm, and edematous.

MICROSCOPIC LESIONS   Mononuclear inflammation of mucosa; focal desquamation; nuclear inclusions with adenovirus, syncytia with RSV; viral pneumonia: mononuclear inflammation of alveolar septa, edema fluid within alveoli.

COMPLICATIONS   Secondary bacterial infections, particularly staphylococcal or pneumococcal pneumonia, which are especially common following viral pneumonia in elderly and infants. Some viruses produce myocarditis.

SIGNS AND SYMPTOMS   Sudden onset of fever, malaise, sore throat, coryza, and muscle pain. Uncomplicated cases clear in a few days but the course is longer if pneumonia develops.

CLINICAL DIAGNOSIS AND OTHER CLINICAL FEATURES   Recognition of the above clinical signs; chest x-rays in viral pneumonia show an interstitial infiltrate pattern.

LABORATORY DIAGNOSIS   Viral throat culture for identification and for epidemiological tracking, especially of influenza viruses; cold agglutinins are occasionally present in adenovirus infections.

PROGNOSIS   Good, unless complicated by bacterial pneumonia.

THERAPY   Supportive care; aspirin should not be used in children to avoid Reye's syndrome.

OTHER INFORMATION   Measles, mumps, herpes, and cytomegalovirus can cause viral pneumonia; these may be diagnosed histologically by their inclusions or by viral culture.

Yellow Fever

DESCRIPTION   A viral hemorrhagic fever characterized by jaundice and renal damage. The liver shows midzonal necrosis.

DISEASE ENTITIES; SYNONYMS AND ACRONYMS   Yellow fever.

INCIDENCE   No endemic areas within the US.

AGE   Any age.

ETIOLOGY, PATHOGENESIS, AND PREDISPOSING FACTORS   Virus is a flavivirus (togavirus, group B arbovirus) transmitted by *Aedes aegypti* mosquitoes between humans in an urban setting or from tree-dwelling monkeys to humans in a jungle setting.

SITES INVOLVED   Viremia following infection; liver and kidneys are the organs most affected.

GROSS LESIONS   Liver: normal size, yellow color, accentuated lobular pattern, bile-staining; kidneys: often swollen and pale. Petechial hemorrhages in skin and organs.

MICROSCOPIC LESIONS   Liver: midzonal necrosis, fat accumulation, and Councilman bodies; with massive necrosis, a single row of hepatocytes adjacent to the portal tracts is usually spared; little inflammation.

COMPLICATIONS   Hepatic failure and/or renal failure; mortality between 5 and 25%.

SIGNS AND SYMPTOMS   Fever, myalgias, and headache followed by jaundice, decreased urine output, leukopenia, hypotension, and hemorrhage; classically, black vomitus.

CLINICAL DIAGNOSIS AND OTHER CLINICAL FEATURES   Jaundice and decreased urine output in a patient with a history of travel or living in an endemic area, i.e., Central or South America, or Africa.

LABORATORY DIAGNOSIS   Serology; viral isolation is only occasionally successful.

PROGNOSIS   Fairly high mortality. Most cases resolve without sequelae.

THERAPY   Prevention of infection through mosquito control programs in endemic areas and vaccination.

OTHER INFORMATION   *A. aegypti* also transmits dengue. Immunization for yellow fever is required for travel to South America and sub-Saharan Africa.

Pathology Facts, by Richard C. Harruff, J.B. Lippincott Company, Philadelphia © 1994.

Chapter 9

Bacterial, Chlamydial, and Rickettsial Infections

(cont'd)

Actinomycosis

DESCRIPTION   Chronic infection with Actinomyces, usually the species *A. israelii*, most frequently involving jaw, thorax or abdomen, and causing swelling, pain, sinus tract formation and purulent drainage.

DISEASE ENTITIES; SYNONYMS AND ACRONYMS   Cervicofacial actinomycosis; pulmonary or thoracic actinomycosis; abdominal or GI actinomycosis; pelvic actinomycosis.

INCIDENCE   Infrequent and sporadic; twice as common in males.

AGE   Any age; more frequent in adolescents and young adults.

ETIOLOGY, PATHOGENESIS, AND PREDISPOSING FACTORS   Actinomyces are gram-positive filamentous bacteria that are commensals of the oral cavity and GI tract; invasion requires a defect in the mucosal barriers, produced by trauma or other disease.

SITES INVOLVED   Cervicofacial (jaw) after trauma, dental work, poor oral hygiene; thoracic, due to aspiration or penetrating injury; abdominal, after appendicitis or other lesion; pelvic, due to intrauterine device.

GROSS LESIONS   Suppuration and fibrosis that spreads through tissues; draining sinus tracts and fistulas frequently develop; colonies of the organism appear as yellow flecks recognized as "sulfur granules."

MICROSCOPIC LESIONS   Abscesses with surrounding fibrosis and chronic inflammation; within the suppuration there are several sulfur granules, which appear as clusters of radiating basophilic filaments.

COMPLICATIONS   Draining sinus tracts and fistulas; lung abscesses; bowel obstruction due to fibrosis and contraction of the wall; pelvic inflammatory disease with tubo-ovarian adhesions.

SIGNS AND SYMPTOMS   Cervicofacial: swelling and induration of jaw, slight tenderness, draining sinuses; pulmonary infection: cough, hemoptysis, weight loss, fever, and night sweats; abdominal infection: pain, distention.

CLINICAL DIAGNOSIS AND OTHER CLINICAL FEATURES   Systemic effects are minimal compared with the marked local inflammation of cervicofacial actinomycosis; chest x-rays show nodular infiltrates with lung involvement; pelvic infections occur with IUD.

LABORATORY DIAGNOSIS   Observation of sulfur granules in exudate draining from sinuses; histologic demonstration of filamentous colonies in tissue; culture of organism, which is anaerobic to microaerophilic.

PROGNOSIS   Infection usually pursues a prolonged, chronic course with low mortality.

THERAPY   Long-term antibiotic treatment with high-dose penicillin; surgical debridement or drainage.

OTHER INFORMATION   Prolonged use of an intrauterine device promotes colonization of the vagina and uterine cervix and increases the risk of pelvic actinomycosis.

Anthrax

DESCRIPTION An acute bacterial infection that usually affects the skin but may also involve the respiratory or intestinal tracts, caused by *Bacillus anthracis*.

DISEASE ENTITIES; SYNONYMS AND ACRONYMS Malignant pustule, malignant edema, woolsorter's disease, ragpicker's disease, charbon.

INCIDENCE Rare in US; occurs in agricultural areas of Europe, Africa, and Asia where animal anthrax is common.

AGE Any age.

ETIOLOGY, PATHOGENESIS, AND PREDISPOSING FACTORS *B. anthracis* is a gram-positive, spore-forming rod that penetrates abraded skin or is inhaled as spores; the organism produces a toxin and its capsule resists phagocytosis.

SITES INVOLVED Skin lesion initially; may spread to regional lymph nodes or progress to septicemia; inhalation of spores causes lung infection (woolsorter's disease).

GROSS LESIONS Skin lesion is initially papular and vesicular; after a few days it is covered with a black eschar. Pulmonary infection produces patchy consolidation.

MICROSCOPIC LESIONS Gram stains of skin lesions show the organism; lung in pulmonary anthrax shows a fibrinous exudate with many organisms but few PMNs.

COMPLICATIONS Septicemia with disseminated intravascular coagulation; respiratory depression due to bacterial toxin; gastrointestinal disease with ulceration, obstruction, perforation, and electrolyte imbalances.

SIGNS AND SYMPTOMS Characteristic skin lesions; respiratory distress in cases with pulmonary infections; diarrhea and ascites in intestinal infections.

CLINICAL DIAGNOSIS AND OTHER CLINICAL FEATURES Recognition of the black eschar surrounded by edema that develops at the site of an abrasion; persons handling infected wool or hides may develop respiratory infection.

LABORATORY DIAGNOSIS Demonstration of the organism in smears from the skin lesion; isolation of organism from blood cultures; serologic demonstration of rising titers of antibodies against the organism.

PROGNOSIS Good prognosis for skin lesions that are localized and treated; poor prognosis for sepsis.

THERAPY Preventive measures include vaccination of animals and persons at high risk, such as veterinarians.

OTHER INFORMATION Infected animals must be quickly buried to avoid contamination of the soil by the carcasses.

Borreliosis

DESCRIPTION   A systemic spirochetal infection characterized by alternating febrile and afebrile periods, caused by *Borrelia recurrentis* in louse-borne disease and other species in tick-borne disease.

DISEASE ENTITIES; SYNONYMS AND ACRONYMS   Relapsing fever.

INCIDENCE   Uncommon in US; endemic and occasionally epidemic regions in Asia, Africa, and South America.

AGE   Any age.

ETIOLOGY, PATHOGENESIS, AND PREDISPOSING FACTORS   Infestation with infected lice, exposure to ticks; parasites contaminate bite wound when the arthropod is crushed; successive waves of spirochetemia produce the characteristic relapsing fever pattern.

SITES INVOLVED   Organism gains access via the arthropod bite then disseminates throughout the bloodstream; heart, meninges, skin, liver, and spleen may be affected.

GROSS LESIONS   There may be multiple small abscesses in the spleen; other organs may show focal hemorrhages.

MICROSCOPIC LESIONS   Midzonal inflammation of liver, focal necrosis; organisms may be seen in liver sinusoids or in the areas of necrosis; microabscesses of spleen.

COMPLICATIONS   Endotoxin shock, consumption coagulopathy; Herxheimer reaction with high fever and shock following antibiotic therapy.

SIGNS AND SYMPTOMS   Fever, myalgias, headache, and lethargy about 1 week after infection; hepatosplenomegaly, skin petechiae, conjunctival hemorrhages. Febrile periods last 2–9 days; afebrile periods, 2–4 days.

CLINICAL DIAGNOSIS AND OTHER CLINICAL FEATURES   Alternating febrile and afebrile periods with 1–10 relapses; indications of coagulopathy.

LABORATORY DIAGNOSIS   Demonstration of spirochetes by examination of a stained blood film or by darkfield microscopy of a blood specimen taking during a febrile period.

PROGNOSIS   Good with treatment; 2–10% mortality if untreated; up to 50% mortality in epidemics.

THERAPY   Tetracycline antibiotics.

OTHER INFORMATION   Antigenic variation explains the relapsing nature of the disease; as specific antibodies clear one wave of spirochetes, another new and antigenically distinct population proliferates.

Botulism

DESCRIPTION Food poisoning causing progressive paralysis, due to consumption of food containing preformed neurotoxin of *Clostridium botulinum*; it may also develop from wounds or in infants with intestinal colonization.

DISEASE ENTITIES; SYNONYMS AND ACRONYMS Food botulism, wound botulism, infant botulism.

INCIDENCE Rare; about 10 adult case per year in US; 100 infant cases.

AGE Infant botulism occurs in babies under 1 year; food or wound botulism may occur at any age.

ETIOLOGY, PATHOGENESIS, AND PREDISPOSING FACTORS *C. botulinum* grows from spores and produces toxin in anaerobic food, wound, or infant intestine; improperly canned food is a common source; the exotoxin blocks synaptic acetylcholine release.

SITES INVOLVED Neurotoxin produces progressive, descending paralysis that first affects cranial nerves, then limbs and trunk; the toxin binds to synaptic vesicles of cholinergic nerves at the neuromuscular junction.

GROSS LESIONS No specific lesions. Secondary pneumonia is likely.

MICROSCOPIC LESIONS None, other than secondary respiratory infections.

COMPLICATIONS Respiratory paralysis that is often fatal; pneumonia. Infant botulism may mimic Sudden Infant Death Syndrome (SIDS).

SIGNS AND SYMPTOMS Cranial nerve paralysis initially, with diplopia, dysarthria, pupil dilatation; progressing to limb and trunk muscle weakness and paralysis.

CLINICAL DIAGNOSIS AND OTHER CLINICAL FEATURES Recognition of characteristic neuromuscular signs; history of eating home-canned foods or occasionally damaged or contaminated commercially canned food; electromyography is confirmatory.

LABORATORY DIAGNOSIS Identification of the toxin in stool or serum or in the suspected food; positive cultures of the organism from stool of an infant or from a wound supports diagnosis of infant or wound botulism.

PROGNOSIS 40% mortality in severe cases; otherwise there is a gradual recovery of muscle strength.

THERAPY Antitoxin to prevent neurotoxin from binding to synapses; antibiotics and debridement of wounds.

OTHER INFORMATION Wound botulism occurs in deep, devitalized wounds; in infant botulism the toxin is released from organisms in the intestine; honey has been implicated in infant botulism; the toxin is heat labile.

Brucellosis

DESCRIPTION A systemic bacterial infection, manifesting as an acute or chronic disease; caused by one of four species of Brucella, a small gram-negative, aerobic coccobacillus.

DISEASE ENTITIES; SYNONYMS AND ACRONYMS Undulant fever, Malta fever, Mediterranean fever.

INCIDENCE Occurs in persons exposed to infected animals; slaughterhouse workers, farmers, and veterinarians.

AGE Any age; more common in adult males.

ETIOLOGY, PATHOGENESIS, AND PREDISPOSING FACTORS Each species of Brucella has a different animal reservoir: *B. abortus,* cattle; *B. suis,* swine; *B. melitensis,* goats; *B. canis,* dogs; exposure to animal tissues and milk cause human infections.

SITES INVOLVED Usually a systemic disease; complications include localization of infection in skeletal system, heart, nervous system, and other organs.

GROSS LESIONS Lymph nodes, spleen, and liver may be enlarged.

MICROSCOPIC LESIONS Proliferation of macrophages and lymphocytes; granulomas that may be centrally necrotic with PMNs or filled with epithelioid cells and resemble sarcoid granulomas.

COMPLICATIONS Endocarditis is the most common cause of death; localized joint infections; osteomyelitis; suppurative vertebral spondylitis; meningitis; peripheral neuritis.

SIGNS AND SYMPTOMS Infection may begin acutely with fever, chills, and pain; or insidiously with fatigue, weight loss, and weakness. Recurrent brucellosis produces multiple bouts of flu-like symptoms.

CLINICAL DIAGNOSIS AND OTHER CLINICAL FEATURES Recognition of the clinical presentation of a patient who is exposed to farm animals or drinks unpasteurized milk.

LABORATORY DIAGNOSIS Isolation of the organism from blood, bone marrow, or other tissues; serologic demonstration of a rise in antibody titer in paired sera.

PROGNOSIS Good with treatment; mortality is low even without treatment; complications cause disabilities.

THERAPY Rifampin and doxycycline for several weeks.

OTHER INFORMATION Dairy herds have been screened for this organism and infected animals eliminated. Occasional cases result from accidental inoculation with Brucella vaccine intended for livestock.

Campylobacter Enteritis

DESCRIPTION   Acute enteric disease characterized by diarrhea, nausea, fever, abdominal pain, and malaise, caused by infection with *Campylobacter jejuni* or *C. coli,* a gram-negative, comma-shaped bacillus.

DISEASE ENTITIES; SYNONYMS AND ACRONYMS   Bacterial diarrhea; vibrionic enteritis; Campylobacteriosis.

INCIDENCE   Very common; causes 5–14% of cases of diarrhea.

AGE   Any age; more common in children and young adults in developed countries.

ETIOLOGY, PATHOGENESIS, AND PREDISPOSING FACTORS   Transmission through water and food, especially milk and poultry; may be passed to humans by contact with infected domestic animals.

SITES INVOLVED   Gastrointestinal tract from jejunum to colon; invasion of mucosa occurs with the most severe infections.

GROSS LESIONS   Mucosa is hyperemic and edematous; there may be focal ulcerations.

MICROSCOPIC LESIONS   Mucosa is infiltrated with mixed inflammatory infiltrates; acute inflammation is associated with ulcers.

COMPLICATIONS   Dehydration; rare sepsis or bowel perforation; infections are usually self-limited.

SIGNS AND SYMPTOMS   Onset 3–5 days after ingestion of contaminated food or water; cramping abdominal pain, nausea, fever, and diarrhea with foul-smelling and occasionally bloody stools.

CLINICAL DIAGNOSIS AND OTHER CLINICAL FEATURES   Recognition of characteristic symptoms, which are similar to other enteropathogenic bacterial enteritis; *C. jejuni* is the most common cause of bacterial diarrhea.

LABORATORY DIAGNOSIS   Isolation of the organism from the stool, which is sometime difficult; the organism grows best at 42°C.

PROGNOSIS   Good; rarely any serious complications.

THERAPY   Fluid and electrolyte therapy; antibiotics are used only in severe cases.

OTHER INFORMATION   *C. fetus* causes systemic campylobacteriosis; *C. pylori* (now *Helicobacter pylori)* is associated with gastritis and gastric ulcers.

Cat Scratch Disease

DESCRIPTION   Cat scratch disease is a self-limited infection producing localized lymphadenitis, caused by an unnamed gram-negative organism, which is introduced into the skin by a cat scratch.

DISEASE ENTITIES; SYNONYMS AND ACRONYMS   Cat scratch fever; benign lymphoreticulosis.

INCIDENCE   Uncommon; worldwide distribution; a common cause of unilateral lymphadenopathy.

AGE   Any age; most common in children in close contact with animals.

ETIOLOGY, PATHOGENESIS, AND PREDISPOSING FACTORS   Organism is inoculated into the skin by claws of a healthy cat and spreads to regional lymph nodes; some cases originate from dog scratch, thorn, or splinter; multiple cases may occur in one family.

SITES INVOLVED   Skin inoculation site and regional lymph nodes draining the skin site; conjunctivitis may develop if eyelid is scratched or occasionally after an animal licks the patient's face.

GROSS LESIONS   Papule, pustule, or crusted, erythematous scratch mark on skin at primary site; regional lymph nodes enlarge several times normal and may become fluctuant.

MICROSCOPIC LESIONS   Acute inflammation at skin site where the organism multiplies in the walls of small blood vessels; lymph nodes show stellate abscesses with suppuration surrounded by granulomatous inflammation.

COMPLICATIONS   Perinaud's syndrome (oculoglandular syndrome); erythema nodosum or multiforme; uncommonly: encephalitis, lytic bone lesions, hepatosplenomegaly, pneumonitis.

SIGNS AND SYMPTOMS   Skin lesion at innoculation site within a few days; regional lymph node enlargement and tenderness within 1–3 weeks after scratch; fever, malaise, headache.

CLINICAL DIAGNOSIS AND OTHER CLINICAL FEATURES   Recognition of localized lymphadenitis in a person in contact with cats; skin lesion may not be present; differential includes tularemia, tuberculosis, brucellosis, and plaque.

LABORATORY DIAGNOSIS   Demonstration of the typical histologic pattern of necrosis and inflammation in a biopsy of affected lymph nodes; organisms may be visualized with silver stains.

PROGNOSIS   Good; the infection is self-limited and usually resolves in 3–4 months.

THERAPY   No specific therapy; surgical drainage of tender fluctuant lymph nodes may be necessary.

OTHER INFORMATION   Skin tests for cat scratch disease are available; however, the antigen is made from infected human nodes and is seldom used due to concerns of transmitting other diseases.

Chancroid

DESCRIPTION   Acute, sexually transmitted disease involving the skin of the genital area and producing painful, necrotizing ulcers, caused by *Hemophilus ducreyi,* a small gram-negative bacillus.

DISEASE ENTITIES; SYNONYMS AND ACRONYMS   Soft chancre; third venereal disease; ulcus molle.

INCIDENCE   Common in tropical climates where the incidence may exceed syphilis; men are more commonly infected.

AGE   Sexually active adolescents and adults.

ETIOLOGY, PATHOGENESIS, AND PREDISPOSING FACTORS   Organism is spread through direct sexual contact with organisms from open lesions; infection is associated with poor personal hygiene.

SITES INVOLVED   Skin of perineum and genital area; penis, vulva; occult lesions on the cervix or vaginal wall.

GROSS LESIONS   Primary lesions are necrotizing ulcers at the genital site; regional lymph nodes are enlarged and suppurative (buboes) and may burst to produce deforming necrosis; multiple ulcers are common.

MICROSCOPIC LESIONS   Ulcers show superficial zone of PMNs and necrotic debris, middle zone of granulation tissue, and deep zone with perivascular lymphocytes and plasma cells; lymph nodes show suppuration and necrosis.

COMPLICATIONS   Disfiguring scarring may occur due to extensive necrosis, which is avoided by prompt recognition and treatment.

SIGNS AND SYMPTOMS   Painful ulcers on the genitalia with enlargement of regional nodes; skin over the nodes may become necrotic and drain through the skin, at which time the person is usually febrile.

CLINICAL DIAGNOSIS AND OTHER CLINICAL FEATURES   Recognition of ulcerative sexually transmitted disease; painful genital ulcers with purulent exudate are highly suggestive of chancroid.

LABORATORY DIAGNOSIS   Demonstration of organisms in Gram stain of drainage fluid; characteristic "school of fish" appearance is due to the parallel arrangement of the organisms; bacterial culture.

PROGNOSIS   Good with therapy.

THERAPY   Antibiotics such as ceftriaxone or erythromycin.

OTHER INFORMATION   Chancroid must be differentiated from other genital ulcers caused by sexually transmitted diseases: syphilis, herpes, lymphogranuloma venereum, granuloma inguinale.

Chlamydial Urogenital Infections

DESCRIPTION   Sexually transmitted infections of the urogenital tract with *Chlamydia trachomatis,* an obligate intracellular gram-negative bacterium.

DISEASE ENTITIES; SYNONYMS AND ACRONYMS   Chlamydial cervicitis or urethritis; nongonococcal urethritis; lymphogranuloma venereum.

INCIDENCE   Urethritis and cervicitis: very common; LGV: uncommon except in tropics.

AGE   Sexually active adults or adolescents.

ETIOLOGY, PATHOGENESIS, AND PREDISPOSING FACTORS   Sexual transmission; Chlamydia are incorporated into phagocytic vacuoles of the infected cell where they multiply and utilize energy sources of the host cell.

SITES INVOLVED   Epithelial cells of urethra, cervix, fallopian tubes, epididymis, prostate, and rectum; LGV involves external genitalia, inguinal lymph nodes, and occasionally rectum or oral region.

GROSS LESIONS   Chlamydia causes urethritis in males, salpingitis or cervicitis in females. Primary lesion of LGV is ulcer on external genitalia with secondary enlargement of inguinal lymph nodes.

MICROSCOPIC LESIONS   Chlamydia-infected cells contain intracytoplasmic inclusions. Lymph nodes in LGV have multiple abscesses with granulomatous pattern.

COMPLICATIONS   Males: epididymitis, infertility, Reiter's syndrome; females: salpingitis, pelvic inflammatory disease, infertility, ectopic pregnancy; LGV: rectal stricture, chronic genital lymphedema.

SIGNS AND SYMPTOMS   Urethritis and cervicitis: similar to gonorrhea with mucoid urethral or cervical discharge; urethral itching, burning on urination. LGV: genital vesicle that soon ulcerates.

CLINICAL DIAGNOSIS AND OTHER CLINICAL FEATURES   Recognition of the urethral or cervical discharge; asymptomatic infections are common in both sexes. LGV needs to be differentiated from other sexually transmitted diseases that present with ulcer.

LABORATORY DIAGNOSIS   Tissue culture of the organism or direct immunofluorescent staining for the organism in scrapings from the cervix or urethra. LGV by serology or culture.

PROGNOSIS   Good with treatment.

THERAPY   Tetracycline antibiotics.

OTHER INFORMATION   Chlamydial urogenital infections currently outnumber the cases of gonorrhea in the US; concurrent infections should be suspected in high-risk patients.

Cholera

DESCRIPTION   Acute diarrheal disease due to gastrointestinal infection with *Vibrio cholerae,* a curved gram-negative bacillus that produces an enterotoxin which activates adenylate cyclase in the bowel mucosa.

DISEASE ENTITIES; SYNONYMS AND ACRONYMS   Endemic cholera, epidemic cholera.

INCIDENCE   Endemic with frequent epidemics in Asia, Africa, India, and most recently, South America.

AGE   Any age; higher mortality in children.

ETIOLOGY, PATHOGENESIS, AND PREDISPOSING FACTORS   Transmitted by feces-contaminated water or food; colonization of small bowel; enterotoxin causes chloride secretion and inhibition of sodium resorption, producing an isotonic fluid diarrhea.

SITES INVOLVED   Organisms colonize small bowel and adhere to mucosal cells but do not invade; enterotoxin activates the adenylate cyclase system in epithelial cells to cause secretion of water and NaCl.

GROSS LESIONS   None; the intestinal mucosa is not invaded; the intestines are filled with large volumes of thin fluid.

MICROSCOPIC LESIONS   None; the intestinal mucosa is histologically normal.

COMPLICATIONS   Dehydration and electrolyte imbalance, which can lead to hypovolemic shock, metabolic acidosis, renal failure, and death.

SIGNS AND SYMPTOMS   Rapidly developing profuse, painless, watery diarrhea, classically called "ricewater stools." Fluid loss may be as much as 1 liter per hour.

CLINICAL DIAGNOSIS AND OTHER CLINICAL FEATURES   Recognition of ricewater stools in a person with potential exposure due to travel in an endemic area; signs of dehydration and hypovolemic shock may develop quickly.

LABORATORY DIAGNOSIS   Isolation of organism in stool culture is diagnostic; organism also may be directly visualized with darkfield microscopy and presumptively identified by antiserum immobilization.

PROGNOSIS   Overall mortality of 50% in untreated cases, highest in infants and children; better with therapy.

THERAPY   Oral fluid/electrolyte replacement; intravenous fluids; tetracycline shortens duration.

OTHER INFORMATION   Cholera cases have been confirmed in South American countries that export food to the US, thus providing a source for cholera to be spread into the US.

Clostridial Food Poisoning

DESCRIPTION   An acute diarrheal disease occurring 6–24 hours after ingestion of meat or gravy contaminated with toxin-producing strains of *Clostridium perfringens*.

DISEASE ENTITIES; SYNONYMS AND ACRONYMS   *C. perfringens* (formerly *C. welchii*) food poisoning, gastroenteritis; necrotizing enteritis, pigbel.

INCIDENCE   Food poisoning is common in US; necrotizing enteritis is rare and complicates malnutrition.

AGE   Any age above infancy.

ETIOLOGY, PATHOGENESIS, AND PREDISPOSING FACTORS   Cooking does not destroy clostridial spores; bacteria grow in slowly cooled food, and large numbers of bacteria may be ingested; enterotoxin A is produced in the small intestine during sporulation.

SITES INVOLVED   Clostridial enterotoxin affects the mucosa of the small intestine to produce fluid accumulation, ileum is particularly affected; in necrotizing enteritis there is necrosis of the small intestine.

GROSS LESIONS   In food poisoning there are no lesions other than fluid accumulation; necrotizing enteritis produces mucosal ulcerations and gas production in the wall.

MICROSCOPIC LESIONS   Minimal changes in food poisoning; in necrotizing enteritis there is necrosis and acute inflammation.

COMPLICATIONS   Food poisoning is usually self-limited without sequelae. Necrotizing enteritis produces peritonitis and septic shock and is often fatal (40% mortality).

SIGNS AND SYMPTOMS   Food poisoning: sudden onset of watery diarrhea and abdominal pain without fever; necrotizing enteritis: abdominal pain, bloody diarrhea, often rapid progression to septic shock.

CLINICAL DIAGNOSIS AND OTHER CLINICAL FEATURES   Recognition of the signs of food poisoning in a person who consumed meats or gravies that were not properly refrigerated; necrotizing enteritis is only seen where people are malnourished.

LABORATORY DIAGNOSIS   Isolation of the organism in suspected foods.

PROGNOSIS   Food poisoning: usually rapid recovery; necrotizing enteritis: often fatal.

THERAPY   Usually unnecessary for food poisoning.

OTHER INFORMATION   Necrotizing enteritis is a condition affecting poorly nourished persons who suddenly feast on meat (pigbel), associated with enterotoxin C; antibiotics and surgical resection are required for therapy.

Clostridial Myonecrosis

DESCRIPTION A rapidly progressive infection that produces necrosis of skeletal muscle, caused by *Clostridium perfringens,* a large gram-positive, anaerobic, spore-forming bacillus that produces myotoxins.

DISEASE ENTITIES; SYNONYMS AND ACRONYMS Gas gangrene; clostridial cellulitis, anaerobic cellulitis; Welch abscess.

INCIDENCE Fairly common complication of wounds that have a great deal of necrotic or ischemic tissue.

AGE Any age.

ETIOLOGY, PATHOGENESIS, AND PREDISPOSING FACTORS Develops in a contaminated wound with low oxygen tension due to penetrating or crush injury; the most important toxin, alpha toxin, is a lecithinase that produces hemolysis and necrosis.

SITES INVOLVED Soft tissues and skeletal muscle; myonecrosis especially involves the muscle with abundant gas formation; in anaerobic cellulitis and Welch abscess there is little muscle necrosis or gas formation.

GROSS LESIONS Overlying skin may be pale, yellow, or gray-brown; the area becomes swollen, cold, and painful with palpable subcutaneous gas bubbles.

MICROSCOPIC LESIONS Coagulative necrosis, edema, gas formation, and many organisms in affected muscles; relatively sparse infiltration of PMNs in the bordering viable muscle.

COMPLICATIONS Disseminated intravascular coagulation; circulatory collapse due to toxemia and shock; hemolysis; renal failure due to hemolysis.

SIGNS AND SYMPTOMS Infection usually becomes evident 2 or more days following a wound or surgery; area becomes painful, edematous, and crepitant; discoloration and blebs of overlying skin; serosanguinous drainage.

CLINICAL DIAGNOSIS AND OTHER CLINICAL FEATURES Recognition of thin, dark, foul-smelling exudate and gas formation in a devitalized, ischemic wound.

LABORATORY DIAGNOSIS Isolation of the organism in anaerobic culture of fluid or tissue from the affected area; gram-positive rods in stained smears of exudate.

PROGNOSIS Poor for myonecrosis, which is often lethal.

THERAPY Debridement of the affected skin tissue; antibiotics such as penicillin.

OTHER INFORMATION Clostridial cellulitis and Welch abscess are relatively benign compared to the highly toxigenic myonecrosis. Sepsis with *C. septicum* may occur with gastrointestinal disease.

Diphtheria

DESCRIPTION   An acute illness usually involving the pharynx, caused by infection with an exotoxin-producing strain of *Corynebacterium diphtheriae*, a gram-positive, aerobic bacillus.

DISEASE ENTITIES; SYNONYMS AND ACRONYMS   Diphtheria.

INCIDENCE   Rare due to childhood vaccination programs; 200–400 cases per year in US.

AGE   Pharyngeal diphtheria usually affects children between 4 and 14 years.

ETIOLOGY, PATHOGENESIS, AND PREDISPOSING FACTORS   Infection of pharynx and other sites occurs in nonimmunized persons living in crowded conditions; transmission is by respiratory droplets; production of cytotoxic exotoxin depends on a bacteriophage.

SITES INVOLVED   Usually the pharynx; nasal and laryngeal tissues may be affected; skin involvement is more common in adults; exotoxin absorbed into the blood affects heart and peripheral nerves.

GROSS LESIONS   Toxin produces a pseudomembrane consisting of patches of gray membrane surrounded by redness. Heart is softened and enlarged. Skin lesions consist of a membrane surrounded by raised edges.

MICROSCOPIC LESIONS   Pseudomembrane is composed of fibrin, PMNs, necrotic debris, and clusters of organisms; epithelium is necrotic and contains many organisms; edema and fatty degeneration of myocardium

COMPLICATIONS   Asphyxia due to aspiration of the pseudomembrane or due to edema of the respiratory tract; heart failure due to myocarditis; paralytic peripheral neuropathy; interstitial nephritis.

SIGNS AND SYMPTOMS   Pharyngitis, laryngitis, fever; hoarseness, cough; cervical lymphadenopathy with "bull-necked" appearance; exudate on pharynx that converts to pseudomembrane; similar pseudomembrane on skin lesions.

CLINICAL DIAGNOSIS AND OTHER CLINICAL FEATURES   Pseudomembrane is distinctive and usually covers the posterior pharynx; bleeding occurs when the pseudomembrane is peeled away; ECG changes indicate myocarditis.

LABORATORY DIAGNOSIS   Culture of the affected area and isolation of a toxin-producing organism; tests for toxin production include guinea pig innoculation and immunodiffusion testing.

PROGNOSIS   5–10% mortality rate with therapy.

THERAPY   Antitoxin and antibiotics such as penicillin or erythromycin; antibiotics alone are ineffective.

OTHER INFORMATION   Diphtheria exotoxin causes local cell necrosis in the pharynx and distant myocarditis; it is a protein with enzymatic activity that blocks ribosomal function.

Escherichia Coli Infection

DESCRIPTION Enteric infections, urinary tract infections, intra-abdominal infections, neonatal meningitis; caused by *Escherichia coli*, a gram-negative, enteric, facultatively anaerobic bacillus.

DISEASE ENTITIES; SYNONYMS AND ACRONYMS *E. coli* enteritis, travelers diarrhea, Montezuma's revenge; many gram-negative infections: pyelonephritis, peritonitis.

INCIDENCE Very common.

AGE Any age; meningitis in neonates is usually due to *E. coli.*

ETIOLOGY, PATHOGENESIS, AND PREDISPOSING FACTORS Enteric infection due to ingestion of contaminated water or food; mechanisms of enteritis: enteroadhesion, enteroinvasion, enterotoxin production; other sites infected by spread via blood or urine.

SITES INVOLVED Enteric infections: intestinal tract; urinary tract infection: bladder or ascending to kidneys; other sites: meninges, peritoneum, blood (sepsis).

GROSS LESIONS Enteroinvasive organisms cause intestinal mucosal ulcerations similar to Shigella. Infection of other sites is characterized by purulent exudate.

MICROSCOPIC LESIONS Enteroinvasive infections: ulceration of mucosa, pseudomembranous exudate; adhesive strains: organisms clinging to surface mucosa; toxigenic strains: no lesions; other sites: suppuration.

COMPLICATIONS Enteric infections: dehydration, hypovolemic shock; infections in other sites: suppuration producing necrosis; any infection can lead to septic shock (endotoxin shock).

SIGNS AND SYMPTOMS Enteritis: diarrhea, fever, dysentery; urinary infections: dysuria, suprapubic pain, fever, flank pain; peritonitis: abdominal pain, rebound tenderness; meningitis: inconsolable infant.

CLINICAL DIAGNOSIS AND OTHER CLINICAL FEATURES Recognition of characteristic presentation in patients with appropriate histories; *E. coli* is the most common cause of traveler's diarrhea, which is variable in severity.

LABORATORY DIAGNOSIS Isolation of organism from stool, urine, CSF, or other site of infection; DNA probes of stool isolates can detect the plasmids carrying the enteropathogenic traits.

PROGNOSIS Depends on site; good for enteric and urinary infections; poor for peritonitis and meningitis.

THERAPY Fluid and electrolyte therapy for diarrhea; antibiotics for urinary and other infections

OTHER INFORMATION *E. coli* is the most common organism causing urinary tract infections and gram-negative infections in general; the ultimate source of the organism is feces.

Gonorrhea

DESCRIPTION Sexually transmitted disease of urethra, epididymis, fallopian tubes, rectum, and pharynx in adults, eyes in neonates; caused by infection with *Neisseria gonorrhoeae*, a gram-negative diplococcus.

DISEASE ENTITIES; SYNONYMS AND ACRONYMS GC, clap, dose, drip; many others.

INCIDENCE Very common; nearly a million cases per year; endemic in poor urban settings.

AGE Sexually active adolescents and young adults; sexually abused children; conjunctivitis in neonates.

ETIOLOGY, PATHOGENESIS, AND PREDISPOSING FACTORS Transmitted by sexual activity; pili of the bacteria mediate their attachment to columnar epithelium and resist phagocytosis; bacterial IgA proteases neutralize secretory antibody.

SITES INVOLVED Anterior urethra in males; cervix, urethra, periurethral and labial glands in females; pharynx and rectum in either sex; conjunctiva in neonates; vulva and vagina in prepubescent females.

GROSS LESIONS Purulent discharge from urethra, vagina, or cervix; Bartholin's gland abscess; untreated infections progress to salpingitis, pelvic inflammatory disease, and epididymitis.

MICROSCOPIC LESIONS Urethral and cervical discharge contains many PMNs and organisms that are frequently intracellular; infected fallopian tubes are filled with purulent exudate; healing produces tubal adhesions.

COMPLICATIONS Disseminated infection with septic arthritis, skin lesions, uncommonly endocarditis or meningitis; male urethral strictures; female sterility, ectopic pregnancy; conjunctivitis leading to blindness.

SIGNS AND SYMPTOMS Constant purulent discharge from urethra or vagina; burning pain on urination; acute abdominal pain indicates pelvic inflammatory disease and/or acute salpingitis.

CLINICAL DIAGNOSIS AND OTHER CLINICAL FEATURES Recognition of characteristic features of infection in a sexually active person; pharyngitis, proctitis, and conjunctivitis are less common; infections are often asymptomatic, especially in females.

LABORATORY DIAGNOSIS Demonstration of diplococcal organism by Gram stain of male urethral discharge; culture of organism from swabs of vagina, cervix, urethra, rectum, or throat.

PROGNOSIS Good with therapy; failures occur with plasmid-mediated penicillinase-producing strains.

THERAPY Penicillin unless the isolate is resistant, then ceftriaxone; silver nitrate eyedrops for neonates.

OTHER INFORMATION Asymptomatic female infections constitute a major reservoir for gonorrhea. Due to high antigen variation among different gonococcal strains, infection does not confer effective immunity.

Granuloma Inguinale

DESCRIPTION   A chronic, progressive, ulcerative, sexually transmitted disease of the genital, inguinal, or anal areas caused by infection with *Calymmatobacterium granulomatis*, a gram-negative bacillus.

DISEASE ENTITIES; SYNONYMS AND ACRONYMS   Donovanosis. The organism was previously named *C. donovani*.

INCIDENCE   Rare in temperate climates; common in tropical climates; more common in men.

AGE   Sexually active adolescents and adults, typically between ages 15 and 40 years.

ETIOLOGY, PATHOGENESIS, AND PREDISPOSING FACTORS   *C. granulomatis* is an intracellular organism that causes local cell necrosis and produces ulcers; it has a low communicability and is spread by sexual contact and autoinoculation.

SITES INVOLVED   Skin in genital, anal, and inguinal regions, especially in skin folds; vulva and vagina may be involved.

GROSS LESIONS   Lesions are relatively painless, soft, raised, ulcerations that are burgundy red; they tend to extend with raised, rolled edges and heal with extensive scar formation.

MICROSCOPIC LESIONS   Margins of the ulcer show epithelial hyperplasia; the base of the ulcer contains microabscesses and macrophages filled with organisms, which can be demonstrated with silver stains.

COMPLICATIONS   Untreated infection may cause extensive destruction, even autoamputation, of external genitalia; secondary infections may occur; lymphatic obstruction due to scarring causes genital lymphedema.

SIGNS AND SYMPTOMS   Development of typical large, raised, red, soft, painless skin ulcers in the perineum or on the genitalia.

CLINICAL DIAGNOSIS AND OTHER CLINICAL FEATURES   Recognition of the genital ulcers, which must be differentiated from syphilis, chancroid, herpes, and LGV.

LABORATORY DIAGNOSIS   Demonstration by special stains of organisms in tissue from biopsy or scrapings of the lesions; the organism is difficult to grow and requires culture in eggs.

PROGNOSIS   No mortality; morbidity includes genital scarring and lymphatic obstruction.

THERAPY   Antibiotics that are effective against intracellular organisms: tetracyclines and chloramphenicol.

OTHER INFORMATION   Male homosexuals constitute a population at high risk for infection. Granuloma inguinale produces the largest ulcers of sexually transmitted diseases.

Hemophilus Influenzae Infection

DESCRIPTION Infection by a fastidious, encapsulated, aerobic, gram-negative bacillus that causes pneumonia, conjunctivitis, epiglottis, otitis, meningitis, and bacteremia.

DISEASE ENTITIES; SYNONYMS AND ACRONYMS Hemophilus pneumonia, otitis media, epiglottitis, meningitis, conjunctivitis.

INCIDENCE Eye and respiratory infections are common; most common cause of meningitis in infants.

AGE Infants between 2 months and 2 years are most susceptible.

ETIOLOGY, PATHOGENESIS, AND PREDISPOSING FACTORS Respiratory transmission of *H. influenzae;* bacteremic spread to other sites; susceptibility to invasion depends on age-dependent production of antibodies to capsule.

SITES INVOLVED Lungs, epiglottis, middle ear, conjunctiva, meninges.

GROSS LESIONS Lungs: consolidation, either lobar or bronchopneumonia pattern; leptomeninges: purulent exudate that extends into subarachnoid space along vessels; epiglottis: swollen, hyperemic, purulent exudate.

MICROSCOPIC LESIONS Pneumonia: alveoli are filled with PMNs; meningitis: fibrin, PMNs, and possibly organisms; epiglottitis: edema, PMNs, and macrophages.

COMPLICATIONS Meningitis leaves permanent deficits in up to 50%, death in 5–10%; epiglottitis can produce airway obstruction; attempts to intubate may induce laryngospasm; Waterhouse-Friderichsen syndrome.

SIGNS AND SYMPTOMS Meningitis is usually preceded by an upper respiratory or middle ear infection, progressing to fever, vomiting, irritability, and/or lethargy; epiglottitis presents acutely with respiratory distress.

CLINICAL DIAGNOSIS AND OTHER CLINICAL FEATURES Recognition of bacterial respiratory infection in an infant or young child; otoscopy; chest x-ray; meningitis must always be ruled out in an infant with a fever and possible meningeal signs.

LABORATORY DIAGNOSIS Demonstration of organism in sputum or spinal fluid by Gram stain, culture; detection of bacterial antigens by fluorescent antibody testing or latex agglutination.

PROGNOSIS Less than 10% mortality in treated severe infections; neurological sequelae can be disabling.

THERAPY Amoxicillin, chloramphenicol; vaccination for prevention.

OTHER INFORMATION *H. influenzae* is a common cause of pneumonia in middle-aged or older adults with chronic obstructive lung disease.

Legionella Pneumonia

DESCRIPTION An acute respiratory infection with *Legionella pneumophila,* a gram-negative, tiny bacillus.

DISEASE ENTITIES; SYNONYMS AND ACRONYMS Legionellosis; Legionnaire's disease; Pontiac fever.

INCIDENCE Occurs as epidemics and sporadic cases with a worldwide distribution.

AGE Older adults with chronic lung disease are particularly susceptible.

ETIOLOGY, PATHOGENESIS, AND PREDISPOSING FACTORS Infection via respiratory tract inhalation; reservoir is primarily aqueous; (e.g., contaminated air conditioning systems, ponds, water systems); immunosuppressed patients are most susceptible.

SITES INVOLVED Organism infects the lower respiratory tract and lungs.

GROSS LESIONS Lungs may show nodular areas of consolidation or may progress to confluent involvement of one or more lobes.

MICROSCOPIC LESIONS Consolidation with an alveolar exudate composed of PMNs, relatively abundant macrophages and fibrin; necrosis of alveolar septa in severe cases.

COMPLICATIONS Respiratory failure; necrotizing pneumonia, lung abscesses.

SIGNS AND SYMPTOMS Presents as a rapidly developing pneumonia with high fever, nonproductive cough, and occasionally diarrhea.

CLINICAL DIAGNOSIS AND OTHER CLINICAL FEATURES Recognition of pneumonia in an older adult with chronic lung or heart disease; x-rays show patchy or diffuse infiltrates, or consolidation of one or more lobes.

LABORATORY DIAGNOSIS Isolation of organism on special media; direct immunofluorescent staining of tissue; confirmation by serology of acute and convalescent serum samples; organism is not seen by Gram stain.

PROGNOSIS 15% mortality in persons requiring hospitalization for respiratory distress.

THERAPY Erythromycin.

OTHER INFORMATION Pontiac fever is a mild form of infection that does not involve pneumonia; many cases are asymptomatic.

Leprosy

DESCRIPTION Chronic progressive bacterial disease of the skin, peripheral nerves, and occasionally the respiratory tract, caused by infection with *Mycobacterium leprae,* an acid-fast intracellular bacillus.

DISEASE ENTITIES; SYNONYMS AND ACRONYMS Hansen's disease; tuberculoid leprosy, lepromatous leprosy, borderline (dimorphous) leprosy.

INCIDENCE Rare in North America; affects 10–12 million worldwide; endemic in several tropical countries.

AGE Any age; usually adults; rare in children under 3 years.

ETIOLOGY, PATHOGENESIS, AND PREDISPOSING FACTORS Transmission requires prolonged intimate contact; infection involves skin and peripheral nerves in cooler distal extremities; cell-mediated immunity is impaired in lepromatous leprosy.

SITES INVOLVED Lepromatous leprosy: diffuse involvement of the skin, eyes, nerves, and upper airway; tuberculoid: predominantly skin, with limited nerve involvement, often ulnar and peroneal nerves.

GROSS LESIONS Lepromatous: multiple and diffuse nodular skin lesions with disfigurement of the hands and face (leonine facies); tuberculoid: single or few lesions, macular or with raised edges.

MICROSCOPIC LESIONS Lepromatous: lesions show diffuse infiltration of foamy macrophages containing many organisms (lepra cells), no granulomas; tuberculoid: epithelioid granulomas with few organisms.

COMPLICATIONS Sensory and motor neuropathy with anesthesia and paralysis; recurrent injury and trophic changes of hands and feet; chronic skin and corneal ulcers; contractures; autoamputation of fingers and toes.

SIGNS AND SYMPTOMS Hypesthetic or anesthetic skin lesions, few and isolated with tuberculoid leprosy, extensive and diffuse with lepromatous leprosy; sensory neuropathy with trophic changes in hands and feet.

CLINICAL DIAGNOSIS AND OTHER CLINICAL FEATURES Recognition of skin lesions with peripheral nerve involvement; peroneal and ulnar nerves are favorite sites; sensory neuropathy precedes motor neuropathy.

LABORATORY DIAGNOSIS Demonstration of organism in smears from slit-skin scrapings or in histologic sections of skin or nerve biopsy; Fite acid-fast stain visualizes organism, which cannot be grown in culture.

PROGNOSIS Usually good with therapy; best for tuberculoid leprosy; therapy decreases shedding of bacillus.

THERAPY Dapsone, alone or combined with rifampin and/or clofazimine; isolation is not required.

OTHER INFORMATION Skin-test reactions to lepromin, an extract from the bacillus, is a measure of the effectiveness of cell-mediated immunity: weak or nonexistent in lepromatous leprosy, strong in tuberculoid leprosy.

Lyme Disease

DESCRIPTION   Infection characterized by skin rash, arthritis, and neurologic changes, caused by *Borrelia burgdorferi,* a spirochete transmitted to humans by deer ticks from the reservoir of deer and small animals.

DISEASE ENTITIES; SYNONYMS AND ACRONYMS   Lyme borreliosis.

INCIDENCE   Endemic in Atlantic coastal states, Minnesota, Wisconsin, California, and Oregon.

AGE   Any age.

ETIOLOGY, PATHOGENESIS, AND PREDISPOSING FACTORS   Transmitted by deer tick, *Ixodes dammini.* Spirochete infects skin at bite site then disseminates via blood, exhibiting tropism for heart, CNS, and joints; immune reactions mediate tissue damage.

SITES INVOLVED   Skin, joints (particularly knees), heart, CNS.

GROSS LESIONS   Skin rash (erythema chronicum migrans) develops around bite and spreads centrifugally; the lesion must be at least 5 cm in diameter to be diagnostically significant.

MICROSCOPIC LESIONS   Infected tissue shows nonspecific perivascular mononuclear cell inflammation; organisms can be seen in vessel walls with special stains; skin rash shows acanthosis.

COMPLICATIONS   Chronic arthritis; cardiac arrhythmias, including complete heart block; neurologic abnormalities, including motor or sensory disturbances, ataxia, or myelitis.

SIGNS AND SYMPTOMS   Characteristic rash after exposure or potential exposure to ticks; fever, malaise, headache, stiff neck, and myalgias; neurologic and cardiac complications develop weeks or months after rash.

CLINICAL DIAGNOSIS AND OTHER CLINICAL FEATURES   Recognition of migrating skin rash with systemic signs of inflammation in a patient from an endemic region with possible tick exposure; complications may occur after the rash is forgotten.

LABORATORY DIAGNOSIS   Serologic tests are not completely reliable but are more accurate in patients with chronic Lyme disease; some patients remain seronegative.

PROGNOSIS   Good with treatment; patients in the later stages require longer courses or intravenous therapy.

THERAPY   Tetracycline for adults; amoxicillin or erythromycin for children; ceftriaxone for neurologic signs.

OTHER INFORMATION   Disease is more common in late summer and fall. Infected persons may not report a tick bite or rash because the tick is tiny and the rash may not be in an easily visible part of the body.

Meningococcal Infection

DESCRIPTION An acute suppurative disease characterized by meningitis and/or sepsis, caused by infection with *Neisseria meningitidis,* a fastidious gram-negative diplococcus.

DISEASE ENTITIES; SYNONYMS AND ACRONYMS Meningococcal meningitis; meningococcemia; Waterhouse-Friderichsen syndrome.

INCIDENCE Greatest in winter and spring; commonly occurs in epidemics; very common in sub-Saharan mid-Africa.

AGE Usually infants and small children; young adults living in crowded conditions (colleges, military).

ETIOLOGY, PATHOGENESIS, AND PREDISPOSING FACTORS Transmitted by respiratory droplets; organisms colonize nasopharynx and invade mucosa of susceptible persons, leading to septicemia and dissemination to meninges and other sites.

SITES INVOLVED Pia and arachnoid are involved in meningitis; in sepsis (meningococcemia) there are lesions of skin (purpuric rash), adrenal glands (hemorrhage), and occasionally other sites (often myocarditis).

GROSS LESIONS Meningitis: purulent exudate involving leptomeninges extending along blood vessels; meningococcemia: hemorrhages in skin, adrenal glands (Waterhouse-Friderichsen syndrome), and other organs.

MICROSCOPIC LESIONS Meningeal exudate contains PMNs and fibrin; diplococci are present in exudate and within PMNs; adrenal glands show acute hemorrhage and necrosis.

COMPLICATIONS Septic shock due to meningococcemia; acute adrenal insufficiency due to hemorrhage; communicating hydrocephalus due to organization of meningeal exudate; dural sinus thrombosis.

SIGNS AND SYMPTOMS Meningitis presents acutely with headache, fever, and stiff neck; meningococcemia presents with rash, fever, tachycardia, and hypotension that often progresses to endotoxin shock.

CLINICAL DIAGNOSIS AND OTHER CLINICAL FEATURES Recognition of signs; infection of pharynx may produce no symptoms or mild pharyngitis; invasion of blood causes symptoms ranging from mild to fulminant meningococcemia that may be fatal within hours.

LABORATORY DIAGNOSIS Granulocytosis with left shift; high PMN count in CSF; isolation of meningococcus from blood or CSF; identification of bacterial antigens in CSF; Gram stain often demonstrates the organisms in CSF.

PROGNOSIS Less than 10% mortality for treated meningitis; high mortality for meningococcemia.

THERAPY Penicillin and supportive therapy; chemoprophylaxis for close contacts with rifampin.

OTHER INFORMATION A vaccine for groups A, C, Y, and W-135 is available; it has been given to military recruits and high-risk patients but is not recommended for routine administration.

Mycoplasma Pneumonia

DESCRIPTION   Infection with *Mycoplasma pneumoniae,* which causes pneumonia with diffuse or patchy interstitial pulmonary infiltrates.

DISEASE ENTITIES; SYNONYMS AND ACRONYMS   Atypical pneumonia, PPLO, walking pneumonia.

INCIDENCE   Common cause of community-acquired pneumonia; outbreaks often occur in groups like the military.

AGE   Any age; more common in adults.

ETIOLOGY, PATHOGENESIS, AND PREDISPOSING FACTORS   Transmission is primarily by droplet spread and rapidly infects people living in close contact. The organism lacks a cell wall but is larger than a virus and multiplies by dividing.

SITES INVOLVED   Lungs and lower airways.

GROSS LESIONS   Most commonly unilateral lower lobe pneumonia with red firm pulmonary parenchyma in affected areas.

MICROSCOPIC LESIONS   Usually there is a patchy interstitial pneumonia; bronchial mucosa is congested and edematous; inflammatory response consists of perivascular lymphocytes initially and PMNs later in the infection.

COMPLICATIONS   Respiratory failure is uncommon. Rarely, the infection involves the heart, brain, and/or joints.

SIGNS AND SYMPTOMS   Gradual onset of cough that is initially nonproductive; then fever, malaise, rhinorrhea, and development of productive cough.

CLINICAL DIAGNOSIS AND OTHER CLINICAL FEATURES   Recognition of symptoms of pneumonia; chest x-rays show "fluffy" interstitial infiltrate pattern; disease manifestations are often less than what would be expected with the degree of lung involvement.

LABORATORY DIAGNOSIS   Serologic detection of complement fixing antibodies; cold agglutinins are present in about one half of patients; WBC is usually normal.

PROGNOSIS   Good.

THERAPY   Tetracycline or erythromycin.

OTHER INFORMATION   X-ray pattern, subacute onset, nonproductive cough, negative Gram stain, and sputum culture differentiate atypical pneumonia from the more common bacterial pneumonias.

Nocardiosis

DESCRIPTION A chronic bacterial infection, usually involving the lungs, caused by *Nocardia asteroides,* a branching, aerobic, gram-positive organism that is weakly acid-fast.

DISEASE ENTITIES; SYNONYMS AND ACRONYMS Pulmonary nocardiosis; cutaneous or subcutaneous nocardiosis, mycetoma, maduromycosis; disseminated nocardiosis.

INCIDENCE Uncommon; occurs sporadically; more likely to occur in immunosuppressed patients.

AGE Any age; often in older adults with chronic lung disease.

ETIOLOGY, PATHOGENESIS, AND PREDISPOSING FACTORS Immunosuppression due to therapy or other diseases increases susceptibility; Nocardia is a soil organism that is probably inhaled in contaminated dust.

SITES INVOLVED Lungs are the usual site of primary infection; organisms may spread through the blood and cause abscesses in the brain, subcutaneous tissues, and other organs.

GROSS LESIONS Lung lesions consist of necrotic centers within regions of consolidation; fibrinous pleuritis, pleural effusions, or empyema may develop.

MICROSCOPIC LESIONS Consolidation of alveoli with exudate of PMNs and fibrin; focal necrosis of lung parenchyma; organisms grow extensively in the consolidated tissue but cannot be visualized without special stains.

COMPLICATIONS Progressive lung disease with abscesses, respiratory failure; dissemination to other sites producing metastatic abscesses; brain abscesses occur in many cases.

SIGNS AND SYMPTOMS Fever, chills, night sweats, cough, and weight loss; signs of disseminated infection are related to localized abscesses, such as neurologic signs and seizures with brain abscess.

CLINICAL DIAGNOSIS AND OTHER CLINICAL FEATURES Recognition of progressive necrotizing lung disease in a susceptible patient that is not due to any of the common organisms; x-rays show nodular infiltrates with or without abscesses.

LABORATORY DIAGNOSIS Demonstration of the filamentous organism in sputum, bronchial aspirate, or tissue from biopsy or autopsy; the organism is difficult to culture because it grows slowly on aerobic media.

PROGNOSIS High mortality for infections other than those limited to skin and subcutaneous tissues.

THERAPY Sulfa antibiotics for up to a year; amikacin or ampicillin are added if there is no response.

OTHER INFORMATION *Nocardia brasiliensis* causes a chronic infection of the lower leg, called mycetoma or maduromycosis, which occurs in South and Central America.

Pertussis

DESCRIPTION   An acute infection of the respiratory system caused by *Bordetella pertussis,* a small gram-negative coccobacillus.

DISEASE ENTITIES; SYNONYMS AND ACRONYMS   Whooping cough.

INCIDENCE   Low incidence in countries with active immunization programs.

AGE   More common in children.

ETIOLOGY, PATHOGENESIS, AND PREDISPOSING FACTORS   Transmission by droplet inhalation; bacteria attach to bronchial mucosa and release a toxin; nonimmunized persons are susceptible; IgA in immune persons prevents bacterial attachment.

SITES INVOLVED   Upper and lower respiratory tract; organism has a strong tropism for brush border of bronchial epithelium.

GROSS LESIONS   Bronchial infection causes production of thick mucus; secondary bacterial pneumonia may produce consolidation.

MICROSCOPIC LESIONS   Bronchial epithelium shows necrosis and is covered by a thick, purulent exudate containing many pertussis bacilli.

COMPLICATIONS   Secondary bacterial pneumonia; subcutaneous emphysema; convulsions due to hypoxia and fever; bronchiectasis leading to chronic lung disease.

SIGNS AND SYMPTOMS   Onset as a cold-like illness that progresses to paroxysms of severe coughing episodes that have a distinctive gasping, inspiratory "whoop."

CLINICAL DIAGNOSIS AND OTHER CLINICAL FEATURES   Recognition of respiratory disease with severe coughing episodes in a susceptible nonimmunized child; chest x-rays show pneumonia in up to a fourth of the younger patients; cough may persist 2 months.

LABORATORY DIAGNOSIS   Isolation of the causative organism from nasopharyngeal cultures during the first 2 weeks of infection; infection causes a striking peripheral lymphocytosis.

PROGNOSIS   Good; most deaths occur in young children, but mortality rate is low.

THERAPY   Erythromycin in the early stages of infection shortens the course and infectious period.

OTHER INFORMATION   Pertussis is included in the childhood DPT vaccination; the rate of vaccination has been declining due to widespread publicity of rare adverse reactions to the vaccination.

Plague

DESCRIPTION   A zoonotic infection cause by *Yersinia pestis,* a gram-negative bacillus that is transmitted to humans by the rat flea.

DISEASE ENTITIES; SYNONYMS AND ACRONYMS   Bubonic plague; black death.

INCIDENCE   Isolated cases occur in the southwestern US, Africa, South America, and Asia.

AGE   Any age.

ETIOLOGY, PATHOGENESIS, AND PREDISPOSING FACTORS   Bites of infected fleas; reservoir of organism in wild rodents; contact with wild rodents or transmission of infected fleas to domestic rats creates the potential for human infection.

SITES INVOLVED   Two forms: bubonic and pneumonic. Bubonic: regional lymph nodes draining the area of the flea bite are first involved, then sepsis; pneumonic: lungs are involved due to sepsis or primary infection.

GROSS LESIONS   Bubonic: enlarged lymph nodes (buboes) are necrotic and suppurative; pneumonic: lungs show patchy bronchopneumonia or lobar consolidation.

MICROSCOPIC LESIONS   Lymph nodes are suppurative, necrotic, and contain numerous organisms; lungs are involved with necrotizing bronchopneumonia.

COMPLICATIONS   Death in 50–90% of untreated cases; systemic infection occurs in either form, with sepsis, shock, and disseminated intravascular coagulation; systemic and pneumonic plague are usually fatal.

SIGNS AND SYMPTOMS   Fever, chills, nausea; swollen tender lymph nodes; purpura and ecchymoses; in pneumonic form: fever, cough, and dyspnea progressing rapidly to respiratory failure.

CLINICAL DIAGNOSIS AND OTHER CLINICAL FEATURES   Recognition of lymphadenitis and systemic signs in a patient who has been in an endemic area and may have been in contact with rodents.

LABORATORY DIAGNOSIS   Demonstration of organisms by direct examination of Gram-stained sputum or material aspirated from a bubo; examination using fluorescent antibody staining is more specific; bacterial culture.

PROGNOSIS   Systemic and pneumonic infections are usually fatal; about 50% mortality for bubonic plague.

THERAPY   Streptomycin, tetracycline, or chloramphenicol; despite therapy toxic shock may still occur.

OTHER INFORMATION   Infection can be spread by droplet transmission from persons with pneumonic plague; strict isolation is required; infected corpses must be handled with extreme caution.

Pneumococcal Infections

DESCRIPTION Pneumonia and other infections (sepsis, meningitis) caused by *Streptococcus pneumoniae*, a gram-positive, aerobic diplococcus, which has a polysaccharide capsule that contributes to its virulence.

DISEASE ENTITIES; SYNONYMS AND ACRONYMS Pneumococcal pneumonia, lobar pneumonia; bacteremia, sepsis; pneumococcal meningitis; pneumococcal otitis media.

INCIDENCE Very common; 10–25% of pneumonias are caused by pneumococcus; common cause of death in elderly.

AGE Most common in the very young and the elderly.

ETIOLOGY, PATHOGENESIS, AND PREDISPOSING FACTORS Respiratory transmission; often follows viral respiratory infection; alcoholism, neurologic impairment, cigarette smoking, aspiration of oral contents; splenectomized patients are highly susceptible.

SITES INVOLVED Initially lungs; exudate within alveoli with either a lobar or bronchopneumonia pattern; invasion of blood to produce bacteremia; hematogenous spread to other sites, particular meninges of brain.

GROSS LESIONS Pneumonia: starts with congestion and edema (red hepatization); progresses to consolidation (gray hepatization); returns to normal in 2–3 weeks (resolution). Meningitis: purulent exudate in meninges.

MICROSCOPIC LESIONS Red hepatization: vasodilatation, vascular congestion, edema, red cells in alveoli; gray hepatization: PMNs and fibrin in alveoli, many organisms; resolution: digestion and clearing of exudate.

COMPLICATIONS Fibrinopurulent pleuritis that produces pleural adhesions with healing; empyema; occasionally lung abscess; bacteremia, sepsis; meningitis, rarely brain abscess; septic arthritis.

SIGNS AND SYMPTOMS Acute onset of fever, chills, pleuritis, and dyspnea, with cough productive of purulent sputum that may be blood-tinged; often follows viral upper respiratory infection.

CLINICAL DIAGNOSIS AND OTHER CLINICAL FEATURES Recognition of abrupt onset of symptoms typical of pneumonia; physical examination is characteristic; chest x-ray may show a lobar or a bronchopneumonia pattern.

LABORATORY DIAGNOSIS Sputum culture; Gram-stained sputum shows large numbers of diplococci along with PMNs; bacteremia in 25% of pneumococcal pneumonia; PMNs and diplococci in CSF in cases of meningitis.

PROGNOSIS Usually good with treatment; 5–20% mortality rate for those with significant underlying diseases.

THERAPY Penicillin; resistance to penicillin occurs but is still very uncommon.

OTHER INFORMATION Pneumococcal capsule resists phagocytosis; opsonization without specific antibody is inefficient; polysaccharide vaccine is recommended for susceptible patients (elderly, asplenic patients).

Rheumatic Fever

DESCRIPTION An acute inflammatory disease with systemic manifestations and particular involvement of the heart valves, which follows an upper respiratory infection with group A beta-hemolytic Streptococcus.

DISEASE ENTITIES; SYNONYMS AND ACRONYMS Acute rheumatic fever, rheumatic carditis; rheumatic heart disease, rheumatic valve disease, rheumatic valvulitis.

INCIDENCE Several outbreaks in US since 1985; previously declining incidence; common in developing countries.

AGE Most common in children; peak incidence between 5 and 15.

ETIOLOGY, PATHOGENESIS, AND PREDISPOSING FACTORS Pharyngitis caused by group A Streptococcus induces autoimmune reaction involving antibodies that cross-react with cardiac proteins; rheumatic fever follows pharyngitis by 1–5 weeks.

SITES INVOLVED All layers of heart (pancarditis: pericarditis, myocarditis, endocarditis) with most important involvement of valves (endocarditis); also joints, skin, and subcutaneous tissues.

GROSS LESIONS Joints are swollen and inflamed; myocardium is soft; fibrinous pericarditis is often present; valves are edematous, fibrin may be deposited along their margins; subcutaneous nodules may be present.

MICROSCOPIC LESIONS Aschoff bodies in myocardium consist of mononuclear inflammatory cells and Anitschkow myocytes; skin nodules resemble Aschoff bodies, with fibrinoid necrosis surrounded by palisades of macrophages.

COMPLICATIONS Relapse rate of 20% within 5 years; relapses increase the risk of heart damage that leads to rheumatic heart disease, with mitral or aortic stenosis or insufficiency due to progressive valve scarring.

SIGNS AND SYMPTOMS Major Jone's criteria: carditis, arthritis, chorea, erythema marginatum, and subcutaneous nodules; minor criteria: fever, arthralgias, history of rheumatic fever, EKG changes and lab tests.

CLINICAL DIAGNOSIS AND OTHER CLINICAL FEATURES Presence of symptoms that include 2 major or 1 major and 2 minor of Jone's criteria; the carditis produces cardiac dilatation with murmur, a third heart sound and prolongation of the P-R interval.

LABORATORY DIAGNOSIS Tests in the minor criteria include: elevated RBC sedimentation rate (ESR), C-reactive protein, leukocytosis; elevation of the serum antistreptolysin O (ASO) titer indicates recent strep infection.

PROGNOSIS Acute mortality is low; scarring of heart valves causes long-term morbidity and mortality.

THERAPY Penicillin for pharyngitis prevents most cases; prophylactic antibiotics following rheumatic fever.

OTHER INFORMATION Rheumatic valve disease, particularly mitral stenosis, is the most common indication for valve replacement surgery.

Rickettsial Infections—Typhus Group

DESCRIPTION   Endemic typhus is an acute febrile illness with a macular rash caused by *Rickettsia typhi;* epidemic typhus is caused by *R. prowazekii* and is transmitted between humans via body lice.

DISEASE ENTITIES; SYNONYMS AND ACRONYMS   Murine (endemic) typhus; louse-borne (epidemic) typhus; Brill-Zinsser disease.

INCIDENCE   Rare; endemic regions in US are the Southeastern and Gulf states.

AGE   Any age.

ETIOLOGY, PATHOGENESIS, AND PREDISPOSING FACTORS   *R. typhi:* transmitted by mouse fleas; *R. prowazekii:* transmitted by human body lice; parasites are passed in arthropod feces, which contaminate the bite wound and provide access to the blood.

SITES INVOLVED   Organisms infect and multiply within endothelial cells of capillaries in the brain, heart, skin, and other organs.

GROSS LESIONS   Pink macular rash on skin; few gross visceral lesions; moderate to marked splenomegaly in severe cases.

MICROSCOPIC LESIONS   Microthrombi occluding capillaries; perivascular "cuffing" with mononuclear cells; occasionally diffuse myocarditis with mononuclear cells.

COMPLICATIONS   Heart failure; coma; recurrence with *R. prowazekii* causes a milder disease called Brill-Zinsser disease.

SIGNS AND SYMPTOMS   Sudden onset of fever, chills and headache; macular rash usually develops in 4–8 days and may become hemorrhagic; stupor or coma develop in severe cases.

CLINICAL DIAGNOSIS AND OTHER CLINICAL FEATURES   Recognition of systemic disease with a rash suggestive of vasculitis; typhus must be differentiated from Rocky Mountain spotted fever. Cardiac decompensation may occur suddenly.

LABORATORY DIAGNOSIS   Serologic demonstration of antibodies; Weil-Felix agglutination reaction can be used but is outdated.

PROGNOSIS   Mortality rate increases with age; therapy reduces mortality.

THERAPY   Tetracycline or chloramphenicol.

OTHER INFORMATION   Louse-borne typhus has caused major epidemics in wartime due to unsanitary conditions and crowding; scrub typhus, or Tsutsugamushi disease, is a mite-borne typhus in the eastern hemisphere.

Rocky Mountain Spotted Fever

DESCRIPTION   A severe infection with *Rickettsia rickettsii*, transmitted by ticks, that involves endothelial cells and produces a vasculitis.

DISEASE ENTITIES; SYNONYMS AND ACRONYMS   RMSF.

INCIDENCE   Uncommon; 649 cases in US in 1990; mostly in southeastern, central, and mid-Atlantic States.

AGE   Highest rate in children, ages 5–9.

ETIOLOGY, PATHOGENESIS, AND PREDISPOSING FACTORS   Caused by a gram-negative intracellular organism transmitted by bites of ticks in endemic wooded areas. Endothelial cells are infected, which produces vasculitis.

SITES INVOLVED   Blood vessels, especially endothelial cells, are invaded by the organism; platelets aggregate and clotting factors are activated, leading to thrombus formation; any organ can be affected.

GROSS LESIONS   Foci of hemorrhage in kidneys, heart, meninges, and skin; skin rash is maculopapular and often purpuric.

MICROSCOPIC LESIONS   Vasculitis with necrosis; microthrombi in vessels of involved organs. Purpuric skin lesions show thrombi and extravasated red blood cells; occasionally there are microinfarcts of the brain.

COMPLICATIONS   Consumption of platelets and clotting factors leads to disseminated intravascular coagulation (DIC).

SIGNS AND SYMPTOMS   Fever, intense headache, and myalgia within 2 weeks of exposure; rash that begins peripherally and involves palms and soles; nonproductive cough.

CLINICAL DIAGNOSIS AND OTHER CLINICAL FEATURES   Recognition of skin rash with signs of systemic infection in a person with history of tick exposure in an endemic region; rash is often purpuric or petechial, indicating vasculitis.

LABORATORY DIAGNOSIS   Specific serology is now available; Weil-Felix, or febrile agglutinins, were used previously. Thrombocytopenia and abnormal clotting tests indicate coagulopathy.

PROGNOSIS   10% mortality despite antibiotic treatment.

THERAPY   Tetracycline in adults; chloramphenicol in children.

OTHER INFORMATION   Humans are infected incidentally, outside of the organism's normal life cycle; person-to-person transmission does not occur; infected ticks can transmit the organism to their progeny.

Salmonellosis

DESCRIPTION   Acute nontyphoidal diseases of the gastrointestinal tract caused by species of Salmonella, usually *S. choleraesuis* or *S. enteritidis*; several different serotypes occur, e.g., *S. typhimurium*.

DISEASE ENTITIES; SYNONYMS AND ACRONYMS   Salmonella enteritis, gastroenteritis; Salmonella food poisoning; Salmonella septicemia.

INCIDENCE   There are an estimated 5 million cases per year in the US.

AGE   Any age; the very young and the very old are most seriously affected.

ETIOLOGY, PATHOGENESIS, AND PREDISPOSING FACTORS   Infection is acquired by ingesting food or water contaminated by animal feces (e.g., poultry, turtles); persons with decreased gastric acidity are more susceptible.

SITES INVOLVED   Infection involves the small intestine, usually with limited mucosal invasion; occasionally blood is invaded (especially with *S. choleraesuis),* causing septicemia and spread to other organs.

GROSS LESIONS   Depends on the severity of the disease; intestinal mucosal erythema or superficial ulcers.

MICROSCOPIC LESIONS   Mixed inflammatory infiltrate in mucosa; shallow erosions; mild infections produce no lesions.

COMPLICATIONS   Dehydration and electrolyte imbalance, which can be life-threatening in the very young or very old; sepsis; metastatic infections in multiple organs and tissues.

SIGNS AND SYMPTOMS   Usually sudden onset of headache, nausea, vomiting, abdominal pains, and diarrhea accompanied by fever.

CLINICAL DIAGNOSIS AND OTHER CLINICAL FEATURES   Recognition of the above; symptoms are variable and range from minimal nausea to severe diarrhea with bloody stools and tenesmus.

LABORATORY DIAGNOSIS   Isolation of the organism from blood or feces.

PROGNOSIS   Usually good; persons with AIDS are at risk for recurrent sepsis with non-typhoid Salmonella.

THERAPY   Fluid and electrolyte therapy; antibiotics are withheld because they prolong the carrier state.

OTHER INFORMATION   Persons with sickle cell disease have a high rate of Salmonella osteomyelitis. Hospitalized patients with Salmonella must be placed under enteric precautions.

Shigellosis

DESCRIPTION   An acute enteric disease (dysentery), characterized by diarrhea and fever, caused by species of Shigella, which are gram-negative aerobic bacilli.

DISEASE ENTITIES; SYNONYMS AND ACRONYMS   Bacillary dysentery.

INCIDENCE   Common; worldwide distribution; infection may be produced by ingestion of 10–100 organisms.

AGE   Any age; most fatal cases occur in children between ages 6 months and 10 years.

ETIOLOGY, PATHOGENESIS, AND PREDISPOSING FACTORS   4 species: *S. dysenteriae, S. flexneri, S. boydii,* and *S. sonnei;* a virulence plasmid confers intestinal invasiveness; transmitted by contaminated water and "food, fingers, feces, and flies."

SITES INVOLVED   Colon and distal small bowel; Shiga enterotoxin activates adenylate cyclase of the intestinal epithelial cells, producing secretion of NaCl and water; the organisms invade the intestinal mucosa.

GROSS LESIONS   Hyperemia of intestinal mucosa; focal mucosal ulcers with pseudomembranous exudate; blood, mucus, and pus in the stools.

MICROSCOPIC LESIONS   Early edema of lamina propria; later, mucosal ulcers covered with pseudomembrane composed of PMNs, fibrin, and cellular debris.

COMPLICATIONS   Dehydration, hypovolemic shock; sepsis; toxic megacolon; hemolytic-uremic syndrome.

SIGNS AND SYMPTOMS   Range from mild or profuse diarrhea to severe dysentery with tenesmus, fever, chills, bloody diarrhea with mucus and pus in the stools, and abdominal pain.

CLINICAL DIAGNOSIS AND OTHER CLINICAL FEATURES   Recognition of the above signs and symptoms; tenesmus and bloody diarrhea with mucus are characteristic of dysentery; proctosigmoidoscopy shows hyperemic mucosa with exudate.

LABORATORY DIAGNOSIS   Isolation of the organism from stool or rectal swabs; leukocytes present in microscopic examination of stool, stained with methylene blue, is suggestive of shigellosis.

PROGNOSIS   Up to 20% mortality in cases requiring hospitalization, mostly in children; relapses are common.

THERAPY   Fluid and electrolyte therapy; antibiotics such as ampicillin; antidiarrheals are contraindicated.

OTHER INFORMATION   Outbreaks of shigellosis occur when there is crowding or poor hygiene such as occurs in jails, mental institutions, group homes for children, or day-care facilities.

Staphylococcal Infections

DESCRIPTION Suppurative infections caused by species of Staphylococcus, usually *S. aureus,* which is a gram-positive coccus that grows in clusters in liquid culture.

DISEASE ENTITIES; SYNONYMS AND ACRONYMS Staphylococcal abscesses, pneumonia, osteomyelitis, endocarditis; carbuncles, furuncles, pyoderma, impetigo.

INCIDENCE Very common.

AGE Any age; outbreaks of staphylococcal infections have occurred in hospital nurseries.

ETIOLOGY, PATHOGENESIS, AND PREDISPOSING FACTORS *S. aureus* is coagulase positive and causes abscesses; skin defects provide entry; *S. saprophyticus* is a urinary tract pathogen; *S. epidermidis* is occasionally pathogenic.

SITES INVOLVED Skin: boils, furuncles, carbuncles, abscesses, impetigo, cellulitis; lung: pneumonia, abscesses; skeletal: osteomyelitis, septic arthritis; heart valves: endocarditis; blood: sepsis.

GROSS LESIONS Infections are suppurative and usually localized (abscesses); skin lesions are deep and begin in hair follicles; endocarditis is characterized by adherent fibrin vegetations and destruction of valves.

MICROSCOPIC LESIONS Suppuration and liquefaction necrosis; abscesses show central PMNs and necrotic debris with surrounding fibrosis; in endocarditis, clumps of bacteria grow in the fibrin vegetations.

COMPLICATIONS Untreated skin infections can become systemic to produce infective endocarditis and visceral abscesses or osteomyelitis; staphylococcal sepsis is potentially lethal.

SIGNS AND SYMPTOMS Fever, chills; red, swollen skin lesions with abscesses that are likely to drain; new heart murmur indicates endocarditis; cough, dyspnea, purulent sputum indicates pneumonia.

CLINICAL DIAGNOSIS AND OTHER CLINICAL FEATURES Recognition of cutaneous abscesses or other sites of suppurative infection; staphylococcal pneumonia often complicates viral respiratory infections, especially influenza.

LABORATORY DIAGNOSIS Culture of the organism from pus or drainage; Gram stain is usually accurate; isolation of the organism in blood cultures confirms endocarditis; antibiotic sensitivity testing is important.

PROGNOSIS Usually good with treatment; endocarditis and osteomyelitis may have serious sequelae.

THERAPY Drainage of abscesses; antibiotics; penicillinase production and methicillin resistance are common.

OTHER INFORMATION *S. aureus* may cause acute-onset food poisoning. Toxic shock syndrome is linked to superabsorbent tampon use and causes rash, fever and hypotension due to a staphylococcal toxin.

Streptococcal Infections

DESCRIPTION Suppurative infections caused by species of Streptococcus, a gram-positive coccus that grows in chains in liquid culture; group A streptococci cause immunologic complications in heart and kidneys.

DISEASE ENTITIES; SYNONYMS AND ACRONYMS Streptococcal pharyngitis; scarlet fever; erysipelas; neonatal sepsis; poststreptococcal complications.

INCIDENCE Very common.

AGE Any age; pharyngitis and skin infections are most common in children.

ETIOLOGY, PATHOGENESIS, AND PREDISPOSING FACTORS Most infections are due to hemolytic species, especially group A (*S. pyogenes*); bacterial DNase and hyaluronidase promote spreading infections; immune reactions cause poststreptococcal complications.

SITES INVOLVED Skin and pharynx: infections are caused by group A organisms; neonatal sepsis is due to group B; heart valves are infected usually with *S. viridans.*

GROSS LESIONS Skin infections tend to spread (e.g., erysipelas); impetigo is similar to staphylococcal infection but more often shows lymphangitis; in pharyngitis there is mucosal hyperemia and purulent exudate.

MICROSCOPIC LESIONS Suppuration; necrosis is less likely than with staph infection because abscesses are uncommon; heart valve lesions are less destructive with strep endocarditis compared with *S. aureus* endocarditis.

COMPLICATIONS Potentially lethal sepsis can develop with any infection; nonsuppurative postinfectious complications: poststreptococcal glomerulonephritis; acute rheumatic fever, rheumatic heart disease.

SIGNS AND SYMPTOMS Fever, chills; pharyngitis: sore throat, enlarged cervical nodes; impetigo: red skin lesions with "honey crust"; erysipelas: diffuse hyperemia and swelling of skin; endocarditis: new heart murmur.

CLINICAL DIAGNOSIS AND OTHER CLINICAL FEATURES Recognition of spreading skin infections; scarlet fever is produced by erythrogenic toxin that may produce toxic-strep syndrome; glomerulonephritis and rheumatic fever are prevented by antibiotics.

LABORATORY DIAGNOSIS Isolation of organism from infected region or blood in endocarditis; grouping is based on capsular antigens; *S. viridans* are ungroupable; Enterococcus is a related but separate genus.

PROGNOSIS Usually good with therapy; toxic-strep syndrome is a type of shock syndrome with high mortality.

THERAPY Antibiotic therapy (usually penicillin); therapy prevents long-term sequelae in heart and kidneys.

OTHER INFORMATION Puerperal sepsis, or childbed fever, is due to group A Streptococci and was a cause of high maternal mortality before the germ theory was accepted, thanks to I. Semmelweiss.

Syphilis

DESCRIPTION   A sexually transmitted disease caused by infection with *Treponema pallidum,* which occurs in three stages: primary, secondary, and tertiary syphilis; congenital infections also occur.

DISEASE ENTITIES; SYNONYMS AND ACRONYMS   Lues; great pox.

INCIDENCE   15 cases per 100,000 population per year; increasing annually.

AGE   Sexually active adults and teens; congenital infections in neonates and infants.

ETIOLOGY, PATHOGENESIS, AND PREDISPOSING FACTORS   Treponema pallidum is a spirochete transmitted through sexual contact with mucocutaneous lesions or transplacentally; infection involves blood vessels in many organs.

SITES INVOLVED   Primary lesion (chancre): genitalia; secondary lesions: skin and mucosal surfaces, genitalia, palms, and soles; tertiary lesions: aorta, CNS; gummas in viscera.

GROSS LESIONS   Chancre: painless, rubbery ulcer; lesions of secondary syphilis: maculopapular rash, condyloma lata; tertiary: tree-barking of aorta, dilatation of root; gummas: nodules with central necrosis.

MICROSCOPIC LESIONS   Lymphoplasmacytic vasculitis with endothelial cell swelling and proliferation (endarteritis obliterans); secondary ischemic damage of affected tissues; gummas: granulomas with central necrosis.

COMPLICATIONS   Late lesions of tertiary syphilis; cardiovascular syphilis: aortitis, aneurysm of thoracic aorta, heart failure due to aortic insufficiency; neurosyphilis: dementia, general paresis, tabes dorsalis.

SIGNS AND SYMPTOMS   Primary: chancre; secondary: skin rash that includes the palms and soles, condyloma lata; latent periods are asymptomatic; tertiary: sensory loss in legs, paresis, aortic valve murmur.

CLINICAL DIAGNOSIS AND OTHER CLINICAL FEATURES   Painless genital ulcer or diffuse rash in a sexually active person; tertiary syphilis occurs decades after initial infection; testing for other concurrent sexually transmitted diseases is advisable.

LABORATORY DIAGNOSIS   Serology; reagin tests such as VDRL or RPR; confirmation with more specific tests such as FTA-ABS (fluorescent treponemal antibody-absorbed serum); darkfield microscopy.

PROGNOSIS   Good if treated early; tertiary syphilis causes irreversible heart failure, dementia, disability.

THERAPY   Penicillin, doxycycline, or tetracycline.

OTHER INFORMATION   The chancre and lesions of secondary syphilis contain numerous organisms and are very infectious. Congenital syphilis causes fetal death or manifestations of infection that occur after birth.

Tetanus

DESCRIPTION   An acute neuromuscular disease characterized by muscle spasms and severe uncontrolled contractions, caused by the exotoxin, tetanospasmin, produced by *Clostridium tetani*.

DISEASE ENTITIES; SYNONYMS AND ACRONYMS   Lockjaw; tetanus neonatorum.

INCIDENCE   Uncommon in developed countries due to immunization programs.

AGE   Any age; neonates of nonimmunized women may become infected through the umbilical stump.

ETIOLOGY, PATHOGENESIS, AND PREDISPOSING FACTORS   Contamination by clostridial spores of a puncture wound or deep laceration; tetanospasmin ascends through nerves to anterior horn cells and crosses the synapse to block inhibitory transmitter release.

SITES INVOLVED   Organism grows within a wound with low oxygen tension; exotoxin is released from that site and gains access to the CNS to block inhibitory neurons; thus, motor neurons and muscles are hyperexcitable.

GROSS LESIONS   There may be necrosis and suppuration in the initial wound; in 10% of cases the wound is small and not detected. The CNS and muscles show no changes.

MICROSCOPIC LESIONS   Primary wound may show necrosis and PMN infiltrates; inflammation is due to other bacteria, not *C. tetani*; anterior horn neurons of spinal cord may show mild edema and chromatolysis.

COMPLICATIONS   Asphyxia due to prolonged spasms of respiratory muscles; fractures of thoracic vertebrae and other sites due to forceful contractions; aspiration pneumonia due to spasm of neck muscles.

SIGNS AND SYMPTOMS   Often begins with pain and stiffness in the jaw, back, or abdomen and progresses to generalized muscle spasms; classically: trismus, risus sardonicus, and opisthotonos.

CLINICAL DIAGNOSIS AND OTHER CLINICAL FEATURES   Recognition of fully established syndrome is not difficult; early signs may be misinterpreted; external stimuli precipitate seizures and muscle spasms that can produce respiratory arrest.

LABORATORY DIAGNOSIS   CBC, blood chemistries, and spinal fluid are normal. The organism is recovered in cultures of the infection site in less than 30% of cases.

PROGNOSIS   There is a 30–90% mortality with the higher rates in very young and elderly patients.

THERAPY   Minimize external stimuli; antitoxin; muscle relaxants; airway support; vaccine prophylaxis.

OTHER INFORMATION   Tetanus occurs in IV drug abusers due to contaminated drugs. Antitoxin (tetanus immune globulin) does not neutralize toxin already bound in the CNS. Survivors of tetanus require immunization.

Tuberculosis

DESCRIPTION   A chronic disease that affects the lungs and may disseminate to involve other organs, characterized by granulomas and cavity formation, caused by infection with *Mycobacterium tuberculosis.*

DISEASE ENTITIES; SYNONYMS AND ACRONYMS   Pulmonary TB; primary TB; secondary, reactivation TB; cavitary TB; miliary TB; TB pneumonia; consumption.

INCIDENCE   About 12/100,000 in US; higher in urban poor; much higher in undeveloped countries.

AGE   Any age; clinical disease is most common in the very old, in the very young, and in the immunosuppressed.

ETIOLOGY, PATHOGENESIS, AND PREDISPOSING FACTORS   *M. tuberculosis* is an aerobic, acid-fast bacillus that is spread by the respiratory route; organism grows in alveoli, spreads by lymphatics and bloodstream, and stimulates cell-mediated immunity.

SITES INVOLVED   Primary infection involves lung, usually limited to a subpleural nodule and hilar lymph nodes (Ghon complex); secondary (reactivation) TB involves apex of lungs; dissemination can involve any organ.

GROSS LESIONS   Typically confluent granulomas with central caseous necrosis and cavitation (cavitary TB); occasionally lobar consolidation (TB pneumonia); in miliary TB there are myriad 1–2 mm granulomas.

MICROSCOPIC LESIONS   Granulomas with central caseous necrosis surrounded by epithelioid cells, Langhan's giant cells, lymphocytes, plasma cells, and fibroblasts.

COMPLICATIONS   Secondary TB represents reactivation of healed primary TB due to immune deterioration; progressive lung destruction; pulmonary hemorrhage; pleural effusion or empyema; extrapulmonary spread.

SIGNS AND SYMPTOMS   Primary TB is usually asymptomatic and heals spontaneously; secondary TB usually presents with productive cough, hemoptysis, fever, night sweats, and weight loss.

CLINICAL DIAGNOSIS AND OTHER CLINICAL FEATURES   Recognition of lung infection with systemic manifestations; skin tests identify infected persons; x-rays often show apical cavitation; atypical presentations occur with anergy and extrapulmonary TB.

LABORATORY DIAGNOSIS   Identification of acid-fast organism in sputum or tissue; isolation of organism by culturing sputum or other material; routine cultures grow slowly; rapid results are provided with radioactive labels.

PROGNOSIS   Usually good with therapy; high mortality in miliary TB; AIDS patients often do poorly.

THERAPY   Long-term multidrug therapy; resistant strains are increasing; INH for skin test converters.

OTHER INFORMATION   Extrapulmonary TB includes meningitis, osteomyelitis (e.g., Pott's disease is vertebral TB); renal, gastrointestinal, and genital TB. There is increasing incidence in AIDS patients.

Tularemia

DESCRIPTION Acute, febrile, zoonotic infection that presents with typhoidal, pneumonic, oculoglandular, or ulceroglandular forms, caused by *Francisella tularensis,* a nonmotile, aerobic, gram-negative bacillus.

DISEASE ENTITIES; SYNONYMS AND ACRONYMS Rabbit fever, Ohara disease.

INCIDENCE Occurs in North America, Japan, Asia; higher incidence during rabbit-hunting season.

AGE Any age.

ETIOLOGY, PATHOGENESIS, AND PREDISPOSING FACTORS Transmitted through contact with small animals and arthropod bites; skin infection: transcutaneous route; pneumonic infection: inhalation of bacteria; enteric infection: consumption of uncooked meat.

SITES INVOLVED Ulceroglandular form: skin ulcer, enlarged regional lymph nodes; oculoglandular form: conjunctival ulcer; pneumonic form: lung infection; typhoidal form: intestinal infection.

GROSS LESIONS Skin or conjunctival ulcer at site of inoculation; enlarged lymph nodes; enlarged, congested spleen; pulmonary consolidation with focal necrotic cavities.

MICROSCOPIC LESIONS Lymph nodes show stellate necrosis and suppuration; pulmonary and disseminated lesions are centrally necrotic with suppurative and granulomatous inflammation; lesions may resemble tubercles.

COMPLICATIONS Pneumonia with respiratory failure; toxin-related shock; osteomyelitis; blindness if the oculoglandular form progresses to infect the globe and optic nerve.

SIGNS AND SYMPTOMS Primary skin pustule that ulcerates; enlarged, fluctuant regional lymph nodes that may form draining sinus tracts; conjunctival pustule or ulcer; pneumonia; triad of fever, organomegaly, and toxemia.

CLINICAL DIAGNOSIS AND OTHER CLINICAL FEATURES Recognition of skin or conjunctival ulcer and lymphadenitis in a patient who was potentially exposed to rabbits or ticks; chest x-rays may show consolidation; presentation is often similar to plague.

LABORATORY DIAGNOSIS Usually serologic; direct fluorescent antibody staining of material from an ulcer or lymph node. The organism may be grown in culture but represents a hazard to laboratory workers.

PROGNOSIS The fatality rate is less than 10%, with most mortality from the pneumonic or typhoidal forms.

THERAPY Streptomycin is the drug of choice; tetracycline and chloramphenicol are also effective.

OTHER INFORMATION Manifestations of infection are highly variable and depend on mode of transmission; differential includes bubonic plague and cat-scratch disease.

Typhoid Fever

DESCRIPTION   Typhoid fever is an acute, systemic illness caused by *Salmonella typhi,* which is a gram-negative, nonencapsulated, flagellated rod.

DISEASE ENTITIES; SYNONYMS AND ACRONYMS   Enteric fever.

INCIDENCE   Occurs worldwide. There are less than 500 sporadic cases per year in the US.

AGE   Any age.

ETIOLOGY, PATHOGENESIS, AND PREDISPOSING FACTORS   The infection is usually acquired from food or water contaminated by feces or urine from a chronic carrier or a convalescing person. Humans are the only reservoir for the organism.

SITES INVOLVED   Organisms invade the small intestinal mucosa and multiply in reticuloendothelial cells of Peyer's patches, lymph nodes, spleen, and liver. Bloodstream invasion occurs via the thoracic duct.

GROSS LESIONS   Infection of Peyer's patches in terminal ileum causes necrosis of overlying mucosa, producing oval ulcerations that are oriented along the long axis of the bowel; liver and spleen are enlarged.

MICROSCOPIC LESIONS   Ileal ulcers show necrosis bordered by mononuclear cells; PMNs are absent; typhoid nodules, which are collections of macrophages and lymphocytes, may be present in liver, spleen and lymph nodes.

COMPLICATIONS   Intestinal perforation and peritonitis; myocarditis; thrombi in small blood vessels in various organs; cardiac arrhythmias.

SIGNS AND SYMPTOMS   Illness begins with fever, malaise, rose spots on the skin, headache, and constipation or diarrhea; fever increases during invasion of intestinal mucosa; afternoon temperature spikes are typical.

CLINICAL DIAGNOSIS AND OTHER CLINICAL FEATURES   Recognition of the above signs and symptoms; rose spots are usually on the anterior chest; there is bradycardia with the fever, rather than tachycardia.

LABORATORY DIAGNOSIS   Isolation of the organism from blood during the acute phase of the illness, or from the urine or feces of a patient in convalescent phase.

PROGNOSIS   Antibiotic therapy decreases the mortality to less than 1%.

THERAPY   Antibiotics such as chloramphenicol, ampicillin, and trimethoprim-sulfamethoxazole.

OTHER INFORMATION   Decreased gastric acid increases susceptibility. Chronic carriers that remain a source of contamination (e.g., Typhoid Mary) often have persistent infection in the gallbladder.

Pathology Facts, by Richard C.
Harruff, J.B. Lippincott
Company, Philadelphia © 1994.

Chapter 10

Fungal Infections

Aspergillosis

DESCRIPTION Infection with Aspergillus, a saprophytic, spore-forming fungus. Disease takes one of three forms: mycetoma; invasive aspergillosis; and allergic bronchopulmonary aspergillosis (ABA).

DISEASE ENTITIES; SYNONYMS AND ACRONYMS Aspergilloma, fungus ball; acute aspergillosis, pulmonary aspergillosis, disseminated aspergillosis; ABA.

INCIDENCE The invasive form is common in immunocompromised patients.

AGE Any age; mycetoma is more common in older adults with chronic cavitary lung disease.

ETIOLOGY, PATHOGENESIS, AND PREDISPOSING FACTORS Most common species: *A. fumigatus, A. niger,* and *A. flavus;* spores are transmitted by air and inhaled to infect lung; pulmonary cavities, immunosuppression, and necrotic skin (burns) favor infection.

SITES INVOLVED Mycetoma grows in lung cavities caused by previous disease; invasive aspergillosis begins in the lung or gut and may spread to other organs; ABA is an allergy to spores that produces asthma attacks.

GROSS LESIONS Invasive aspergillosis: necrotizing bronchopneumonia, abscesses; dissemination produces multiple abscesses and infarcts in viscera; mycetoma: black shaggy mass in lung cavities or ectatic bronchi.

MICROSCOPIC LESIONS Invasive form: hyphae in tissue, variable inflammation, vascular thrombi with hyphae due to angioinvasion; mycetoma: solid mass of hyphae; ABA: mucus plugs in bronchi.

COMPLICATIONS Infection of nasal sinuses that spreads to face, brain, or eye; disseminated infection commonly causes death in immunocompromised patients (e.g., bone marrow recipients); mycetoma: pulmonary hemorrhage.

SIGNS AND SYMPTOMS Pulmonary aspergillosis: pneumonia with cough, chest pain, fever; mycetoma: cough, hemoptysis; ABA: asthma attacks, wheezing, cough, fever.

CLINICAL DIAGNOSIS AND OTHER CLINICAL FEATURES Recognition of infection in immunosuppressed patient; bone marrow transplant patients must be monitored; x-rays show nodular densities that may cavitate; endoscopic biopsy for confirmation.

LABORATORY DIAGNOSIS Isolation of organism from the affected tissue; histologic demonstration of organism in tissue from biopsy; aspergillus has septate hyphae with acute angle branching visualized by silver stains.

PROGNOSIS Poor for invasive aspergillosis; disseminated infections are often fatal.

THERAPY Amphotericin B and other antifungal drugs; surgical excision for mycetoma.

OTHER INFORMATION Patients with ABA treated with steroids may develop invasive pulmonary aspergillosis. Sputum cultures are unlikely to diagnose invasive aspergillosis; thus, biopsies are required.

Blastomycosis

DESCRIPTION Infection with *Blastomyces dermatitidis*, characterized by pulmonary granulomas; skin and other organs are also infected.

DISEASE ENTITIES; SYNONYMS AND ACRONYMS North American blastomycosis; pulmonary blastomycosis; cutaneous blastomycosis, Gilchrist's disease.

INCIDENCE Uncommon; there are several endemic areas inside the US where most of the cases occur.

AGE Any age; rare in children.

ETIOLOGY, PATHOGENESIS, AND PREDISPOSING FACTORS Inhalation of conidia from dust of contaminated soil; infection is more common in men who work outdoors; infection may be asymptomatic, acute, or chronic.

SITES INVOLVED Lung primarily, especially upper lobes; hematogenous dissemination to other sites; skin is frequently involved; skeletal and genitourinary infections are fairly common.

GROSS LESIONS Consolidation of lungs and occasional cavitation; hilar lymph node enlargement. Skin lesions begin as papules that progress to verrucous plaques and ulcers.

MICROSCOPIC LESIONS Combination of both suppurative and granulomatous inflammation with necrosis and scattered Langhan's giant cells; epidermis in affected region shows pseudoepitheliomatous hyperplasia.

COMPLICATIONS Progressive pulmonary or disseminated disease, which is eventually fatal if not successfully treated. Pulmonary fibrosis occurs with healing; the lesions less often cavitate.

SIGNS AND SYMPTOMS Many infections are asymptomatic; acute blastomycosis: fevers, chills, cough, chest pain, dyspnea; chronic: weight loss, fevers, hemoptysis; skin lesions that are verrucous and/or ulcerative.

CLINICAL DIAGNOSIS AND OTHER CLINICAL FEATURES Recognition of pulmonary infection; x-ray shows patchy infiltrates with acute disease, upper lobe nodules in chronic disease; skin or lung biopsy may be required for diagnosis.

LABORATORY DIAGNOSIS Culture of the dimorphic fungus from sputum or tissue biopsy; histologic demonstration of organism in tissue, where the yeast form displays a double contoured wall and broad-based budding.

PROGNOSIS Usually good with treatment; immunosuppressed patients may succumb to progressive infection.

THERAPY Amphotericin B for severe infections; ketoconazole; cavities rarely require surgical resection.

OTHER INFORMATION Dissemination often causes osteomyelitis and/or septic arthritis; infections of the male genitourinary system may occur.

Candidiasis

DESCRIPTION Infection, usually of the oral cavity or vagina, with a Candida species, usually *C. albicans,* which causes an inflammatory, pruritic infection characterized by thick, white discharge.

DISEASE ENTITIES; SYNONYMS AND ACRONYMS Moniliasis; vaginal candidiasis, candidal vaginitis; oral candidiasis, thrush; mucocutaneous candidiasis.

INCIDENCE Common, particularly in predisposed individuals; common in AIDS patients.

AGE Any age; thrush is common in bottle-fed infants.

ETIOLOGY, PATHOGENESIS, AND PREDISPOSING FACTORS Broad-spectrum antibiotics alter normal flora and promote yeast overgrowth; other predisposing factors: diabetes, oral contraceptives, pregnancy, steroid therapy, chemotherapy, immunodeficiency.

SITES INVOLVED Oral mucosa (thrush); vaginal mucosa (vaginitis); skin in moist skin folds; disseminated infections occur with immunosuppression; sepsis and endocarditis may occur with IV drug abuse or IV catheters.

GROSS LESIONS Involved mucosa is covered by a whitish creamy pseudomembrane that covers an erythematous surface; in endocarditis there are large fibrin vegetations attached to the valves.

MICROSCOPIC LESIONS The pseudomembrane is composed of masses of yeast organisms that invade the superficial layers of epithelium.

COMPLICATIONS IV drug abusers who use unsterile needles or patients with indwelling intravenous catheters may develop candidal endocarditis with potential embolization leading to brain abscesses.

SIGNS AND SYMPTOMS Thrush: white plaques on oral mucosa; vaginal candidiasis: creamy discharge, pruritis, dyspareunia; mucocutaneous candidiasis: pruritic, eczematous skin lesions that may become chronic.

CLINICAL DIAGNOSIS AND OTHER CLINICAL FEATURES Recognition of typical lesions; underlying diabetes or immunodeficiency should not be overlooked; infections are trivial in normal people but life-threatening in immunosuppressed patients.

LABORATORY DIAGNOSIS Demonstration of the organism in smears of scrapings from the pseudomembrane in superficial infections; isolation of the organism in cultures from tissue or blood in cases of sepsis and dissemination.

PROGNOSIS Good for mucocutaneous infections; poor for endocarditis and disseminated candidiasis.

THERAPY Topical nystatin or miconazole for superficial infections; amphotericin B for systemic infections.

OTHER INFORMATION Isolating this organism from the sputum or vagina is not diagnostic because the organism is a part of the normal oral and vaginal flora.

Coccidioidomycosis

DESCRIPTION Infection with *Coccidioides immitis*, which produces a disease that is frequently subclinical but may present as a diffuse pneumonia; the disease is endemic in Southwestern US.

DISEASE ENTITIES; SYNONYMS AND ACRONYMS San Joaquin Valley fever, Valley fever, desert fever.

INCIDENCE Endemic in Southwestern US where the infection rate may exceed 80% in some areas.

AGE Any age; adolescents account for about half of symptomatic infections.

ETIOLOGY, PATHOGENESIS, AND PREDISPOSING FACTORS Inhalation of dust or aerosols containing *C. immitis* arthrospores, which are highly infectious; organism grows to form spherules filled with endospores; infection occasionally disseminates via blood.

SITES INVOLVED Primary infection is in lung, usually subpleural in middle or lower lobes; dissemination can involve skin, bone, meninges, thyroid, and peritoneum.

GROSS LESIONS Primary lesion in lung is usually a solitary area of consolidation that may be up to 3 cm in diameter.

MICROSCOPIC LESIONS Caseating granulomas containing spherules; when spherules release their endospores, PMNs are attracted by the endospores and suppuration is superimposed; abscesses may form.

COMPLICATIONS Dissemination, especially in nonwhite patients, immunosuppressed patients, and pregnant women; pulmonary cavitation with progressive infections; metastatic infections.

SIGNS AND SYMPTOMS Primary infection may be asymptomatic or a flu-like illness with fever, chills, cough, pleuritic chest pain, and arthralgias; erythematous skin rash or erythema nodosum.

CLINICAL DIAGNOSIS AND OTHER CLINICAL FEATURES Recognition of pulmonary disease in a patient traveling or living in an endemic area; x-rays show nodular infiltrates, pleural effusion; skin test with coccidioidin; occasionally biopsy is required.

LABORATORY DIAGNOSIS Culture of organism from sputum or tissue; histologic demonstration of spherules filled with endospores in tissue sections stained with silver; the fungus is dimorphic and has hyphae in culture.

PROGNOSIS Usually good for uncomplicated cases; poor for disseminated infections.

THERAPY Amphotericin B for disseminated or progressive pulmonary infections.

OTHER INFORMATION Most cases heal completely without treatment; progressive pulmonary disease produces cavitation, hemoptysis, night sweats, and weight loss similar to TB; healed lesions produce coin lesions on x-ray.

Cryptococcosis

DESCRIPTION Infection with *Cryptococcus neoformans,* a yeast-like fungus with a thick mucopolysaccharide capsule, that causes pneumonia and meningitis, usually in immunocompromised patients.

DISEASE ENTITIES; SYNONYMS AND ACRONYMS European blastomycosis.

INCIDENCE Sporadic cases worldwide; common in AIDS patients; occasionally occurs in normal persons.

AGE Any age; most commonly in the adult male AIDS population.

ETIOLOGY, PATHOGENESIS, AND PREDISPOSING FACTORS Transmitted by respiratory route; pigeon nests and droppings are major reservoirs; infection is most likely in patients with immunodeficiency, steroid therapy, malignant lymphoma, or Hodgkin's disease.

SITES INVOLVED Initial infection is in lung; in susceptible individuals there is hematogenous spread to other organs, most often meninges and brain, less often skin, bones, and kidney.

GROSS LESIONS Consolidation of lung with mucoid texture; scattered granulomas or abscesses; meningitis has a mucoid exudate, most prominent at base of brain; occasionally mucoid masses are present within brain.

MICROSCOPIC LESIONS Lung lesions contain many organisms and few inflammatory cells; older lesions tend to form granulomas; in meningitis there may be huge numbers of organisms and few inflammatory cells.

COMPLICATIONS Pneumonia: lung abscesses, respiratory failure; hematogenous dissemination with miliary disease; meningitis: seizures, hydrocephalus, visual and cranial nerve defects, high mortality.

SIGNS AND SYMPTOMS Pneumonia: low-grade fever, pleuritic chest pains, cough, malaise; meningitis: headache, fever, stiff neck, usually slowly progressive neurologic deterioration.

CLINICAL DIAGNOSIS AND OTHER CLINICAL FEATURES Cryptococcal pneumonia is usually indolent but may progress rapidly to respiratory failure in AIDS patients; similarly, meningitis is usually slowly progressive with asymptomatic intervals.

LABORATORY DIAGNOSIS Demonstration of organisms in India ink prep of CSF, in stained smears of CSF, or in histologic sections of tissue; isolation of organism in culture.

PROGNOSIS Mortality of 100% for untreated meningitis; 40% for treated meningitis; poor for AIDS patients.

THERAPY Amphotericin B in combination with flucytosine.

OTHER INFORMATION Because pigeon droppings and nests are highly contaminated, large quantities of pigeon "guano" should probably be chemically treated, or at least wetted down to decrease aerosolization.

Dermatophyte Infections

DESCRIPTION Infections of skin, nails, or hair, caused by three species of fungi that are tropic for the keratinized tissues. Also called dermatophytosis.

DISEASE ENTITIES; SYNONYMS AND ACRONYMS Tinea corporis or circinata (ringworm); t. capitis (scalp ringworm); t. pedis (athlete's foot); t. cruris (jock itch).

INCIDENCE Very common; more common in men and in hot climates.

AGE Any age; tinea capitis is common in children; tinea pedis in youth; and tinea unguium in adults.

ETIOLOGY, PATHOGENESIS, AND PREDISPOSING FACTORS Three species cause most infections: Microsporum (skin and hair), Trichophyton (hair, skin, and nails), Epidermophyton (skin and nails); spread by direct contact or fomites.

SITES INVOLVED Tinea pedis: skin of feet; tinea barbae: bearded area of face; tinea capitis: scalp; tinea corporis: neck, trunk, or extremities; tinea cruris: groin skin; tinea unguium: fingernails, toenails.

GROSS LESIONS T. corporis: annular, scaly or vesicular, central clearing; t. capitis: patchy hair loss; t. unguium: thickened nails, yellow discoloration; t. pedis: scaly or vesicular soles, fissures between toes.

MICROSCOPIC LESIONS Hyperkeratosis or parakeratosis; acute or chronic inflammation; spongiosis; fungal hyphae in superficial keratin layer.

COMPLICATIONS Trichophyton infection of feet may be associated with sterile maculopapular or vesicular lesions on the hands, known as an "id" or dermatophytid reaction; occasional secondary bacterial infection.

SIGNS AND SYMPTOMS Alopecia involving scalp in school children; circular pattern of pruritic, scaly, or vesicular rash on chest, back, arms, or inner thighs; painful cracks between toes; discoloration of nails.

CLINICAL DIAGNOSIS AND OTHER CLINICAL FEATURES Recognition of alopecia or circular scaly or vesicular rash on skin; differential includes alopecia areata, seborrheic dermatitis, atopic dermatitis, contact dermatitis.

LABORATORY DIAGNOSIS Microscopic examination of skin scrapings or nail clippings in solution of KOH; fungal cultures of skin or nails.

PROGNOSIS Usually responds to therapy; severe infections may occur in immunocompromised patients.

THERAPY Topical drying agents; topical antifungal agents; oral griseofulvin for nail infections.

OTHER INFORMATION Tinea versicolor, caused by *Malassezia furfur*, produces hypopigmented macules; cutaneous candidiasis occurs in moist skin folds.

Histoplasmosis

DESCRIPTION Systemic fungal infection with *Histoplasma capsulatum* causing an acute pulmonary disease, which usually heals but occasionally progresses or disseminates to involve several organs.

DISEASE ENTITIES; SYNONYMS AND ACRONYMS American histoplasmosis; acute or chronic histoplasmosis; disseminated histoplasmosis.

INCIDENCE Endemic in the Mississippi and Ohio River valleys where there is a high rate of infection.

AGE Any age; particularly children and adults who are active outdoors.

ETIOLOGY, PATHOGENESIS, AND PREDISPOSING FACTORS Inhalation of spores derived from soil containing feces of birds or bats; spores are ingested by macrophages; intracellular infection induces cell-mediated immunity.

SITES INVOLVED Primary infection involves the lungs and hilar lymph nodes; disseminated infection may involve liver, spleen, heart, meninges, GI tract, adrenal glands, and other endocrine glands.

GROSS LESIONS Consolidated nodules with central caseation that eventually become sclerotic and calcify; 1–3 cm lesions occur in lung and hilar lymph nodes; 1–2-mm sclerotic nodules are common in liver and spleen.

MICROSCOPIC LESIONS Granulomas with epithelioid cells, Langhan's giant cells, and organisms within macrophages; caseation necrosis is common; in disseminated infection, organisms are present in cells throughout RE system.

COMPLICATIONS Respiratory failure with severe acute infection; chronic cavitary lesions in lung; disseminated infections are often fatal, especially in infants and AIDS patients.

SIGNS AND SYMPTOMS Infection is frequently asymptomatic or causes a mild respiratory illness similar to a cold; occasionally severe acute respiratory disease; chronic pulmonary infections are similar to TB clinically.

CLINICAL DIAGNOSIS AND OTHER CLINICAL FEATURES Recognition of pulmonary infection in patient from endemic region; x-rays show patchy infiltrates, multiple small nodules, or a single large nodule; erythema nodosum may occur with acute infection.

LABORATORY DIAGNOSIS Culture of biphasic fungus from blood, sputum, or tissue; histologic demonstration of small, encapsulated intracellular organism with silver stain; serology showing rise in titer in paired sera.

PROGNOSIS Usually good except in disseminated infections.

THERAPY Amphotericin B for severe or disseminated infections; ketoconazole.

OTHER INFORMATION Histoplasmosis resembles TB, clinically and pathologically; the healed pulmonary and lymph node foci are similar to the Ghon complex; local epidemics have originated near dusty construction sites.

Pneumocystis Carinii Pneumonia

DESCRIPTION   Opportunistic infection of lung that produces a bilateral pneumonia in severely immunosuppressed patients, caused by infection with *Pneumocystis carinii.*

DISEASE ENTITIES; SYNONYMS AND ACRONYMS   Interstitial plasma cell pneumonia.

INCIDENCE   Common only in severe immune deficiency; affects about half of all AIDS patients.

AGE   Any age with immune deficiency, including malnourished and premature infants.

ETIOLOGY, PATHOGENESIS, AND PREDISPOSING FACTORS   Pneumocystis is ubiquitous and possibly causes subclinical infection in normal persons; active infection in AIDS may be due to reactivation of a latent infection or a newly acquired infection.

SITES INVOLVED   Lungs; slight inflammation in alveolar septa and prominent acellular exudate in alveolar spaces; dissemination to other organs may occur, especially with aerosolized pentamidine prophylaxis.

GROSS LESIONS   Bilateral lungs are heavy, congested, airless and diffusely consolidated; less often there is nodular or unilateral consolidation.

MICROSCOPIC LESIONS   Characteristic feature is foamy, acellular, eosinophilic exudate within alveoli; special stains (e.g., silver) demonstrate numerous parasitic cysts within the exudate.

COMPLICATIONS   Respiratory distress, respiratory failure and death; occasional pulmonary fibrosis; dissemination to other organs (e.g., spleen) is increasingly common due to aerosolized pentamidine prophylaxis.

SIGNS AND SYMPTOMS   Fever, progressive dyspnea, increased respiratory rate, peripheral cyanosis, and nonproductive cough in a patient with immunodeficiency or belonging to a group at high risk for AIDS.

CLINICAL DIAGNOSIS AND OTHER CLINICAL FEATURES   Recognition of presentation in a patient with immunodeficiency; most cases now occur in AIDS; x-rays show bilateral perihilar infiltrates; other infections need to be excluded.

LABORATORY DIAGNOSIS   Demonstration of organisms in lung biopsy or cytologic preparations from bronchoalveolar lavage, using Gomori methenamine-silver stain for cysts or Giemsa stain for trophozoites.

PROGNOSIS   Fatal if untreated; aggressive therapy is usually successful.

THERAPY   Trimethoprim-sulfamethoxazole, pentamidine; steroids; aerosolized pentamidine for prophylaxis.

OTHER INFORMATION   The organism is now classified as a fungus because DNA studies show greater homology with fungi than with protozoa. (See also pg. 180.)

Pathology Facts, by Richard C.
Harruff, J.B. Lippincott
Company, Philadelphia © 1994.

Chapter 11

Protozoan Infections

African Trypanosomiasis

DESCRIPTION A systemic disease endemic to Africa that usually involves the central nervous system, caused by the flagellated protozoans, *Trypanosoma brucei, gambiense* or *rhodesiense*, transmitted by the tsetse fly.

DISEASE ENTITIES; SYNONYMS AND ACRONYMS West African sleeping sickness (*T. gambiense*); East African or Rhodesian sleeping sickness (*T. rhodesiense*).

INCIDENCE Endemic in Africa where up to 2% are infected; visitors to game preserves may return infected.

AGE Any age.

ETIOLOGY, PATHOGENESIS, AND PREDISPOSING FACTORS Transmitted by the bite of the tsetse fly; organism multiplies in fly's gut and salivary gland; East African type occurs along streams; West African type is common in savannas and woodlands.

SITES INVOLVED Initially skin, where chancre develops at bite site; with hemolymphatic spread, lymph nodes and blood are involved; via the blood, CNS involvement (brain and meninges) is common.

GROSS LESIONS The bite site becomes swollen with a central red papule; spleen and lymph nodes are enlarged during the systemic stage; in the stage of brain invasion, the leptomeninges may be thickened.

MICROSCOPIC LESIONS Skin chancre: edema, mononuclear cell inflammation, organisms and endothelial cell proliferation; spleen and lymph nodes: histiocytic hyperplasia; CNS: mononuclear cell meningoencephalitis.

COMPLICATIONS Coma and neurologic deterioration; disseminated intravascular coagulation; myocarditis and rapid progression are typical of rhodesiense infection; non-Africans often have rapid progression.

SIGNS AND SYMPTOMS Painful chancre at bite site; systemic infection: fever, headache, painless lymphadenopathy; rash is apparent on light skin; CNS involvement: wasting, somnolence, apathy; coma in fatal cases.

CLINICAL DIAGNOSIS AND OTHER CLINICAL FEATURES Recognition of chancre, systemic signs, and CNS changes in an inhabitant or traveler to an endemic region; onset of CNS disease may be delayed for years with gambiense infection.

LABORATORY DIAGNOSIS Demonstration of organism in blood, CSF, or lymph node aspirate; serology tests (ELISA) for specific antibodies; elevated IgM; antigenic shifts are typical and result in immune evasion.

PROGNOSIS Untreated, infection with either organism is fatal.

THERAPY Suramin for rhodesiense infection; pentamidine for gambiense infection and for prophylaxis.

OTHER INFORMATION Man is major reservoir for *T. gambiense*; deer and cattle also harbor *T. rhodesiense*; disease may be mistaken for malaria in visitors; disease control is aimed at control of fly vector.

Amebiasis

DESCRIPTION Infection of colon with *Entamoeba histolytica,* an amebic protozoan with infective precyst and cyst stages, causing diseases ranging from an asymptomatic carrier state to amebic dysentery.

DISEASE ENTITIES; SYNONYMS AND ACRONYMS Amebic dysentery, amebic colitis, ameboma, amebic abscess, amebiasis.

INCIDENCE Fairly common with higher incidence in areas with poor sanitation and overcrowding.

AGE Any age; rare under 2 years of age; more common in adult males, especially homosexuals.

ETIOLOGY, PATHOGENESIS, AND PREDISPOSING FACTORS Organism is transmitted through contaminated water, raw vegetables, food handlers, fecal-oral and oral-anal contact. Cysts are infective; trophozoites are killed by gastric acid.

SITES INVOLVED Ameba resides in lumen of colon and produces disease by invading mucosa; spread via portal blood may produce liver abscess, which can rupture into pleural space or peritoneum.

GROSS LESIONS Multiple mucosal ulcers, which are slightly raised and are covered with a shaggy exudate; ameboma presents a pericolonic mass containing amebas and inflammatory tissue.

MICROSCOPIC LESIONS Ulcers extend under the adjacent intact mucosa to produce the classical "flask-shaped ulcers." Amebas may be abundant or few within the base of the ulcer.

COMPLICATIONS Perforation of bowel with peritonitis; liver abscess with pleural, peritoneal, or pericardial rupture; bowel obstruction by ameboma; skin ulcers around perineum or genitalia.

SIGNS AND SYMPTOMS Dysentery: cramping abdominal pain with tenesmus, bloody diarrhea, fever, chills, nausea, vomiting; colitis: episodes of diarrhea with abdominal pain alternating with constipation.

CLINICAL DIAGNOSIS AND OTHER CLINICAL FEATURES Manifestations include dysentery, colitis, and asymptomatic cyst-passers; differential includes inflammatory bowel disease, diverticular disease, bacillary dysentery, appendicitis, colon carcinoma.

LABORATORY DIAGNOSIS Demonstration of amebic trophozoites or cysts in stool specimen; erythrophagocytosis indicates virulence; serologic tests for antiamebic antibodies are positive for years after active infection.

PROGNOSIS Good, for uncomplicated cases that are treated; complications may be fatal.

THERAPY Metronidazole is the drug of choice.

OTHER INFORMATION Chlorination does not kill all cysts, but filtration systems do remove them. Skin lesions on the perineum or genitalia may develop with sexual transmission.

Chagas Disease

DESCRIPTION   Systemic disease with acute and chronic manifestations of myocarditis, caused by infection with *Trypanosoma cruzi*, a flagellated protozoan, which is endemic in South and Central America.

DISEASE ENTITIES; SYNONYMS AND ACRONYMS   American trypanosomiasis. Vector is also called kissing bug or assassin bug.

INCIDENCE   Common only in Central and South America; in some areas it is a major cause of death.

AGE   Acute form: children, most severe in ages under 5 years; chronic: presents in young adults.

ETIOLOGY, PATHOGENESIS, AND PREDISPOSING FACTORS   Transmitted by reduviid bug, which bites exposed skin while subject is asleep; trypanosomes in bug's feces enter the wound and spread via blood to infect tissue cells.

SITES INVOLVED   Chagoma appears transiently at the skin bite site; trypanosomes preferentially parasitize mesenchymal cells, particularly heart, esophagus, colon, stomach, ureters, and occasionally bronchi.

GROSS LESIONS   Cardiac enlargement with 4-chamber dilatation; dilated cardiomyopathy; dilatation of esophagus (megaesophagus) or colon (megacolon).

MICROSCOPIC LESIONS   Acute: leishmanial forms within myocardial cells, myocardial necrosis, acute inflammation; chronic: lymphocytic myocarditis, focal fibrosis. GI tract: possibly decreased myenteric plexus.

COMPLICATIONS   Progressive heart failure; heart block, other arrhythmias, sudden death; left ventricular mural thrombus with systemic embolism; left ventricular apex aneurysm; pulmonary embolism.

SIGNS AND SYMPTOMS   Acute: fever, erythematous nodule at bite site (chagoma), edema of eye if the conjunctiva is invaded (Romana's sign); chronic: cardiac enlargement and other signs of heart failure.

CLINICAL DIAGNOSIS AND OTHER CLINICAL FEATURES   One of the most common causes of heart failure in South/Central America; ECG may show heart block or an arrhythmia; cardiac enlargement on x-ray; infections in children are accompanied by a rash.

LABORATORY DIAGNOSIS   Acute infections: parasites are present in the blood smear; chronic disease: positive serologic test; in xenodiagnosis, a reduviid bug is allowed to bite the patient with a suspected infection.

PROGNOSIS   Disease remains dormant in 90% of cases; others progress to chronic disease.

THERAPY   None approved in this country; nifurtimox is available from the CDC on an investigational basis.

OTHER INFORMATION   Once infected, the patient is likely to harbor viable organisms for life. Some cases of Chagas disease have been transmitted through blood transfusions or transplanted organs.

Cryptosporidiosis

DESCRIPTION Infection of the gastrointestinal tract with Cryptosporidium, a protozoan parasite that causes severe diarrhea in persons with immune deficiencies and a limited illness in healthy persons.

DISEASE ENTITIES; SYNONYMS AND ACRONYMS Cryptosporidiosis.

INCIDENCE Up to 20% of AIDS patients acquire this infection during the course of their illness.

AGE Any age; more likely to be diagnosed in adults.

ETIOLOGY, PATHOGENESIS, AND PREDISPOSING FACTORS Fecal-oral transmission via water or person-to-person; the organism is a common veterinary pathogen that may infect people in contact with animals.

SITES INVOLVED The organism attaches to the brush border of small intestinal mucosa, especially the terminal ileum and cecum. Biliary tract and appendix may also be involved.

GROSS LESIONS Intestinal mucosa usually appears normal; Peyer's patches may appear prominent; mesenteric lymph nodes may be enlarged.

MICROSCOPIC LESIONS Blunting of villi; mixed inflammatory cell infiltrates, including eosinophils, in lamina propria; organisms are visible as small round projections on the brush border of the mucosal epithelium.

COMPLICATIONS Secretory (watery) diarrhea leading to dehydration and electrolyte abnormalities; malabsorption and weight loss, especially in AIDS where cryptosporidiosis may contribute to cachexia.

SIGNS AND SYMPTOMS Diarrhea with intermittent cramping abdominal pain; malaise, fever, nausea, and vomiting are less common. In AIDS patients, the diarrhea is often profuse and watery.

CLINICAL DIAGNOSIS AND OTHER CLINICAL FEATURES In normal persons, the disease spontaneously remits in 1–2 weeks. In AIDS, the disease is usually relentless; respiratory tract involvement occasionally occurs in AIDS.

LABORATORY DIAGNOSIS Demonstration of oocysts in a stool sample by using special stains such as auramine-rhodamine or a modified acid-fast stain.

PROGNOSIS Good in healthy persons; poor in AIDS patients.

THERAPY Support; maintenance of hydration and nutrition; no specific chemotherapy is available.

OTHER INFORMATION The coccidial parasite *Isospora belli* causes a treatable intestinal disease that is clinically indistinguishable from cryptosporidiosis.

Giardiasis

DESCRIPTION   Acute or chronic disease of the small intestine caused by infection with *Giardia lamblia,* a protozoan organism with trophozoites and infective cyst forms.

DISEASE ENTITIES; SYNONYMS AND ACRONYMS   Giardial enteritis; beaver fever.

INCIDENCE   The most common GI protozoan pathogen in US; most common in settings with poor sanitation.

AGE   Any age; children in day-care centers; elderly in institutions.

ETIOLOGY, PATHOGENESIS, AND PREDISPOSING FACTORS   Fecal-oral transmission by ingestion of cysts in contaminated water, especially from open reservoirs or cold streams. Routine chlorination does not kill Giardia cysts but boiling does.

SITES INVOLVED   Proximal small intestine, where the trophozoites adhere to the luminal surface of the epithelial cells and interfere with absorption; they occasionally migrate into the bile or pancreatic ducts.

GROSS LESIONS   No significant gross lesion.

MICROSCOPIC LESIONS   Mucosa may appear normal, or there may be blunting of villi; trophozoites can be seen adhering to the brush border of the mucosal epithelial cells.

COMPLICATIONS   Malabsorption, especially fat malabsorption with steatorrhea and deficiency of fat-soluble vitamins; disaccharidase deficiency.

SIGNS AND SYMPTOMS   Infection is often asymptomatic; in symptomatic cases, there are diarrhea, bloating, cramping abdominal pain, fever, and fatigue; weight loss occurs with chronic infections.

CLINICAL DIAGNOSIS AND OTHER CLINICAL FEATURES   Following acute giardial enteritis, there is a chronic phase of giardiasis with loose greasy stools, flatulence, and malaise; malabsorption is likely to develop in this chronic phase.

LABORATORY DIAGNOSIS   Demonstration of cysts or trophozoites in stool samples, duodenal aspirates or small intestinal biopsy; fecal fat content may be increased, indicating malabsorption.

PROGNOSIS   Usually good, except for the few cases that develop severe malnutrition.

THERAPY   Metronidazole (Flagyl) or quinacrine.

OTHER INFORMATION   Campers and backpackers in the mountains may contract giardiasis by drinking out of streams that are often contaminated by beavers, which are one of the wild animal reservoirs for Giardia.

Leishmaniasis

DESCRIPTION   Generalized visceral or localized cutaneous or mucocutaneous disease caused by infection with one of four species of the intracellular protozoan parasite, Leishmania.

DISEASE ENTITIES; SYNONYMS AND ACRONYMS   Visceral leishmaniasis: kala-azar; cutaneous leishmaniasis: tropical sore, espundia, Chiclero ulcer, uta, Baghdad ulcer.

INCIDENCE   Endemic regions in India, China, South and Central America, Middle East, and Africa.

AGE   Any age; more common in young people.

ETIOLOGY, PATHOGENESIS, AND PREDISPOSING FACTORS   Transmitted by the bite of phlebotomus sandfly; kala-azar is caused by *L. donovani;* mucocutaneous disease is caused by *L. major, L. mexicana, L. braziliensis,* and *L. tropicana.*

SITES INVOLVED   Reticuloendothelial cells (macrophages and endothelial cells); kala-azar: spleen, liver, bone marrow, lymph nodes, and skin; mucocutaneous disease: skin and/or mucosa, no visceral involvement.

GROSS LESIONS   Spleen, lymph nodes, and liver are enlarged in kala-azar. In cutaneous disease, the lesion is initially a papule that expands gradually to produce a shallow ulcer; multiple skin lesions may occur.

MICROSCOPIC LESIONS   Abundant foamy macrophages filled with parasites characterize all infected sites. Skin lesions show granulomatous inflammation and undergo necrosis.

COMPLICATIONS   Replacement of marrow by infected macrophages produces anemia, leukopenia, and thrombocytopenia, with infections and bleeding; immunosuppression; destructive skin lesions; perforation of nasal septum.

SIGNS AND SYMPTOMS   Visceral: fever, gradual or abrupt in onset, weakness, weight loss, diarrhea, hepatosplenomegaly, lymphadenopathy; cutaneous: indolent ulcers, single or multiple.

CLINICAL DIAGNOSIS AND OTHER CLINICAL FEATURES   Recognition of cutaneous ulcer or visceral involvement in an inhabitant or traveler to an endemic region; splenomegaly in kala-azar is often massive.

LABORATORY DIAGNOSIS   Kala-azar: demonstration of parasites in smears from bone marrow or lymph node aspirates; liver and spleen punctures are often recommended but are hazardous procedures; culture on special media.

PROGNOSIS   Untreated kala-azar may be fatal; treatment improves survival; skin ulcers heal very slowly.

THERAPY   Pentavalent antimony (e.g., sodium stibogluconate); amphotericin B, pentamidine.

OTHER INFORMATION   Many infections are subclinical or latent; these may become reactivated and progressive in malnutrition and in patients with AIDS.

Malaria

DESCRIPTION An acute and chronic disease, transmitted by mosquitoes, caused by infection of the circulating red blood cells with one or more of the human malaria protozoan parasites of the species Plasmodium.

DISEASE ENTITIES; SYNONYMS AND ACRONYMS Malignant tertian malaria, algid malaria, cerebral malaria; blackwater fever; benign tertian malaria; quartan malaria.

INCIDENCE Common in tropical and subtropical areas but almost completely eradicated in the US.

AGE Any age.

ETIOLOGY, PATHOGENESIS, AND PREDISPOSING FACTORS Exposure to mosquitoes of the genus Anopheles in an endemic area is necessary for infection. *P. falciparum* causes malignant tertian malaria; the other species are *P. ovale, P. malariae,* and *P. vivax.*

SITES INVOLVED Parasites multiply in mosquito's salivary gland; after transmission to human by mosquito bite, parasites infect and replicate within hepatocytes, then infect erythrocytes.

GROSS LESIONS Liver and spleen are enlarged, congested, and possibly discolored due to hemolysis induced by parasite; in cerebral malaria there is cerebral edema with petechiae in the white matter.

MICROSCOPIC LESIONS Malaria pigment (hemozoin) in hepatic Kupffer cells, splenic macrophages and parasitized red cells; parasites within red cells; ring hemorrhages around cerebral blood vessels in cerebral malaria.

COMPLICATIONS Pneumonia, ARDS; massive hemolysis with hemoglobinuria and acute renal failure; splenic rupture; hypoglycemia; encephalopathy, seizures, and coma in cerebral malaria; chronic anemia with heart failure.

SIGNS AND SYMPTOMS Cyclic fever spikes (quartan: 72-hour cycle, tertian: 48-our cycle), accompanied by chills and sweating, malaise, headache, and nausea; hepatosplenomegaly, mild jaundice, pallor, tachycardia.

CLINICAL DIAGNOSIS AND OTHER CLINICAL FEATURES Cyclic fever is less common than described; any fever in an endemic region is suspicious, especially if splenomegaly is present; falciparum causes the worst complications; the others may relapse.

LABORATORY DIAGNOSIS Demonstration of parasites within red cells in stained blood smears; hemolytic anemia with hyperbilirubinemia and reticulocytosis; serologic tests for antibodies are not useful for acute infections.

PROGNOSIS Good for all but falciparum malaria, which has a 10% mortality in untreated persons.

THERAPY Several antimalarial drugs are available. Chemoprophylaxis is important for travelers.

OTHER INFORMATION Malaria control depends on vector (mosquito) control using insecticides, repellents, and eliminating standing water where larvae hatch. Malaria is occasionally transmitted through blood transfusion.

Toxoplasmosis

DESCRIPTION   A systemic infection with *Toxoplasma gondii,* an intracellular protozoan whose final host is the domestic cat; human infection is usually due to contact with cats and their feces.

DISEASE ENTITIES; SYNONYMS AND ACRONYMS   Congenital toxoplasmosis, ocular toxoplasmosis, lymphadenopathic toxoplasmosis; toxoplasmosis in immunosuppressed host.

INCIDENCE   Very common; infections are frequently asymptomatic.

AGE   Any age; transplacental passage of acute maternal infection causes fetal brain damage.

ETIOLOGY, PATHOGENESIS, AND PREDISPOSING FACTORS   Infection is acquired by oral ingestion of food or water; two forms of organism: tachyzoites multiple rapidly in acute infections; bradyzoites replicate slowly and become encysted in tissue cells.

SITES INVOLVED   After ingestion, trophozoites invade intestinal mucosa and spread via lymphatics and blood to multiple organs: brain, eye (retina), heart, lungs, etc.

GROSS LESIONS   Lesions in neonates include cerebral calcifications, hydrocephalus, microcephaly, chorioretinitis, and microphthalmia; encephalitis, meningitis or brain abscesses occur in immunosuppressed adults.

MICROSCOPIC LESIONS   Parasites in tissue may appear as tachyzoites or encysted bradyzoites; aggregates of unencapsulated organisms constitute pseudocysts; often there are necrosis and granulomatous inflammation.

COMPLICATIONS   Transplacental infection may lead to chorioretinitis and blindness, brain damage with mental retardation, giant cell hepatitis, or adrenal necrosis; AIDS patients may develop cerebral infections.

SIGNS AND SYMPTOMS   Infection may be asymptomatic or causes mild fever with lymphadenopathy that often involves posterior cervical nodes; encephalitis, pneumonia, myocarditis, and retinitis is uncommon in normal adults.

CLINICAL DIAGNOSIS AND OTHER CLINICAL FEATURES   Maternal infections acquired during mid-pregnancy cause severe congenital disease. Generalized lymphadenopathy is the most common presentation in normal children and adults.

LABORATORY DIAGNOSIS   Usually by serologic tests for IgM or IgG antibodies. Organisms occasionally can be demonstrated histologically in lymph node biopsy.

PROGNOSIS   Insignificant infection in normal subjects; devastating CNS infection in neonates and AIDS patients.

THERAPY   Sulfadiazine or pyrimethamine; prophylaxis may be indicated for AIDS patients.

OTHER INFORMATION   Pregnant women should not clean the cat's litter box in order to avoid the risk of primary maternal infection with transplacental transmission to the fetus.

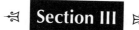

Systemic
Pathology

Pathology Facts, by Richard C.
Harruff, J.B. Lippincott
Company, Philadelphia © 1994.

Chapter 12

Cardiovascular System

Aneurysms

DESCRIPTION   Localized dilatation of a blood vessel. Common types are atherosclerotic, syphilitic, mycotic, congenital (berry), and dissecting aneurysms.

DISEASE ENTITIES; SYNONYMS AND ACRONYMS   Luetic aneurysm; dissecting hematoma; medial defect aneurysm.

INCIDENCE   Atherosclerotic, berry, and dissecting aneurysms are common; the others are not.

AGE   Berry aneurysms affect young or middle age adults. The others affect the elderly.

ETIOLOGY, PATHOGENESIS AND PREDISPOSING FACTORS   Weakening of the vessel wall: by atherosclerosis; syphilitic vasculitis; congenital defect in media (berry); cystic medial necrosis (dissecting); bacterial infection (mycotic).

SITES INVOLVED   Atherosclerotic: abdominal aorta; syphilitic: thoracic aorta; berry: circle of Willis or its branches; dissecting: thoracic aorta; mycotic: any site, commonly cerebral, mesenteric, renal arteries, aorta.

GROSS LESIONS   Atherosclerotic: fusiform; berry: saccular; syphilitic: dilatation of aortic root, "tree-barking" of intima; dissecting: intimal tear extends into media and then produces a false lumen along the aorta.

MICROSCOPIC LESIONS   Syphilitic: inflammation and obliteration of vasa vasorum with degeneration of elastica; dissecting: cystic degeneration of elastica; berry: smooth muscle defect in media; mycotic: acute inflammation.

COMPLICATIONS   Rupture is a potentially fatal outcome of all types; subarachnoid hemorrhage, hemothorax, hemopericardium with tamponade; syphilitic aneurysm causes aortic insufficiency and heart failure.

SIGNS AND SYMPTOMS   Often silent until rupture. Pulsatile mass in abdomen with atherosclerotic aneurysm; aortic insufficiency with syphilitic; severe headache with leaking berry aneurysm.

CLINICAL DIAGNOSIS AND OTHER CLINICAL FEATURES   Palpation of pulsatile abdominal mass; suspicion regarding severe headache; chest pain without myocardial infarction; lumbar puncture, x-rays, arteriography, CT and MRI scans for investigation.

LABORATORY DIAGNOSIS   VDRL for syphilis, otherwise laboratory is of little help. Frequently, aneurysms are discovered only at autopsy, particularly a ruptured berry aneurysm or a dissecting aortic aneurysm.

PROGNOSIS   High mortality after aneurysm ruptures; surgical treatment before rupture provides good prognosis.

THERAPY   Surgical clipping of berry aneurysm; resection of aortic aneurysms and synthetic fiber graft.

OTHER INFORMATION   Patients with the hereditary collagen disorder Marfan's syndrome are predisposed to develop dissecting aortic aneurysm.

Angiosarcoma

DESCRIPTION   Malignant neoplasm of blood vessel origin.

DISEASE ENTITIES; SYNONYMS AND ACRONYMS   Hemangiosarcoma.

INCIDENCE   Rare; males and females affected.

AGE   Any age.

ETIOLOGY, PATHOGENESIS, AND PREDISPOSING FACTORS   Hepatic angiosarcomas have been associated with occupational exposure to arsenic, vinyl chloride, and Thorotrast.

SITES INVOLVED   Skin, breast, and liver are most common primary sites; metastases may involve any secondary site; primary angiosarcomas of heart are recognized.

GROSS LESIONS   Initially small, demarcated, red nodules of skin. Advanced, they are large, pale gray, fleshy, unencapsulated masses with central necrosis and hemorrhage.

MICROSCOPIC LESIONS   Variable degrees of differentiation, ranging from recognizable blood vessels with large anaplastic endothelial cells to undifferentiated sarcomas with giant cells and frequent mitoses.

COMPLICATIONS   Local invasion and disseminated metastatic spread.

SIGNS AND SYMPTOMS   Primary skin tumors present as painless red nodules. Advanced lesions and those originating in the liver cause mass effects, tissue destruction, and organ dysfunction similar to other cancers.

CLINICAL DIAGNOSIS AND OTHER CLINICAL FEATURES   Recognition of primary skin lesion that first appears innocent and then becomes aggressive; skin biopsy and biopsy of liver or other involved site is required for diagnosis.

LABORATORY DIAGNOSIS   Histologic examination of biopsy. Advanced, anaplastic lesions may be difficult to differentiate from other sarcomas; immunohistochemical techniques may establish vascular origin.

PROGNOSIS   Often poor, especially for the hepatic angiosarcoma, which is highly malignant.

THERAPY   Surgical excision, radiation therapy, and chemotherapy.

OTHER INFORMATION   Hemangiopericytoma and angioblastomatosis (von Hippel-Lindau syndrome) are other examples of aggressive vascular tumors.

Atherosclerosis

DESCRIPTION   Degenerative disease of large elastic and medium-sized arteries characterized by intimal proliferation with lipid deposition, resulting in narrowing of the vessel lumen.

DISEASE ENTITIES; SYNONYMS AND ACRONYMS   Arteriosclerosis, hardening of the arteries, atherosclerotic cardiovascular disease, ASCVD, AS, CAD

INCIDENCE   High, especially in developed countries; predominantly males and postmenopausal females.

AGE   Middle age to elderly; younger ages are affected if they have a familial hyperlipidemia.

ETIOLOGY, PATHOGENESIS, AND PREDISPOSING FACTORS   Modifiable risk factors: high saturated fat and cholesterol diet, cigarette smoking, obesity, hypertension, physical inactivity. Inherited factors: abnormal lipoproteins and lipoprotein receptors.

SITES INVOLVED   Elastic arteries: aorta (especially abdominal portion), carotid arteries. Muscular arteries: coronary, cerebral, iliac, femoral, renal, mesenteric arteries.

GROSS LESIONS   Characteristic lesion is atheroma, an elevated fibrofatty plaque arising within intima, yellow to gray in color. Advanced lesions may calcify, involve the media, and compromise the lumen.

MICROSCOPIC LESIONS   Early atheroma: foamy macrophages within intimal proliferation of smooth muscle cells. Developed: fibrous cap, necrotic lipid core, cholesterol crystals. Complicated: presence of secondary changes.

COMPLICATIONS   Complications of atheroma: thrombosis; plaque hemorrhage, rupture, or ulceration; calcification; aneurysm. Organ complications: infarction, gangrene, ischemic atrophy, rupture of aneurysm.

SIGNS AND SYMPTOMS   Depends on the organ involved: heart attacks, strokes, leg gangrene, bowel infarcts, etc.

CLINICAL DIAGNOSIS AND OTHER CLINICAL FEATURES   Depends on the organ system involved. In general, there is pain and dysfunction referable to the region supplied by an occluded artery. Angiography may identify the exact site of stenosis.

LABORATORY DIAGNOSIS   Depends on organ involved. In general, studies are aimed at documenting tissue necrosis by elevation of certain enzymes (CK, SGOT, SGPT, LDH).

PROGNOSIS   Depends on site and extent of necrosis. Advanced AS is usually eventually fatal.

THERAPY   Surgical: angioplasty, bypass; medical: cholesterol-lowering drugs.

OTHER INFORMATION   Diseases of AS related to specific organs: ischemic heart disease, myocardial infarct, cerebral infarct, peripheral vascular disease, aortic aneurysm, intestinal infarct.

Cardiomyopathy

DESCRIPTION   Intrinsic disease of heart muscle not caused by another heart or systemic disease; classified as: congestive (dilated) cardiomyopathy, hypertrophic cardiomyopathy, or restrictive cardiomyopathy.

DISEASE ENTITIES; SYNONYMS AND ACRONYMS   Primary cardiomyopathy, CMP; idiopathic hypertrophic subaortic stenosis, IHSS, asymmetric septal hypertrophy.

INCIDENCE   Fairly common cause of nonischemic heart disease.

AGE   Any age; often seen in young adults.

ETIOLOGY, PATHOGENESIS, AND PREDISPOSING FACTORS   Congestive CMP: previous viral myocarditis, alcoholism, drugs (adriamycin), toxins, idiopathic; hypertrophic CMP: sporadic or autosomal dominant (e.g., mutation of myosin); restrictive CMP: see below.

SITES INVOLVED   Heart, myocardium; in certain forms of restrictive CMP (amyloidosis), there is infiltration of the interstitium; the gene for hypertrophic CMP is carried on chromosome 14.

GROSS LESIONS   Congestive: cardiac enlargement with globoid dilatation involving all chambers. Hypertrophic: cardiac hypertrophy, particularly septum, which bulges into the left ventricular outflow tract.

MICROSCOPIC LESIONS   Congestive: variable and nonspecific changes; focal fibrosis. Hypertrophic: specific change of myofiber disarray; hypertrophic fibers.

COMPLICATIONS   Progressive heart failure, especially with congestive CMP; hypertrophic CMP is a cause of sudden death, often occurring with exercise; mural thrombosis and pulmonary embolism occur in congestive CMP.

SIGNS AND SYMPTOMS   Signs of heart failure: ankle edema, pulmonary edema. Hypertrophic CMP may present as chest pain and/or syncope during strenuous exercise.

CLINICAL DIAGNOSIS AND OTHER CLINICAL FEATURES   Diagnosis requires exclusion of other causes of cardiac dysfunction; thus catheterization to assess arteries and valves, echocardiography, and electrocardiography are performed.

LABORATORY DIAGNOSIS   No specific tests. Occasionally an endomyocardial biopsy is examined histologically to exclude active myocarditis.

PROGNOSIS   Both may terminate in heart failure, especially congestive CMP.

THERAPY   Excision of the septal bulge (for hypertrophic CMP); cardiac transplant.

OTHER INFORMATION   Restrictive CMP, also called infiltrative or obliterative CMP, includes several entities, such as cardiac amyloidosis and endomyocardial fibrosis.

Congental Heart Disease

DESCRIPTION   Heart disease caused by an anatomic defect in the heart that develops in utero and is present at birth.

DISEASE ENTITIES; SYNONYMS AND ACRONYMS   Ventricular septal defect, patent ductus arteriosus, atrial septal defect, pulmonic stenosis, coarctation of aorta, etc.

INCIDENCE   Between 0.3 and 1% of all live births.

AGE   Develops during embryonic period, within the first trimester; present at birth.

ETIOLOGY, PATHOGENESIS, AND PREDISPOSING FACTORS   Usually undetermined. Maternal rubella infection during the first trimester and the drug thalidomide are proven causes. Other viruses, drugs, and maternal diseases are suspected causes.

SITES INVOLVED   Ventricular septum, atrial septum, ductus arteriosus, origin of pulmonary artery, pulmonary valve, aorta, aortic valve, relative origin and separation of great arteries, tricuspid valve.

GROSS LESIONS   Abnormal communication between left and right chambers; abnormal origin or malformation of aorta and/or pulmonary artery; malformation of valves.

MICROSCOPIC LESIONS   Microscopic changes are usually not evident, although focal infarcts and areas of fibrosis may be present in some types.

COMPLICATIONS   Heart failure, pulmonary edema, pneumonia, hypoxia, cyanosis, sudden death.

SIGNS AND SYMPTOMS   Cyanosis, dyspnea, pulmonary edema, fatigue, heart murmur.

CLINICAL DIAGNOSIS AND OTHER CLINICAL FEATURES   Detection of heart murmur; recognition of cyanosis, dyspnea, or fatigue; electrocardiography, echocardiography, and cardiac catheterization.

LABORATORY DIAGNOSIS   Arterial blood gases with low oxygen saturation may be present.

PROGNOSIS   Depends on the type of malformation; septal defects can be repaired successfully.

THERAPY   Corrective surgery; treatment of heart failure.

OTHER INFORMATION   Prenatal screening for maternal rubella antibodies is important in reducing this cause of congenital heart disease.

Heart Failure

DESCRIPTION   Condition in which the heart is unable to pump sufficient blood to supply the body's needs. There may be failure of both sides of the heart or predominantly right or left heart failure.

DISEASE ENTITIES; SYNONYMS AND ACRONYMS   Congestive heart failure, CHF; left heart failure, right heart failure.

INCIDENCE   Common complication of ischemic and hypertensive heart disease.

AGE   Most common in elderly; congenital heart disease and cardiomyopathy cause CHF in young patients.

ETIOLOGY, PATHOGENESIS, AND PREDISPOSING FACTORS   Ischemic, hypertensive, congenital, or valvular heart diseases; nutritional, endocrine, or metabolic heart diseases; myocarditis and other inflammatory heart diseases; cardiomyopathy.

SITES INVOLVED   In CHF, all organs suffer congestion, edema, and chronic and/or acute hypoxia. Right heart failure causes visceral congestion and pedal edema; left heart failure causes pulmonary edema.

GROSS LESIONS   Cardiac enlargement due to a combination of dilatation and hypertrophy. Pulmonary edema, nutmeg liver, dependent edema, pleural effusion.

MICROSCOPIC LESIONS   Pink proteinaceous material in lung alveoli; alveolar capillary congestion with "heart failure" cells. Centrilobular congestion and possibly centrilobular necrosis in liver.

COMPLICATIONS   Pulmonary edema with respiratory failure; bronchopneumonia; pulmonary embolism.

SIGNS AND SYMPTOMS   Dyspnea, orthopnea, cyanosis, jugular venous distension, enlarged liver, pedal edema, frothy pink sputum, rales on lung auscultation, enlarged heart.

CLINICAL DIAGNOSIS AND OTHER CLINICAL FEATURES   Recognition of typical presentation; enlarged cardiac silhouette on chest x-ray; ECG evidence of cardiac hypertrophy; decreased cardiac output; increased central venous and pulmonary artery pressures.

LABORATORY DIAGNOSIS   Arterial blood gas measurements indicating low oxygen saturation; enzyme elevations indicating myocardial and/or liver necrosis.

PROGNOSIS   Poor if untreated.

THERAPY   Treatment of underlying disease; diuretics, digoxin, nitrites, antiarrhythmatics.

OTHER INFORMATION   Cor pulmonale refers to pure right heart failure due to lung disease or disease of pulmonary arteries; heart failure is not a disease—it is a clinical condition due to a primary heart disease.

Hemangioma

DESCRIPTION Benign tumor of blood vessels.

DISEASE ENTITIES; SYNONYMS AND ACRONYMS Capillary hemangioma, juvenile (strawberry) hemangioma, cavernous hemangioma, glomangioma.

INCIDENCE Common.

AGE Any age. The juvenile type is seen in infants and usually spontaneously regresses.

ETIOLOGY, PATHOGENESIS, AND PREDISPOSING FACTORS Unknown; neoplastic in origin. Rare multiple hemangiomatous syndromes, von Hippel-Lindau disease and Sturge-Weber disease, are inherited.

SITES INVOLVED Skin, subcutaneous tissue, mucous membranes, and internal viscera, including liver, spleen, and brain.

GROSS LESIONS In skin: bright red, usually flat and circumscribed lesions; known as "birth mark," "port wine stain." In viscera: dark red, bloody, circumscribed, soft mass, ranging up to several centimeters.

MICROSCOPIC LESIONS Masses of closely packed, well-formed blood vessels of various sizes, lined by endothelium, within connective tissue stroma; red cells in vessel lumens; thrombosis and fibrosis are secondary changes.

COMPLICATIONS Occasionally, hemangiomas in viscera may enlarge or rupture, causing hemorrhage; in brain they may cause neurologic dysfunction. Rare splenic hemangiomas may cause thrombocytopenia.

SIGNS AND SYMPTOMS Cutaneous hemangiomas are visible. Visceral hemangiomas are usually silent unless there is a complication.

CLINICAL DIAGNOSIS AND OTHER CLINICAL FEATURES Recognition of the distinctive skin lesion. In visceral lesions, hemangioma is a common differential diagnosis for a benign tumor and a common incidental finding on CT scan of liver.

LABORATORY DIAGNOSIS Histologic examination of a biopsy or the resected tumor; subclassification is based on the size of the blood vessels (e.g., capillary, cavernous).

PROGNOSIS Rarely serious unless there is bleeding, location in brain, or platelet consumption.

THERAPY Surgical resection is rarely necessary except for cosmetic purposes.

OTHER INFORMATION Glomangioma is a variant, noted for its painfulness, arising from the glomus body and found in fingers and toes. Pyogenic granuloma is a variant resembling granulation tissue.

Hypertensive Heart Disease

DESCRIPTION   Heart disease caused by systemic arterial hypertension characterized by left ventricular hypertrophy; if hypertension persists, the heart eventually fails and dilates.

DISEASE ENTITIES; SYNONYMS AND ACRONYMS   Hypertensive cardiovascular disease, HCVD; left ventricular hypertrophy, LVH.

INCIDENCE   Common; prevalence of hypertension is 20–30%; more common in blacks; more common in females.

AGE   Any adult age; usually middle age; increasing incidence with age.

ETIOLOGY, PATHOGENESIS, AND PREDISPOSING FACTORS   Increased workload stimulates the myocardium to hypertrophy; the increased muscle mass functions poorly; hypertension is either primary (essential) or secondary to endocrine or renal disease.

SITES INVOLVED   Heart, left ventricle myocardium; with heart failure, lungs and viscera are secondarily involved due to congestion.

GROSS LESIONS   Cardiac enlargement (cardiomegaly) initially due to left ventricular hypertrophy; as the heart fails, the cardiac enlargement is due to both hypertrophy and dilatation of the chambers.

MICROSCOPIC LESIONS   Thickened myocardial fibers with prominent hyperchromatic nuclei; focal interstitial fibrosis is often present.

COMPLICATIONS   Congestive heart failure develops in up to 40% of cases. Other complications of hypertension are sudden death, intracerebral hemorrhage, renal failure, dissecting aneurysm, ruptured berry aneurysm.

SIGNS AND SYMPTOMS   Initial symptoms are the same as described for Hypertensive Vascular Disease; often there are no symptoms until the onset of heart failure; chest pain is likely due to superimposed atherosclerosis.

CLINICAL DIAGNOSIS AND OTHER CLINICAL FEATURES   Hypertension, defined by WHO as systolic pressure greater than 140 mm Hg and/or diastolic pressure greater than 90 mm Hg; ECG changes of LVH; cardiac enlargement on x-ray.

LABORATORY DIAGNOSIS   No tests are specific for essential hypertension. Elevated renin in a single renal vein or elevated cortisol, aldosterone or catecholamines are findings that indicate secondary hypertension.

PROGNOSIS   Hypertension is life-threatening if untreated; antihypertensive treatment prolongs survival.

THERAPY   Antihypertensive drugs, salt restriction, diuretics; digoxin for heart failure.

OTHER INFORMATION   Hypertensive cardiovascular disease is frequently compounded by ischemic heart disease; a particularly serious combination because the increased muscle mass is supplied by stenotic arteries.

Hypertensive Vascular Disease

DESCRIPTION   Alterations in small arteries and arterioles due to sustained elevated systemic blood pressure. Arteriosclerosis and arteriolosclerosis are the specific lesions.

DISEASE ENTITIES; SYNONYMS AND ACRONYMS   High blood pressure, hypertension, HTN, HCVD.

INCIDENCE   Very common, especially in Americans of African descent.

AGE   Usually presents in middle age.

ETIOLOGY, PATHOGENESIS, AND PREDISPOSING FACTORS   Primary or essential hypertension has no established etiology. Chronic renal failure, renal artery stenosis, endocrine disease or tumors (pheochromocytoma) are causes of secondary hypertension.

SITES INVOLVED   Small arteries and arterioles of the kidney, brain, and retina are the most significant sites of involvement.

GROSS LESIONS   Primary lesions are not appreciable grossly; secondary lesions consist of cardiac hypertrophy, cerebral hemorrhage, and arteriolonephrosclerosis.

MICROSCOPIC LESIONS   Hyaline, or benign, arteriolosclerosis is the lesion of mild hypertension. Malignant arteriolosclerosis, with fibrinoid necrosis and onion-skinning of the vessel wall accompanies severe hypertension.

COMPLICATIONS   Heart failure, cerebral hemorrhage (stroke), and renal failure are direct complications. Hypertension is a major risk factor for atherosclerosis.

SIGNS AND SYMPTOMS   There are usually no symptoms with mild hypertension. Cardiac or neurologic symptoms, or development of one of the complications may bring serious cases of hypertension to medical attention.

CLINICAL DIAGNOSIS AND OTHER CLINICAL FEATURES   WHO defines hypertension as systolic blood pressure greater than 140 mm Hg, diastolic pressure greater than 90 mm Hg, or both. Cardiac hypertrophy on x-ray or by ECG may also be present.

LABORATORY DIAGNOSIS   Differences in renal vein renin levels indicate renal artery stenosis. Elevated catecholamines, aldosterone, or thyroid hormones may be present in hypertension secondary to endocrine diseases.

PROGNOSIS   Morbidity and mortality are increased with hypertension. Treatment prolongs life.

THERAPY   Salt restriction, diuretics, antisympathetic agents, and angiotensin antagonists.

OTHER INFORMATION   The etiology of essential hypertension involves imbalance in control mechanisms of cardiac output, renal function, peripheral resistance, and sodium regulation; genetic factors may be important.

Infective Endocarditis

DESCRIPTION   Infection of the heart valves by bacteria or fungi; often categorized as either acute or subacute infective endocarditis, depending on the clinical course, organism, and condition of the valves.

DISEASE ENTITIES; SYNONYMS AND ACRONYMS   IE; acute bacterial endocarditis, ABE; subacute bacterial endocarditis, SBE.

INCIDENCE   Moderately common in predisposed persons.

AGE   Any age; depends on predisposing condition.

ETIOLOGY, PATHOGENESIS, AND PREDISPOSING FACTORS   Abnormal valves (e.g., congenital or rheumatic heart disease, prosthetic valves); immune suppression (diabetes, AIDS, therapeutic); IV drug abuse; *Staphylococcus aureus* causes the most severe damage.

SITES INVOLVED   Most commonly mitral valve, followed by the aortic; tricuspid valve may be infected in IV drug abusers.

GROSS LESIONS   Warty-appearing vegetations on the valve surfaces, particularly at the lines of closure. Valve perforations may develop, and the infective process may burrow into the myocardium, forming an abscess.

MICROSCOPIC LESIONS   Vegetations are composed of masses of fibrin and platelets adherent to the valve endocardium. Bacterial colonies are often present, actively growing in the fibrin.

COMPLICATIONS   Valve perforation leading to insufficiency and heart failure; myocardial abscess; arrhythmias; septic embolus with secondary abscesses in brain, lung, spleen; acute glomerulonephritis.

SIGNS AND SYMPTOMS   Fever without obvious site of infection; heart murmur that was not heard before or has changed from previous exams; skin lesions, fingernail splinter hemorrhages, Roth spots on fundoscopic exam.

CLINICAL DIAGNOSIS AND OTHER CLINICAL FEATURES   High level of suspicion in a susceptible individual. Echocardiography is used most often to confirm diagnosis.

LABORATORY DIAGNOSIS   Positive blood culture. Bacteremia may be transient, so that two to four blood samples should be taken.

PROGNOSIS   Valve damage is severe with virulent organisms; antibiotics often control less virulent ones.

THERAPY   Specific antibiotics.

OTHER INFORMATION   All patients with known defective or prosthetic valves, or with congenital heart disease, need to be treated prophylactically with antibiotics before any dental or surgical procedures.

Kaposi's Sarcoma

DESCRIPTION   Malignant tumor of vascular origin frequently associated with AIDS.

DISEASE ENTITIES; SYNONYMS AND ACRONYMS   KS; classical Kaposi's sarcoma; Kaposi's sarcoma associated with AIDS.

INCIDENCE   Common in AIDS patients. Non–AIDS-associated KS is rare.

AGE   AIDS type: young adult to middle aged males. Non-AIDS type: elderly males (60–70 years).

ETIOLOGY, PATHOGENESIS, AND PREDISPOSING FACTORS   Behaves as a malignant neoplasm but may be due to a viral infection in patients with severe immune deficiency; cytomegalovirus has been implicated.

SITES INVOLVED   Multiple simultaneous sites of skin; oral mucosa; mucosa of gastrointestinal tract; widespread involvement of viscera may occur.

GROSS LESIONS   Slightly raised purple to brown skin nodules from 1 mm to 1 cm in size, present on several body sites, hands and feet most commonly but not exclusively.

MICROSCOPIC LESIONS   Varies from a tumor composed of tightly packed, slit-like blood vessels with an inflammatory cell component to a highly cellular form with little resemblance to vascular tissue.

COMPLICATIONS   Bleeding from lesions involving mucosa; gastrointestinal involvement. Visceral lesions may cause problems but their significance is usually overshadowed by the underlying AIDS.

SIGNS AND SYMPTOMS   Multiple purple or brown flat or raised skin lesions. Other manifestations of HIV infection (fever, weight loss, lymphadenopathy) may be present.

CLINICAL DIAGNOSIS AND OTHER CLINICAL FEATURES   Recognition of distinctive skin lesions in a patient at risk for HIV infection.

LABORATORY DIAGNOSIS   Histologic examination of biopsied lesion. Work-up should include testing for HIV infection and search for opportunistic infections.

PROGNOSIS   The lesions themselves occasionally present a serious problem; however, AIDS is fatal.

THERAPY   Chemotherapy, radiation therapy; treatment of HIV infection.

OTHER INFORMATION   Prior to AIDS, Kaposi's sarcoma was rare and affected elderly men of Eastern European and other ethnic backgrounds; another form is endemic in Africa and affects children.

Lymphangioma

DESCRIPTION   Benign neoplasm of lymphatic vessels.

DISEASE ENTITIES; SYNONYMS AND ACRONYMS   Capillary lymphangioma; cystic or cavernous lymphangioma, cystic hygroma.

INCIDENCE   Uncommon.

AGE   Cystic lymphangioma (cystic hygroma) occurs in infants.

ETIOLOGY, PATHOGENESIS, AND PREDISPOSING FACTORS   Unknown; neoplastic.

SITES INVOLVED   Skin, subcutaneous tissue, mediastinum, retroperitoneum, spleen. Cystic lymphangiomas usually involve the neck and axilla.

GROSS LESIONS   A resected cystic lymphangioma appears as a soft, spongy, pink multicystic mass that exudes watery fluid from its cut surface and ranges in size up to 15 cm.

MICROSCOPIC LESIONS   Multiple rounded spaces within connective tissue, lined by endothelium; red cells are absent from the lumens of the vessels; lymphocytes may be present in the stroma.

COMPLICATIONS   The cystic variety may compress and distort important structures of the axilla, neck or mediastinum, and cause functional disturbances.

SIGNS AND SYMPTOMS   Capillary lymphangioma may appear as a pink fleshy nodule on the skin surface. The cystic type causes a subcutaneous swelling or tumor.

CLINICAL DIAGNOSIS AND OTHER CLINICAL FEATURES   Recognition of a neck or axillary swelling or mass in an infant.

LABORATORY DIAGNOSIS   Histologic examination of an excised lesion.

PROGNOSIS   Usually good, although the cystic type is difficult to resect and may recur.

THERAPY   Surgical excision.

OTHER INFORMATION   Lymphangioma circumscriptum involves the superficial skin and presents as a group of watery vesicles.

Lymphatic Obstruction

DESCRIPTION   Interruption of the flow of lymph fluid through lymphatic channels, resulting in lymphedema.

DISEASE ENTITIES; SYNONYMS AND ACRONYMS   Lymphedema, lymphangiectasia, elephantiasis, Milroy's disease.

INCIDENCE   Commonly seen after surgery for carcinoma of the breast.

AGE   Middle-aged to elderly in females (same as for breast cancer).

ETIOLOGY, PATHOGENESIS, AND PREDISPOSING FACTORS   Mechanical obstruction by scar tissue, tumor cells, pressure from adjacent tumors, parasites, radiation-induced fibrosis; severance by surgical incisions or wounds. Familial (Milroy's).

SITES INVOLVED   Depends on site of obstructed lymphatics; usually upper extremity following mastectomy. Lower extremity is involved with elephantiasis due to lymphatic obstruction by filaria.

GROSS LESIONS   Skin is swollen and doughy with prominence of hair follicles, producing "peau d'orange" overlying a breast cancer. Subcutaneous tissue is edematous with thin clear fluid.

MICROSCOPIC LESIONS   Lymphatic channels are dilated. Tissue components, particularly in connective tissue, are widely separated by interstitial edema.

COMPLICATIONS   Marked enlargement and distortion of the affected part; gradual increase in the subcutaneous fibrous tissue.

SIGNS AND SYMPTOMS   Edema following mastectomy or after injury or surgery involving axilla or groin; leg or scrotal edema in a resident of a region endemic for Filaria bancrofti.

CLINICAL DIAGNOSIS AND OTHER CLINICAL FEATURES   Lymphedema due to lymphatic obstruction is a prime consideration in cases of localized edema without inflammation; lymphangiography would rarely be necessary for confirmation.

LABORATORY DIAGNOSIS   Rarely necessary due to characteristic clinical features. Biopsy of inguinal lymph nodes in persons from regions endemic for filariasis may show dead parasites with inflammation in lymphatics.

PROGNOSIS   Disfiguring, sometimes painful; not life-threatening. Postmastectomy lymphedema usually resolves.

THERAPY   Usually not effective. Compressive dressings may retard fluid accumulation within tissues.

OTHER INFORMATION   Venous obstruction and a deep hematoma may cause similar swellings of an extremity following trauma.

Myocardial Infarction

DESCRIPTION   Myocardial necrosis due to inadequate blood delivered by the coronary arteries to meet the metabolic demands of the heart; most commonly caused by coronary atherosclerosis with or without thrombosis.

DISEASE ENTITIES; SYNONYMS AND ACRONYMS   Ischemic heart disease, coronary heart disease, atherosclerotic heart disease, MI, IHD, CAD, ASHD.

INCIDENCE   Very common in males and postmenopausal females; leading mortality for US and developed countries.

AGE   Usually after age 50–60; postmenopausal women.

ETIOLOGY, PATHOGENESIS, AND PREDISPOSING FACTORS   Coronary atherosclerosis is by far the most common cause; less often, coronary vasospasm, arteritis, dissecting aneurysm, coronary anomaly, intramyocardial artery, anemia, CO or CN poisoning.

SITES INVOLVED   Transmural infarct usually involves left ventricle in region of distribution of artery occluded: LAD-anterior wall and septum; right-posterior wall and septum; circumflex-lateral wall.

GROSS LESIONS   Twelve hours: no myocardial change; 24 hours: pallor or reddish mottling; 3–5 days: demarcated yellow region with hyperemic border; 2–3 weeks: soft, gelatinous; months: white scar, firm, thin wall.

MICROSCOPIC LESIONS   Twelve to 18 hours: myocardial eosinophilia; 1–3 days: loss of nuclei and cross striations, PMN exudate; 1 week: PMN exudate subsides; 3 weeks: granulation tissue with progressing fibrosis; 3 months: scar.

COMPLICATIONS   Arrhythmias (most common cause of death), cardiogenic shock, ventricular rupture, mitral insufficiency, heart failure, ventricular aneurysm, mural thrombosis and embolism, pericarditis.

SIGNS AND SYMPTOMS   Crushing precordial pain with radiation; diaphoresis, dyspnea, gastrointestinal symptoms; not relieved by rest or nitroglycerin. Angina pectoris pain is similar but is relieved by rest or nitrites.

CLINICAL DIAGNOSIS AND OTHER CLINICAL FEATURES   Characteristic chest pain, EKG changes (appearance of Q waves, ST segment, and T wave changes), and serum enzyme elevations.

LABORATORY DIAGNOSIS   Elevations in serum enzymes: creatine kinase (CK or CPK) MB isoenzyme; lactic dehydrogenase (LDH), predominantly LDH-1 isoenzyme; aspartate aminotransferase (AST—also called SGOT).

PROGNOSIS   Fairly good if patient reaches hospital; most deaths occur outside hospital due to arrhythmias.

THERAPY   Surgical: balloon angioplasty, coronary artery bypass graft; medical: many agents.

OTHER INFORMATION   IHD also includes angina pectoris, chronic IHD, and sudden death. A subendocardial infarct differs from transmural: limited to the inner third, circumferential, and related to systemic hypotension.

Myocarditis

DESCRIPTION   Any inflammatory condition of the heart, excluding those related to ischemic heart disease, due to infectious and noninfectious causes; most commonly due to viral infection.

DISEASE ENTITIES; SYNONYMS AND ACRONYMS   Viral myocarditis, Chagas disease, Fiedler's myocarditis, rheumatic myocarditis.

INCIDENCE   Present in less than 1% of autopsies.

AGE   Any age.

ETIOLOGY, PATHOGENESIS, AND PREDISPOSING FACTORS   Usually Coxsackie or other virus; less often bacteria or fungus; Trypanosoma cruzi (Chagas); hypersensitivity disease (SLE, drug reaction); radiation; sarcoidosis; idiopathic (giant cell myocarditis).

SITES INVOLVED   Myocardium of heart; endocardium may also be involved; lungs and viscera show secondary congestion due to heart failure.

GROSS LESIONS   Flabby, dilated heart with foci of epicardial, myocardial, and endocardial petechial hemorrhages.

MICROSCOPIC LESIONS   Diffuse infiltration by mononuclear inflammatory cells, particularly lymphocytes; focal myofiber necrosis; variable numbers of PMNs; focal fibrosis. Granulomatous inflammation present in some types.

COMPLICATIONS   Heart failure, arrhythmias, sudden death. Some cases progress to dilated (congestive) cardiomyopathy.

SIGNS AND SYMPTOMS   Chest pain, palpitations, fatigue, dyspnea; onset may follow a viral upper respiratory illness.

CLINICAL DIAGNOSIS AND OTHER CLINICAL FEATURES   Evidence of cardiac dysfunction with normal coronary arteries and valves by catheterization and echocardiography; possibly electrocardiographic changes.

LABORATORY DIAGNOSIS   Elevated ESR; presence of antibodies to Coxsackie virus or other etiologic agent; lymphocytosis; examination of endomyocardial biopsy showing inflammation.

PROGNOSIS   Usually resolves; many cases progress to dilated cardiomyopathy with heart failure.

THERAPY   Treatment of infection or systemic disease; control of heart failure; cardiac transplant.

OTHER INFORMATION   Acute rheumatic heart disease is a special category of myocarditis caused by hypersensitivity to streptococcal antigens.

Nonbacterial Thrombotic Endocarditis

DESCRIPTION   Accumulation of sterile (noninfected) fibrin vegetations on the heart valves and other sites of the endocardium in patients with conditions causing hypercoagulability of the blood.

DISEASE ENTITIES; SYNONYMS AND ACRONYMS   NBTE, marantic endocarditis, noninfective endocarditis.

INCIDENCE   Uncommon except in predisposed individuals.

AGE   Any age, most common in elderly because of increased predisposing factors.

ETIOLOGY, PATHOGENESIS, AND PREDISPOSING FACTORS   Increased blood coagulability; frequently associated with neoplasms, particularly adenocarcinoma of the pancreas; DIC; wasting or terminal conditions.

SITES INVOLVED   Heart valves, frequently on the surface opposite the lines of closure. Mitral valve is often involved. Other sites of the endocardium may also be involved.

GROSS LESIONS   Rows of small vegetations along the edges of valve cusps or leaflets with no indication of inflammation or perforation of the valve.

MICROSCOPIC LESIONS   Clumps of fibrin adherent to the valve endocardium with no evidence of bacterial growth.

COMPLICATIONS   Embolization of fibrin thrombi; infarcts in other organs; infective endocarditis.

SIGNS AND SYMPTOMS   Often overlooked or insignificant in a seriously ill patient; occasionally presents with stroke or other sequelae of embolization; mimics infective endocarditis.

CLINICAL DIAGNOSIS AND OTHER CLINICAL FEATURES   Recognition of embolic complications; detection of heart murmur; echocardiography.

LABORATORY DIAGNOSIS   No specific laboratory tests; coagulation tests may be normal or show elevated fibrin split products.

PROGNOSIS   Depends on the complication, such as cerebral infarct or infective endocarditis.

THERAPY   Anticoagulation may be indicated in some cases; otherwise, treatment of underlying disease.

OTHER INFORMATION   A similar lesion develops in systemic lupus erythematosus: Libman-Sacks endocarditis. In this condition, the fibrin deposition is initiated by inflammation of the endocardium.

Polyarteritis Nodosa

DESCRIPTION   An inflammatory disease that usually affects small and medium-sized arteries, characterized by acute inflammation and necrosis of the media and secondary thrombosis of the vessel.

DISEASE ENTITIES; SYNONYMS AND ACRONYMS   Periarteritis nodosa, PN.

INCIDENCE   Uncommon; more common in men.

AGE   Middle age; 20–60 years.

ETIOLOGY, PATHOGENESIS, AND PREDISPOSING FACTORS   Related to immune complex deposition in vessel walls; highly associated with hepatitis B antigen; occurs with autoimmune diseases, serum sickness, drug allergies, HIV infection, IV amphetamine abuse.

SITES INVOLVED   Multisystemic and highly variable. Kidneys, heart, skeletal muscle, skin, and mesentery most commonly; other organs may also be involved.

GROSS LESIONS   Nodular swellings distributed along the length of the affected artery; aneurysms may develop. Secondary lesions consist of infarcts and hemorrhages.

MICROSCOPIC LESIONS   Fibrinoid necrosis of the media with a mixture of inflammatory cells extending to the adventitia. Secondary thrombosis and aneurysm may be present. Healed lesions show fibrosis of the media.

COMPLICATIONS   Myocardial, cerebral, and intestinal infarcts; seizures, hemiplegia; hemorrhage from ruptured aneurysm; necrotizing glomerulonephritis leading to renal failure; hypertension.

SIGNS AND SYMPTOMS   Fever, malaise, myalgia, arthralgia; subcutaneous nodules; vague, multisystem, multiorgan involvement that is not typical for other diseases; occasionally presents with infarction of a major organ.

CLINICAL DIAGNOSIS AND OTHER CLINICAL FEATURES   High index of suspicion is required to make the diagnosis. A major indicator is the multisystem involvement; other autoimmune diseases may be present; hepatitis B infection is likely.

LABORATORY DIAGNOSIS   Elevation of ESR; presence of HBs antigen; antinuclear antibodies; definitive diagnosis requires biopsy (skin or kidney) and histologic demonstration of the vascular lesions.

PROGNOSIS   Usually poor.

THERAPY   Corticosteroids and other immunosuppressive agents.

OTHER INFORMATION   Hypersensitivity angiitis is a related vasculitis that affects smaller blood vessels and more often presents with a rash.

Rheumatic Heart Disease

DESCRIPTION Heart disease initiating as acute pancarditis of rheumatic fever that subsequently progresses to chronic valvular heart disease due to fibrosis, thickening, and fusion of the valve leaflets.

DISEASE ENTITIES; SYNONYMS AND ACRONYMS Rheumatic fever, rheumatic carditis, rheumatic valvulitis, mitral stenosis, RHD.

INCIDENCE Increasingly uncommon since the introduction of penicillin; some studies shows a recent increase.

AGE Acute RHD: childhood and youth; chronic RHD: late middle age (40–60).

ETIOLOGY, PATHOGENESIS, AND PREDISPOSING FACTORS Cross reaction of antistreptococcal antibodies with cardiac sarcolemmal and valvular glycopeptides. Follows pharyngitis with group A beta-hemolytic Streptococcus by about 2 weeks.

SITES INVOLVED Acute RHD involves pericardium, myocardium, and endocardium—a pancarditis. Chronic RHD involves the heart valves, frequently the mitral valve, followed by the aortic.

GROSS LESIONS Acute: cardiac enlargement, dilatation; fibrinous pericarditis. Chronic: fibrosis and calcification of valves; fusion of commissures and chordae; mitral stenosis with "fish-mouth" deformity.

MICROSCOPIC LESIONS Acute: myocarditis with Aschoff bodies—perivascular collections of mononuclear cells, Anitschkow cells, and Aschoff myocytes; fibrin deposits at valve edges. Chronic: fibrous scarring of valves.

COMPLICATIONS Acute: heart failure; chronic: mitral stenosis leading to heart failure; pulmonary edema; atrial fibrillation; mural thrombi; aortic stenosis with left ventricular hypertrophy; infective endocarditis.

SIGNS AND SYMPTOMS Acute: arthritis, fever, subcutaneous nodules, erythema marginatum, cardiac enlargement, heart murmurs or friction rub, chorea. Chronic: progressive heart failure due to mitral or aortic stenosis.

CLINICAL DIAGNOSIS AND OTHER CLINICAL FEATURES Acute: manifestations of rheumatic fever as specified by the Jones criteria. Chronic: valve disease, by auscultation, echocardiography and cardiac catheterization, with a history of rheumatic fever.

LABORATORY DIAGNOSIS Acute: elevated erythrocyte sedimentation rate (ESR), C-reactive protein, antistreptococcal antibodies, pharyngeal culture positive for group A Streptococcus. Chronic: no specific findings.

PROGNOSIS Varies from complete recovery after the acute phase to serious progressive scarring of heart valves.

THERAPY Penicillin, therapeutically and prophylactically; commissurotomy, prosthetic valve replacement.

OTHER INFORMATION Rheumatic heart disease represents an autoimmune disease caused by antibodies against an infective organism cross-reacting with the body's own tissue.

Rickettsial Vasculitis

DESCRIPTION   Inflammation of small blood vessels, caused by rickettsial infection.

DISEASE ENTITIES; SYNONYMS AND ACRONYMS   Rocky mountain spotted fever, RMSF; typhus.

INCIDENCE   Uncommon in US. Typhus may occur in epidemics during disasters.

AGE   Any age.

ETIOLOGY, PATHOGENESIS, AND PREDISPOSING FACTORS   Infection of the endothelial cells by intracellular rickettsiae, which are transmitted by various arthropods.

SITES INVOLVED   Small blood vessels of skin, kidney, heart, brain, liver, testes, and other organs.

GROSS LESIONS   Petechial hemorrhages involving multiple affected organs, most obviously seen as a hemorrhagic skin rash.

MICROSCOPIC LESIONS   Acute inflammation with necrosis of vessel wall. Older lesions show a mononuclear infiltrate which extends to the perivascular tissue.

COMPLICATIONS   Vascular thrombosis and hemorrhagic infarcts involving multiple organs, most critically the heart and brain.

SIGNS AND SYMPTOMS   Headaches, high fevers, generalized aching, and skin rash, depending on the particular rickettsial infection.

CLINICAL DIAGNOSIS AND OTHER CLINICAL FEATURES   Recognition of presenting signs and symptoms in a patient from an endemic region.

LABORATORY DIAGNOSIS   Culture of organism; elevated antibody titers; demonstration of organism in biopsy material.

PROGNOSIS   High mortality if untreated.

THERAPY   Tetracycline antibiotics.

OTHER INFORMATION   The highly variable manifestations of RMSF may cause unfortunate delay in making a correct diagnosis. See also the specific diseases in Section II: Infectious Diseases.

Temporal Arteritis

DESCRIPTION   Multifocal granulomatous vasculitis involving the temporal and cranial arteries; occasionally other arteries are involved.

DISEASE ENTITIES; SYNONYMS AND ACRONYMS   Giant cell arteritis.

INCIDENCE   Approximately 1% for population aged 80 years; the most common vasculitis in US.

AGE   Average age is 70 years; incidence increases with age.

ETIOLOGY, PATHOGENESIS, AND PREDISPOSING FACTORS   Possibly related to cell-mediated autoimmunity directed against arterial antigens.

SITES INVOLVED   Temporal arteries and cranial arteries are most commonly involved; less often, other arteries of the head and neck; aorta, branches from aortic arch, and other arteries are rarely involved.

GROSS LESIONS   Affected artery is cord-like, thickened, and nodular; this is particularly prominent externally when the temporal artery is involved.

MICROSCOPIC LESIONS   Granulomatous inflammation of the media with multinucleated giant cells distributed along a fragmented internal elastica; secondary thrombosis may be present. Healing produces fibrosis of the wall.

COMPLICATIONS   Blindness occurs in a minority of cases. Cerebral infarcts and infarcts of other organs occasionally occur.

SIGNS AND SYMPTOMS   Headache and throbbing temporal pain, fever, malaise, weight loss, muscle aches, visual symptoms; enlarged, tender temporal artery.

CLINICAL DIAGNOSIS AND OTHER CLINICAL FEATURES   Recognition of the presenting symptoms and signs; headaches and unilateral visual disturbances are important indicators.

LABORATORY DIAGNOSIS   Biopsy and histologic demonstration of the characteristic lesion. In at least 40% of cases, biopsy is negative because of the focal nature of the disease. ESR is characteristically elevated.

PROGNOSIS   Usually a benign and self-limited disease, resolving in 6–12 months.

THERAPY   Corticosteroids typically produce a rapid response; they may be discontinued after several months.

OTHER INFORMATION   Because the artery biopsy is so often negative, diagnosis is often based on clinical features alone.

Thromboangiitis Obliterans

DESCRIPTION   Disease of young to middle-aged men who smoke heavily, characterized by inflammation and thrombosis of the arteries of the legs, eventually resulting in gangrene.

DISEASE ENTITIES; SYNONYMS AND ACRONYMS   Buerger's disease.

INCIDENCE   Once common, now rare; more common in middle East and Japan.

AGE   Young to middle-aged men.

ETIOLOGY, PATHOGENESIS, AND PREDISPOSING FACTORS   Possibly related to a cell-mediated hypersensitivity against components of tobacco; associated with HLA-A9 and HLA-B5.

SITES INVOLVED   Medium-sized and small arteries of the legs; inflammation spreads to involve adjacent veins.

GROSS LESIONS   Thrombotic occlusion of involved arteries of legs; secondary gangrene of leg.

MICROSCOPIC LESIONS   Early acute inflammation of arteries with microabscesses in the vessel wall. Giant cells are sometimes seen. Thrombosis of the artery is common. Thrombi may organize and canalize.

COMPLICATIONS   Gangrene of the legs.

SIGNS AND SYMPTOMS   Intermittent claudication (cramping) of the legs following exercise. Relationship to smoking is often obvious.

CLINICAL DIAGNOSIS AND OTHER CLINICAL FEATURES   Recognition of the typical pattern of lower extremity ischemia, which must be differentiated from that of atherosclerosis.

LABORATORY DIAGNOSIS   Often the definitive diagnosis is established by histologic examination of the blood vessels in a leg amputated for gangrene.

PROGNOSIS   Survival of the affected limb is poor unless smoking is ceased.

THERAPY   Cessation of smoking. Amputation of gangrenous leg.

OTHER INFORMATION   Leg gangrene is usually caused by atherosclerosis; the lesion of thromboangiitis obliterans is differentiated histologically by microabscesses in the vessel wall.

Varicose Veins

DESCRIPTION   Abnormal dilatation of veins at various sites, leading to tortuosity of the vessel, incompetence of valves, and a propensity to thrombosis.

DISEASE ENTITIES; SYNONYMS AND ACRONYMS   Varicose leg veins; internal and external hemorrhoids (piles); esophageal varices; varicocele.

INCIDENCE   Common; female predominance with varicose leg veins.

AGE   30–50 years and over; increasing incidence with age.

ETIOLOGY, PATHOGENESIS, AND PREDISPOSING FACTORS   Varicose leg veins: obesity, pregnancy, long periods of standing, heart failure; hemorrhoids: pregnancy, constipation; esophageal varices: hepatic cirrhosis.

SITES INVOLVED   Subcutaneous veins of legs; hemorrhoidal plexus of rectum and anal canal, either inside or outside of anal sphincter; submucosal veins of distal esophagus; scrotum (varicocele).

GROSS LESIONS   Dilated and tortuous subcutaneous veins in legs; dilated submucosal veins of rectum or esophagus; mass of dilated veins in scrotum. Thrombosis may be superimposed.

MICROSCOPIC LESIONS   Vein walls are often abnormally thin but may be thickened by fibrosis and smooth muscle hyperplasia; inflammation and thrombosis are commonly present; calcification may occur.

COMPLICATIONS   Thrombosis with inflammation and pain are likely in leg varicosities and in hemorrhoids. Hemorrhoids may cause rectal bleeding. Esophageal varices may rupture and bleed profusely.

SIGNS AND SYMPTOMS   Pain, bleeding, or unsightly dilated tortuous veins, depending on the site involved.

CLINICAL DIAGNOSIS AND OTHER CLINICAL FEATURES   Visual inspection identifies varicose leg veins; esophageal varices are diagnosed by endoscopy or radiographic methods; hemorrhoids, by rectal examination or proctoscopy; varicocele, by palpation.

LABORATORY DIAGNOSIS   Microscopic examination of hemorrhoids that are resected surgically serves to confirm the clinical diagnosis, which is rarely in doubt.

PROGNOSIS   High mortality for ruptured, bleeding esophageal varices.

THERAPY   Surgical resection; sclerotherapy for esophageal varices.

OTHER INFORMATION   Rectal bleeding from hemorrhoids may be confused with bleeding from rectal cancers. An occasional rectal tumor may induce hemorrhoids.

Wegener's Granulomatosis

DESCRIPTION Systemic, necrotizing granulomatous vasculitis that most often affects the respiratory tract and kidneys.

DISEASE ENTITIES; SYNONYMS AND ACRONYMS Granulomatous vasculitis.

INCIDENCE Uncommon; men are affected more than women.

AGE Middle age; fifth and sixth decades.

ETIOLOGY, PATHOGENESIS, AND PREDISPOSING FACTORS Unknown. Most likely an immunologic origin.

SITES INVOLVED Blood vessels of any site can be involved; most often nasopharynx, paranasal sinuses, trachea, lung parenchyma, and kidneys.

GROSS LESIONS Granulomas in the lung that may be up to 5 cm and cause cavities. Ulcers of the nasopharyngeal mucosa.

MICROSCOPIC LESIONS Necrotizing vasculitis involving small arteries and veins, resembling acute lesions of polyarteritis nodosa; granulomas with giant cells and fibrosis; necrotizing glomerulonephritis.

COMPLICATIONS Recurrent pneumonia leading to progressive respiratory insufficiency; upper respiratory tract ulcers; renal failure; infarcts involving any organ.

SIGNS AND SYMPTOMS Persistent bilateral pneumonia, chronic sinusitis; fevers; arthralgia; skin rashes; hematuria and proteinuria.

CLINICAL DIAGNOSIS AND OTHER CLINICAL FEATURES Suspicion regarding upper respiratory disease with systemic symptoms; x-ray evidence of bilateral pneumonitis with nodular pattern; confirmation requires biopsy (lung, kidney, nasopharynx).

LABORATORY DIAGNOSIS Elevation of ESR; histologic examination of biopsy showing granulomatous inflammation involving blood vessels; presence of antineutrophil cytoplasmic antibodies in serum.

PROGNOSIS Poor without treatment; mean survival is 5–6 months; treatment definitely improves survival.

THERAPY Immunosuppressive therapy with cyclophosphamide and steroids.

OTHER INFORMATION Lymphomatoid granulomatosis and so-called isolated angiitis of the CNS are other forms of granulomatous vasculitis.

Pathology Facts, by Richard C.
Harruff, J.B. Lippincott
Company, Philadelphia © 1994.

Chapter 13

Respiratory System

Adult Respiratory Distress Syndrome

DESCRIPTION   A clinical entity characterized by rapidly developing respiratory failure with hypoxemia and pulmonary edema refractory to therapy; often associated with shock and sepsis.

DISEASE ENTITIES; SYNONYMS AND ACRONYMS   ARDS; diffuse alveolar damage, DAD; shock lung, traumatic wet lung.

INCIDENCE   Common following severe trauma or sepsis.

AGE   Any age; often young adults with traumatic injuries.

ETIOLOGY, PATHOGENESIS, AND PREDISPOSING FACTORS   Hypovolemic shock, septic shock, burns, inhalation of toxic fumes, aspiration, fat embolism, viral infections. Postulated mechanisms implicate damage to endothelium and alveolar-capillary membranes.

SITES INVOLVED   Lungs, alveolar walls, and alveolar spaces; alveolar-capillary unit is the site of initial damage (thus, the name "diffuse alveolar damage").

GROSS LESIONS   Initial phases: beefy red, heavy, congested, edematous lungs with regions of alveolar collapse (atelectasis); later phases: heavy, solid, airless lungs.

MICROSCOPIC LESIONS   24–48 hours (exudative phase): edema; 3 days (diffuse alveolar damage): hyaline membranes; 4–7 days (proliferative phase): Type II cell and fibroblast hyperplasia, mononuclear cell infiltrates.

COMPLICATIONS   Severe respiratory failure refractory to oxygen therapy; residual pulmonary fibrosis in survivors.

SIGNS AND SYMPTOMS   Respiratory failure with pulmonary edema following shock or other severe systemic insult; occasionally develops during a viral respiratory illness.

CLINICAL DIAGNOSIS AND OTHER CLINICAL FEATURES   By definition, respiratory failure developing in the proper clinical setting constitutes ARDS; however, other causes, such as bacterial pneumonia and cardiogenic pulmonary edema must be excluded.

LABORATORY DIAGNOSIS   There are no specific tests. Blood gas measurements are used to assess the severity of hypoxemia. Microbiologic cultures may identify or exclude an infectious etiology.

PROGNOSIS   Poor; 50% or greater mortality; 75,000 annually die from ARDS.

THERAPY   Supportive therapy; mechanical ventilation; antibiotic therapy for superimposed pneumonia.

OTHER INFORMATION   ARDS is one of the major complications of shock and involves many of the same mechanisms acting on the alveolar membrane causing loss of surfactant and atelectasis.

Atelectasis

DESCRIPTION   Collapse of normally expanded and aerated lung tissue; most cases are categorized as either obstructive-absorptive or compressive.

DISEASE ENTITIES; SYNONYMS AND ACRONYMS   Collapse of lung.

INCIDENCE   Common in predisposed patients.

AGE   Any age depending on etiology.

ETIOLOGY, PATHOGENESIS, AND PREDISPOSING FACTORS   Obstructive-absorptive type is caused by tumors, mucus, or foreign material obstructing bronchi; the air distally is absorbed. Compressive type is due to air, blood, or fluid filling the pleural space.

SITES INVOLVED   Lung parenchyma, alveoli undergo collapse; pleura, chest wall, and bronchi are sites of defects leading to collapse.

GROSS LESIONS   Visibly collapsed lung within the pleural space appears red, airless, and solid. Pleural space may be filled with air (pneumothorax), blood (hemothorax), or pus (empyema).

MICROSCOPIC LESIONS   Alveolar spaces are collapsed upon themselves; instead of thin-walled septa surrounding airspaces, the parenchyma appears solid.

COMPLICATIONS   Hypoxia, respiratory failure; pneumonia.

SIGNS AND SYMPTOMS   Dyspnea, tachypnea; cyanosis; loss of breath sounds and percussion changes on the affected side.

CLINICAL DIAGNOSIS AND OTHER CLINICAL FEATURES   Suspected in penetrating or other injuries of the chest; physical exam is often accurate. Chest x-ray shows air, blood, or fluid in the pleural space with loss of lung volume and mediastinal shift.

LABORATORY DIAGNOSIS   Blood gas measurements may show decreased oxygen saturation. Histologic examination of bronchial biopsy may be needed to confirm presence of obstructive tumor.

PROGNOSIS   Re-expansion of the lung is often possible; ultimate prognosis depends on underlying disease.

THERAPY   Evacuation of pleural space; removal of bronchial obstruction.

OTHER INFORMATION   Patchy atelectasis occurs in conditions with accumulations of mucus in bronchi (e.g., asthma) and with loss of alveolar surfactant (ARDS, hyaline membrane disease of the newborn).

Bronchial Asthma

DESCRIPTION   Disease of airways characterized by reversible paroxysmal narrowing of bronchi after inhaling allergen or irritant; classified as extrinsic or intrinsic asthma or as asthma due to specific etiology.

DISEASE ENTITIES; SYNONYMS AND ACRONYMS   Intrinsic asthma, extrinsic asthma; status asthmaticus.

INCIDENCE   Common. One third to one half of cases are allergen mediated.

AGE   Most common in children (10% incidence); least common in adolescence; up to 5% incidence in adults.

ETIOLOGY, PATHOGENESIS, AND PREDISPOSING FACTORS   Specific IgE antibodies or nonspecific inhaled irritants provoke mast cell degranulation; histamine, leukotrienes, and other mediators are released to cause bronchospasm and bronchial mucus secretion.

SITES INVOLVED   Lungs, pulmonary bronchi; particularly bronchial smooth muscle and mucus glands.

GROSS LESIONS   In lungs from patients dying in status asthmaticus, bronchi show narrowing and edema of their mucosa; thick mucus fills nearly all bronchi; the lungs are hyperinflated.

MICROSCOPIC LESIONS   Changes in bronchi: mucus gland hyperplasia, mucus filling bronchi, smooth muscle hyperplasia, hyaline thickening of basement membranes, infiltrates of eosinophils in the submucosa.

COMPLICATIONS   Sudden respiratory failure and death; pneumonia; chronic bronchitis (COPD); bronchiectasis.

SIGNS AND SYMPTOMS   Sudden onset of dyspnea with wheezing, often following exposure to airborne allergen or respiratory irritant; occasionally after exercise, rarely after aspirin consumption.

CLINICAL DIAGNOSIS AND OTHER CLINICAL FEATURES   Recognition of the characteristic paroxysmal and reversible airway obstruction; exclusion of other causes of dyspnea (e.g., heart failure, pneumonia). Chest x-ray may show hyperinflated lungs.

LABORATORY DIAGNOSIS   IgE antibodies against specific allergen are found in about half of cases; CBC often shows eosinophilia. Curschmann's spirals, Charcot-Leyden crystals, and eosinophils are typically seen in sputum.

PROGNOSIS   Childhood asthma may disappear; adult asthma progresses to COPD. Status asthmaticus may be fatal.

THERAPY   Bronchodilators, especially theophylline; sympathomimetics; corticosteroids.

OTHER INFORMATION   Most asthma attacks are precipitated by inhalation of allergens or irritants; others are due to viral respiratory infections, especially in children; rare cases are triggered by aspirin or yellow dye.

Bronchiectasis

DESCRIPTION   Permanent abnormal dilatation of bronchi caused by destruction of their supporting structures by chronic necrotizing infection within their lumina.

DISEASE ENTITIES; SYNONYMS AND ACRONYMS   Postinfective bronchiectasis, postobstructive bronchiectasis; bronchiectasis with cystic fibrosis.

INCIDENCE   Uncommon except in the predisposed (e.g., cystic fibrosis, endobronchial tumor).

AGE   Seen early with cystic fibrosis, Kartagener's syndrome; incidence increases with age.

ETIOLOGY, PATHOGENESIS, AND PREDISPOSING FACTORS   Bronchial obstruction by foreign body, tumor, or mucus plugs (asthma); cystic fibrosis with mucus impaction and Pseudomonas infections; postinfective (adenovirus, pertussis); immotile cilia syndrome.

SITES INVOLVED   Bronchi of lungs; in the lower lobes in postinfective bronchiectasis; distal to the site of bronchial obstruction with postobstructive bronchiectasis; generalized in cystic fibrosis.

GROSS LESIONS   Dilated bronchi, peribronchial fibrosis, collapse of intervening lung tissue, mucopurulent exudate in lumina. Categorized as saccular, varicose, or cylindrical.

MICROSCOPIC LESIONS   Fibrosis of bronchial walls and peribronchial tissue; fibrous obliteration of normal bronchial structures, including cartilage; chronic inflammatory cells; squamous metaplasia and dysplasia.

COMPLICATIONS   Recurrent pneumonia, lung abscesses, metastatic infections in other organs (e.g., brain abscess); respiratory failure.

SIGNS AND SYMPTOMS   Chronic productive cough, worse in morning; foul-smelling purulent sputum; hemoptysis; low-grade fever; clubbing of fingers.

CLINICAL DIAGNOSIS AND OTHER CLINICAL FEATURES   To be expected in a patient with cystic fibrosis, immotile cilia syndrome, or previous history of severe pulmonary infection. Bronchograms (chest x-rays with contrast media) are diagnostic.

LABORATORY DIAGNOSIS   Sweat chloride test for cystic fibrosis; electron microscopy of bronchial biopsy for immotile cilia. Microbiologic cultures guide antibiotic therapy.

PROGNOSIS   Often poor; lesions progress unless localized and amenable to resection.

THERAPY   Antibiotics; surgical resection.

OTHER INFORMATION   Kartagener's syndrome (immotile cilia syndrome) consists of chronic sinusitis, situs inversus, male infertility, and bronchiectasis; cilia of the respiratory cells and sperm tails lack dynein arms.

Bronchiolitis

DESCRIPTION   Inflammation of the bronchioles, presenting either as an acute viral infection of the bronchioles or as a chronic condition causing airflow obstruction in the small airways.

DISEASE ENTITIES; SYNONYMS AND ACRONYMS   Acute viral bronchiolitis, bronchiolitis obliterans; chronic bronchiolitis (a component of COPD).

INCIDENCE   Acute: a fairly common infectious disease; chronic: common in smokers.

AGE   Acute: an important respiratory disease in children; chronic: middle age to elderly adults.

ETIOLOGY, PATHOGENESIS, AND PREDISPOSING FACTORS   Acute: viral infections, especially respiratory syncytial virus, also adenovirus and measles; irritant gases or fumes; hypersensitivity reaction. Chronic: cigarette smoking, air pollution.

SITES INVOLVED   Pulmonary bronchioles (the small conducting airways lacking cartilage in their walls that are not directly connected to alveoli).

GROSS LESIONS   The lesion in the small airways is not apparent grossly; inflammation of the larger airways (bronchitis) may be present; chronic bronchiolitis is often associated with emphysema.

MICROSCOPIC LESIONS   Acute: lymphocytes infiltrating bronchiolar mucosa, occasional necrosis with PMNs; chronic: lymphocytes around bronchioles, variable fibrosis, goblet cell metaplasia.

COMPLICATIONS   Acute: bronchiolar obliteration, respiratory failure, pneumonia, postinfective bronchiectasis. Chronic: airflow obstruction in small airways, COPD.

SIGNS AND SYMPTOMS   Acute: rapid development of respiratory distress accompanied by fever, cough, and wheezing; chronic: dyspnea developing over several years, other signs of COPD.

CLINICAL DIAGNOSIS AND OTHER CLINICAL FEATURES   Acute: presentation as acute lower respiratory illness in infants and young children; chronic: small airway obstruction, measured by pulmonary function testing.

LABORATORY DIAGNOSIS   Acute: viral cultures, elevated antibody titers; bacterial cultures may reveal a secondary bacterial infection. Chronic: histologic study of lung resected surgically or obtained at autopsy.

PROGNOSIS   Acute: usually good, a few develop bacterial pneumonia: chronic: poor, as in COPD.

THERAPY   Cessation of smoking; bronchodilators; moist environment ("croup tent") for infants.

OTHER INFORMATION   Bronchiolitis obliterans is a severe form with extensive necrosis of bronchioles during the acute phase and fibrous obliteration during the healing phase.

Carcinoma of Lung

DESCRIPTION   Primary malignant neoplasm of lung, originating from transformed bronchial epithelium. Four types: squamous carcinoma, adenocarcinoma, small cell carcinoma, large cell undifferentiated carcinoma.

DISEASE ENTITIES; SYNONYMS AND ACRONYMS   Bronchogenic carcinoma, lung cancer; epidermoid carcinoma; oat cell carcinoma.

INCIDENCE   Most common cause of cancer death in US. Over 100,000 die annually; male:female = 4:1.

AGE   Middle aged to elderly.

ETIOLOGY, PATHOGENESIS, AND PREDISPOSING FACTORS   Tobacco smoking in general; cigarette smoking in particular. Infrequent causes include uranium mining, asbestos exposure, and possibly some minor contribution by air pollution.

SITES INVOLVED   Most have bronchial origin; a few arise peripherally—usually adenocarcinoma. Common spread is to lung and pleura, regional and mediastinal lymph nodes, adrenals, brain, liver, bone.

GROSS LESIONS   Irregular invasive mass of gray-tan tumor spreading out from bronchus, destroying and replacing normal tissue. Often grows within and spreads around bronchi.

MICROSCOPIC LESIONS   Squamous: intercellular bridges, keratin formation; adenocarcinoma: gland formation, mucin production; small cell: small dark nuclei with little cytoplasm; large cell: no keratin, glands, or mucin.

COMPLICATIONS   Bronchial obstruction with pneumonia, atelectasis, abscesses; invasion of blood vessels with hemorrhage; pleural effusion; destruction of lung; metastases; paraneoplastic syndrome.

SIGNS AND SYMPTOMS   Cough, hemoptysis, recurrent pulmonary infections, clubbing of fingers, Cushing's syndrome, dyspnea, fatigue, weight loss; distant effects due to metastasis.

CLINICAL DIAGNOSIS AND OTHER CLINICAL FEATURES   Clinical symptoms, history of smoking, and chest x-ray evidence of lesion (which may be masked by pneumonia, abscess, or atelectasis) are highly suspicious. Diagnosis is confirmed histologically.

LABORATORY DIAGNOSIS   Cytology of sputum, thoracentesis fluid, or fine needle aspiration; histologic examination of biopsy tissue from bronchoscopy or thoracotomy. Histologic typing is important for therapy and prognosis.

PROGNOSIS   High mortality; overall 5-year survival is 6%.

THERAPY   Pneumonectomy for early cancers; chemotherapy, radiation therapy. Chemotherapy for small cell type.

OTHER INFORMATION   Lung cancer is the most preventable of cancers. Due to the increased incidence of smoking, lung cancer has exceeded breast cancer as the leading cause of cancer death in women.

Chronic Bronchitis

DESCRIPTION Defined clinically as chronic excessive sputum production. This correlates pathologically with hyperplasia and hypertrophy of the mucus-secreting glands in the trachea and bronchi.

DISEASE ENTITIES; SYNONYMS AND ACRONYMS Chronic obstructive pulmonary disease, COPD, COLD.

INCIDENCE Common, especially in cigarette smokers.

AGE Increasing incidence with age.

ETIOLOGY, PATHOGENESIS, AND PREDISPOSING FACTORS Chronic airway irritation caused by tobacco smoking, especially cigarettes, air pollution, dusty occupations. Recurrent infections, especially with *Hemophilus influenzae,* exacerbate the condition.

SITES INVOLVED Bronchi of lungs, especially bronchial mucus glands.

GROSS LESIONS Thick mucus or mucopurulent sputum in bronchi, constantly coughed up by patient; thickening of the bronchial mucosa due to edema.

MICROSCOPIC LESIONS Hyperplasia of bronchial mucus glands, measured by the Reid index; chronic and occasionally acute inflammation; peribronchial fibrosis; squamous metaplasia; goblet cell metaplasia in smallest airways.

COMPLICATIONS Acute bronchitis and bronchopneumonia; episodes of acute respiratory failure as well as chronic progressive respiratory failure. Lung cancer may frequently develop in these patients.

SIGNS AND SYMPTOMS Excessive sputum production for prolonged periods; productive cough; frequent episodes of febrile respiratory illness with respiratory decompensation; cyanosis; "blue bloater" appearance.

CLINICAL DIAGNOSIS AND OTHER CLINICAL FEATURES Excessive sputum production in a cigarette smoker or in a person chronically exposed to air pollution; pulmonary function testing shows airway obstruction; chest x-ray may reveal concurrent pneumonia.

LABORATORY DIAGNOSIS Sputum culture may detect infection; blood gas measurements may show hypoxia and/or hypercapnia. Histologic study of resected lung shows characteristic changes in bronchi.

PROGNOSIS Poor; chronic bronchitis represents a chronic progressive lung disease.

THERAPY Cessation of smoking; avoidance of polluted atmosphere; bronchodilators; antibiotics.

OTHER INFORMATION Chronic bronchitis and bronchiolitis, along with emphysema, comprise chronic obstructive pulmonary disease (COPD); these components are present in variable proportions in a particular patient.

Chronic Interstitial Pneumonias

DESCRIPTION   A group of conditions that may represent a single disease entity or several, characterized by idiopathic progressive interstitial fibrosis eventually leading to end-stage honeycomb lung.

DISEASE ENTITIES; SYNONYMS AND ACRONYMS   Hamman-Rich, fibrosing alveolitis, idiopathic pulmonary fibrosis, usual interstitial pneumonia, UIP.

INCIDENCE   Uncommon.

AGE   Usually becomes symptomatic in the 60s.

ETIOLOGY, PATHOGENESIS, AND PREDISPOSING FACTORS   Idiopathic; 20% are associated with a connective tissue disease (RA, PSS, SLE) and 40% with serum protein abnormalities. An acute viral respiratory illness precedes UIP in a quarter of cases.

SITES INVOLVED   Involvement is variable throughout the lung; some areas may be normal, others are severely fibrotic; subpleural parenchyma in the lower lobes is usually most involved.

GROSS LESIONS   Lungs are retracted with bands of fibrous scar tissue surrounding cyst-like spaces (honeycomb appearance). The pleural surfaces show a nodular "hob-nail" pattern.

MICROSCOPIC LESIONS   Alveoli are obliterated by septal and intra-alveolar fibrosis; bronchioles are dilated; progressive fibrosis produces cystic spaces lined by flattened epithelium; blood vessel walls are thickened.

COMPLICATIONS   Respiratory failure; chronic right heart failure (cor pulmonale).

SIGNS AND SYMPTOMS   Chronic dyspnea and respiratory failure progressing gradually, usually over 5–10 years.

CLINICAL DIAGNOSIS AND OTHER CLINICAL FEATURES   Chronic lung disease by history; fine crackles at lung bases on deep inspiration; interstitial subpleural opacities on chest x-ray; pulmonary function abnormalities indicating restrictive disease.

LABORATORY DIAGNOSIS   Microbiologic cultures to exclude infectious etiology; transbronchial biopsy shows histologic features of interstitial fibrosis; antinuclear antibodies and serum protein abnormalities may be present.

PROGNOSIS   Poor; average survival is 5 years after the disease becomes symptomatic.

THERAPY   Supportive. Corticosteroids are given, usually with little response.

OTHER INFORMATION   Desquamative interstitial pneumonia (DIP) may be a variant of UIP with shorter course, younger patient, better survival and response to steroids. Histologically, alveoli are filled with macrophages.

Chronic Obstructive Pulmonary Disease

DESCRIPTION Chronic lung disease, characterized by airflow obstruction, particularly within the small airways; chronic bronchitis, bronchiolitis, and emphysema are components present in varying proportions.

DISEASE ENTITIES; SYNONYMS AND ACRONYMS Chronic obstructive lung disease (COLD); chronic bronchitis, emphysema.

INCIDENCE Common, especially in smokers; smoking is the most common cause of COPD.

AGE Usually presents at 55–60 years.

ETIOLOGY, PATHOGENESIS, AND PREDISPOSING FACTORS Tobacco smoking, which injures bronchi, bronchioles, and alveolar septa; air pollution; antiproteinase deficiency. Bronchial asthma may progress to COPD.

SITES INVOLVED Bronchi, bronchioles, and alveoli. Chronic bronchitis and bronchiolitis cause airflow obstruction due to increased mucus; emphysema causes even worse obstruction by loss of elasticity of the lungs.

GROSS LESIONS There is admixture of lesions characteristic of both emphysema and chronic bronchitis: hyperinflated lungs with destruction of alveolar septa; bullae; thick mucus secretions in bronchi.

MICROSCOPIC LESIONS Combination of findings for chronic bronchitis and emphysema: increased size and number of bronchial mucus glands; increased size of airspaces; decreased number and thinning of alveolar septa.

COMPLICATIONS Progressive respiratory failure; recurrent infections (acute bronchitis, pneumonia); right heart failure and right ventricular hypertrophy (cor pulmonale); pneumothorax.

SIGNS AND SYMPTOMS Traditionally, the emphysematous patient is a "pink puffer" and the chronic bronchitic is a "blue bloater." In most cases of COPD these two extremes are rarely seen because the two conditions coexist.

CLINICAL DIAGNOSIS AND OTHER CLINICAL FEATURES Pulmonary function testing shows airflow obstruction, particularly on expiration; total lung capacity and functional residual capacity are both increased; hyperexpansion of lungs on x-ray.

LABORATORY DIAGNOSIS Blood gas measurements indicate the level of functional impairment. Microbiologic cultures guide treatment of recurrent infections.

PROGNOSIS Poor; progressive and debilitating disease.

THERAPY Cessation of smoking; bronchodilators, antibiotics; portable oxygen for terminal phases.

OTHER INFORMATION Airway obstruction results from loss of elastic recoil of emphysematous lungs, which causes small airways to collapse on expiration, as well as from the increased mucus within bronchi and bronchioles.

Emphysema

DESCRIPTION Permanent abnormal dilatation of distal pulmonary airspaces with destruction of their walls; the important types are classified as either centrilobular or panlobular emphysema.

DISEASE ENTITIES; SYNONYMS AND ACRONYMS Chronic obstructive pulmonary disease, COPD; centriacinar emphysema; panacinar emphysema.

INCIDENCE Common, especially in cigarette smokers. PiZ allele occurs in 5% of population.

AGE Increasing incidence with age.

ETIOLOGY, PATHOGENESIS, AND PREDISPOSING FACTORS Tobacco (cigarette) smoking is major cause, especially of centrilobular emphysema. Familial antiproteinase (antitrypsin) deficiency, associated with PiZ allele, results in panlobular emphysema.

SITES INVOLVED In centrilobular emphysema, the proximal acinus is most affected; in panlobular, the entire acinus is affected uniformly. Bullae are often present in the apex of the upper lobes.

GROSS LESIONS Airspaces are dilated, best appreciated in perfused lungs cut in thin slices. In centrilobular, the upper lobes are most affected; in panlobular, the lower lobes are worse.

MICROSCOPIC LESIONS Alveolar septa are noticeably diminished in number with increase in size of airspaces. Many septa are abnormally thin; some show retraction balls; there is variable anthracosis.

COMPLICATIONS Respiratory failure; right heart failure and right ventricular hypertrophy (cor pulmonale); recurrent respiratory infections, especially if chronic bronchitis coexists.

SIGNS AND SYMPTOMS Dyspnea with increased respiratory rate; increased anterior to posterior chest diameter (barrel chest); pursed lip breathing; "pink puffer" appearance.

CLINICAL DIAGNOSIS AND OTHER CLINICAL FEATURES Recognition of typical presentation in cigarette smoker. Pulmonary function testing indicates airflow obstruction, worse on expiration. Chest x-ray shows hyperexpanded lungs.

LABORATORY DIAGNOSIS Blood gas measurements indicate the degree of hypoxia and hypercapnia. Serum immunoelectrophoresis may detect a familial deficiency of alpha-1-antitrypsin.

PROGNOSIS Poor; emphysema represents a chronic progressive lung disease.

THERAPY Cessation of smoking; bronchodilators; antibiotics for infections.

OTHER INFORMATION Emphysema and chronic bronchitis are two components of chronic obstructive pulmonary disease (COPD). Airflow obstruction in emphysema is due to the loss of elastic recoil within the lung parenchyma.

Fungal Infections of Lung

DESCRIPTION   Lung infections caused by certain fungi, some of which are by themselves pathogenic, causing disease in normal persons; others are opportunistic, invading only immunocompromised patients.

DISEASE ENTITIES; SYNONYMS AND ACRONYMS   Histoplasmosis, coccidioidomycosis, cryptococcosis, blastomycosis; aspergillosis, mucormycosis, candidiasis.

INCIDENCE   Common; histoplasmosis is endemic in Ohio River Valley; coccidioidomycosis is endemic in Southwest.

AGE   Any age.

ETIOLOGY, PATHOGENESIS, AND PREDISPOSING FACTORS   Pathogenic: *H. capsulatum, C. immitis, C. neoformans, B. dermatitidis;* cause mild disease in normals. Opportunistic: Aspergillus, Mucor, Candida; cause serious disease in immunosuppressed.

SITES INVOLVED   Lesions are usually confined to lungs, but histoplasmosis may disseminate throughout the reticuloendothelial system; cryptococcus causes meningitis; blastomycosis typically has a skin lesion.

GROSS LESIONS   Histoplasmosis, blastomycosis, and coccidioidomycosis cause granulomas in lung similar to tuberculosis; opportunistic fungi cause bronchopneumonia, abscesses, "fungus balls" and often disseminate.

MICROSCOPIC LESIONS   Pathogenic fungi evoke granulomatous inflammation; often there is purulence as well. Opportunistic fungi may elicit little response in the impaired host. Silver stains allow identification.

COMPLICATIONS   Debilitation or any immune suppression allow pathogenic fungi to progress, causing severe lung disease and dissemination to other organs. Infections with opportunistic fungi are often disseminated.

SIGNS AND SYMPTOMS   Cough, chest pain, dyspnea; the disease is often mild and self-limited in healthy persons infected with pathogenic fungi; immunosuppressed patients are likely to present with disseminated infections.

CLINICAL DIAGNOSIS AND OTHER CLINICAL FEATURES   Suspicion of a febrile respiratory illness in a patient from an endemic region; histoplasmosis is often discovered as a calcified granuloma on routine chest x-ray of an asymptomatic individual.

LABORATORY DIAGNOSIS   Culture of organism from sputum or lung biopsy tissue; elevated antibody titers; special silver stains of lung biopsy showing distinctive morphology for each organism.

PROGNOSIS   Good for previously healthy persons; poor for those with opportunistic infection.

THERAPY   Systemic antifungal agents (amphotericin B) for progressive or opportunistic disease.

OTHER INFORMATION   Granulomas of histoplasmosis and blastomycosis, seen on chest x-ray, may mimic a lung tumor. See specific organisms in Section II: Infectious Diseases.

Hypersensitivity Pneumonitis

DESCRIPTION   Inflammatory and fibrosing interstitial lung disease mediated by hypersensitivity response to inhaled dust containing bacterial or fungal spores, or other protein of animal or vegetable origin.

DISEASE ENTITIES; SYNONYMS AND ACRONYMS   Extrinsic allergic alveolitis; farmer's lung, pigeon-breeder's lung, bagassosis, bronchopulmonary aspergillosis.

INCIDENCE   Uncommon; confined to certain predisposed occupational groups.

AGE   The acute form most likely involves young adults; chronic disease, the middle aged to elderly.

ETIOLOGY, PATHOGENESIS, AND PREDISPOSING FACTORS   Dust particles less than 5 microns deposit in the alveoli and elicit immediate and delayed hypersensitivity responses; usually the antigen is from a fungus growing in moldy organic material.

SITES INVOLVED   Lungs; alveoli and bronchioles.

GROSS LESIONS   The acute phase shows nonspecific congestion of lung; fibrosis with honeycombing are present in the late stages.

MICROSCOPIC LESIONS   Early: bronchiolitis; interstitial pneumonia with lymphocytes and plasma cells in alveolar walls; mild DAD; focal granulomas with foreign body giant cells. Late: fibrosis with cystic spaces.

COMPLICATIONS   Respiratory failure with a progressive lung disease; right ventricular failure and right ventricular hypertrophy (cor pulmonale).

SIGNS AND SYMPTOMS   Chest tightness, dyspnea, cough, and mild fever develop a few hours after exposure to aeroallergen. With time, the symptoms become chronic.

CLINICAL DIAGNOSIS AND OTHER CLINICAL FEATURES   Recognition of characteristic pattern of illness following exposure to organic dusts. Chest x-ray may be normal early in the disease; features of interstitial pneumonia are present in the late phase.

LABORATORY DIAGNOSIS   Microbiologic culture to exclude infection; detection of antibodies to an environmental antigen; histology of lung biopsy showing interstitial inflammation and fibrosis; eosinophilia on CBC.

PROGNOSIS   Good if diagnosis is made early and allergen is removed; poor if fibrosis is allowed to progress.

THERAPY   Removal of environmental antigen; steroids.

OTHER INFORMATION   Aspergillosis: aspergillus spores; bagassosis: actinomycetes from moldy sugarcane; farmer's lung: *Micropolyspora faeni* from moldy hay; pigeon-breeder's lung: unknown antigen in droppings or serum.

Lung Abscess

DESCRIPTION   Localized accumulation of purulent exudate within lung with necrosis of underlying parenchyma; arising as a complication of pneumonia, from aspiration of oral contents, or from septic embolus.

DISEASE ENTITIES; SYNONYMS AND ACRONYMS   Necrotizing pneumonia.

INCIDENCE   Common in alcoholics and patients with neurologic dysfunction impairing the gag reflex.

AGE   Any age, depending on etiology; more often in elderly because of increased incidence of strokes.

ETIOLOGY, PATHOGENESIS, AND PREDISPOSING FACTORS   Aspiration of anaerobic bacteria from oral contents along with foreign material or vomitus; septic arterial embolus from heart valve; complication of pneumonia, especially staphylococcal.

SITES INVOLVED   Aspiration type: depends on position of patient; often single and located in right lower lobe due to configuration of bronchi. Septic embolic type: often multiple and involves any lobe.

GROSS LESIONS   Cavity in parenchyma with purulent or liquid center, frequently foul smelling; fibrotic wall of cavity that becomes thicker and firmer in older lesions.

MICROSCOPIC LESIONS   Degenerating PMNs and cellular debris with necrosis of underlying parenchyma surrounded by granulation tissue, fibrous scar tissue, and a mixture of acute and chronic inflammatory cells.

COMPLICATIONS   Sepsis, empyema, metastatic infections; progressive destruction of lung leading to respiratory failure.

SIGNS AND SYMPTOMS   Dyspnea, chest pain, cough productive of foul-smelling sputum; cyanosis, clubbing of fingernails.

CLINICAL DIAGNOSIS AND OTHER CLINICAL FEATURES   Chest x-ray shows circumscribed opacity or cavity, sometimes with air-fluid level; CT and MRI scans demonstrate the central liquefaction; bronchoscopy with biopsy to exclude underlying neoplasm.

LABORATORY DIAGNOSIS   Microbiologic culture of sputum or, preferably, material from bronchoscopy; cytologic examination of sputum and/or bronchoalveolar lavage; histologic examination of bronchoscopic biopsy.

PROGNOSIS   Often cured by antibiotics, leaving a residual lung scar.

THERAPY   Specific antibiotics.

OTHER INFORMATION   Underlying lung cancer should be suspected and excluded as the cause of a lung abscess. Cavitary lesions in the apex of upper lobes are frequently due to tuberculosis rather than bacterial abscess.

Malignant Mesothelioma

DESCRIPTION   Malignant neoplasm originating from mesothelial lining of pleura (much less commonly peritoneum) associated with asbestos exposure.

DISEASE ENTITIES; SYNONYMS AND ACRONYMS   Mesothelioma.

INCIDENCE   Uncommon. Most cases are in men because of occupational exposure.

AGE   Middle age.

ETIOLOGY, PATHOGENESIS, AND PREDISPOSING FACTORS   Asbestos, especially the crocidolite form; occupational exposure is heaviest for those who process and handle the fibers; exposure while washing soiled clothes has caused mesothelioma in housewives.

SITES INVOLVED   Visceral and parietal pleura; peritoneum is much less common.

GROSS LESIONS   Firm, whitish-gray tumor that fills the pleural space and extends into interlobar sulci, compressing the lung as it expands. Invasion and metastases may be present but are not the most common pattern.

MICROSCOPIC LESIONS   Characterized by two components present in varying proportions: an epithelial component forming glands and a connective tissue (fibroblastic) component. This growth pattern is called biphasic.

COMPLICATIONS   Respiratory failure due to restrictive lung disease and actual lung compression.

SIGNS AND SYMPTOMS   Progressive dyspnea, chest pain, weight loss.

CLINICAL DIAGNOSIS AND OTHER CLINICAL FEATURES   History and physical examination indicate lung disease with loss of breath sounds; chest x-ray shows "white-out" of the lung field.

LABORATORY DIAGNOSIS   Cytology of aspirated pleural fluid shows large atypical mesothelial cells. Finding the characteristic biphasic growth pattern histologically in a pleural biopsy establishes the diagnosis.

PROGNOSIS   Hopeless.

THERAPY   No effective therapy exists.

OTHER INFORMATION   Mesothelioma is but one manifestation of asbestosis. More often, asbestosis causes a progressive pulmonary fibrosis.

Pleural Effusion

DESCRIPTION   Collection of fluid within the pleural space, further categorized by the nature or appearance of the fluid.

DISEASE ENTITIES; SYNONYMS AND ACRONYMS   Hydrothorax, pyothorax, empyema, hemothorax, chylothorax.

INCIDENCE   Common, especially with heart failure and lymphatic obstruction due to neoplasm.

AGE   Any age, but more common in elderly due to increased incidence of heart failure and cancer.

ETIOLOGY, PATHOGENESIS, AND PREDISPOSING FACTORS   Heart failure, neoplasm, TB, connective tissue diseases, asbestosis, pneumonia, abscess, lung infarct, chest trauma, obstruction of lymphatics.

SITES INVOLVED   Pleural space; pleural or hilar lymphatics are involved in cases of metastatic tumor.

GROSS LESIONS   Transudate, due to heart failure, is thin and watery; effusion due to tumor or TB has a higher protein content (exudate) and blood; thick purulent exudate constitutes empyema; a chylothorax is milky.

MICROSCOPIC LESIONS   In a transudate due to increased hydrostatic pressure, there are few cells; in exudate due to chronic inflammation, mesothelial cells and lymphocytes predominate; an empyema shows abundant PMNs.

COMPLICATIONS   Compressive atelectasis and respiratory failure; effusions due to tumor tend to reaccumulate rapidly after they are drained.

SIGNS AND SYMPTOMS   Progressive dyspnea; possibly with signs of heart failure; neoplasms often present with effusions; weight loss and fever indicate TB or cancer; individuals with large effusions do not float in water.

CLINICAL DIAGNOSIS AND OTHER CLINICAL FEATURES   Workup often focuses on the two most common causes—heart failure and cancer; bacterial infections and tuberculosis are other considerations; diagnostic thoracentesis obtains fluid for analysis.

LABORATORY DIAGNOSIS   Analysis of pleural fluid for protein, glucose, LDH, cell count and differential; stains and cultures for bacteria, TB, and fungi; cytologic examination to detect neoplastic cells.

PROGNOSIS   Depends on underlying disease; in cancer, recurrent pleural effusion may be the terminal condition.

THERAPY   Treatment of underlying disease; drainage of the pleural fluid; obliteration of the pleural space.

OTHER INFORMATION   Pleural effusion is readily visualized by a lateral decubitus x-ray. Pleural effusion in TB is more likely with primary TB than with secondary TB.

Pneumoconiosis

DESCRIPTION   Chronic lung disease caused by inhalation of inorganic dusts and characterized by lung fibrosis that is either nodular, as in silicosis, or diffuse and interstitial, as in asbestosis.

DISEASE ENTITIES; SYNONYMS AND ACRONYMS   Silicosis, coal pneumoconiosis, anthracosilicosis, progressive massive fibrosis, PMF, asbestosis, berylliosis, talcosis.

INCIDENCE   Occurs in occupational groups: miners, sandblasters, stonecutters, asbestos workers, insulators.

AGE   Increasing incidence with age due to cumulative effects of exposure.

ETIOLOGY, PATHOGENESIS, AND PREDISPOSING FACTORS   Inorganic dust inhalation; particles 2 microns or less deposit in alveoli and are ingested by macrophages; fibroblast stimulating factor secreted by activated macrophages mediates excessive fibrosis.

SITES INVOLVED   Lung parenchyma and small airways; pleura (especially with asbestosis); hilar lymph nodes (silicosis). Progressive massive fibrosis usually involves the upper lobes.

GROSS LESIONS   Silicosis: 2–4-mm firm nodules throughout lungs; in PMF, nodules are greater than 1 cm. Asbestosis: interstitial fibrosis progressing to honeycombing. Coal pneumoconiosis: fibrosis and anthracosis.

MICROSCOPIC LESIONS   Silicosis: dense collagenous nodules with mononuclear cells at periphery. Asbestosis: septa thickened by fibrosis; asbestos (ferruginous) bodies. Coal pneumoconiosis: abundant black pigment.

COMPLICATIONS   Simple coal pneumoconiosis and simple nodular silicosis produce only mild abnormalities. PMF and asbestosis produce severe obstructive and restrictive disease with cor pulmonale.

SIGNS AND SYMPTOMS   Progressive dyspnea, respiratory failure; signs of right heart failure. Rheumatoid arthritis coexisting with nodular pneumoconiosis is called Caplan's syndrome.

CLINICAL DIAGNOSIS AND OTHER CLINICAL FEATURES   History of exposure (which may be minimal with asbestosis); physical exam indicating lung disease; x-ray showing either nodular or interstitial fibrosis; pulmonary function test abnormalities.

LABORATORY DIAGNOSIS   Sputum cytology; histologic examination of lung biopsy; cultures for bacteria, TB, and fungi to exclude infectious disease; TB shows increased incidence in silicosis.

PROGNOSIS   Poor; once the disease becomes symptomatic, it is progressive and disabling.

THERAPY   Supportive, such as oxygen therapy; avoidance of further exposure is usually too late to help.

OTHER INFORMATION   Mesothelioma is the neoplastic complication of asbestosis. In smokers, pneumoconiosis is often difficult to differentiate from COPD.

Pneumocystis Carinii Pneumonia

DESCRIPTION   Opportunistic infection of lung by the fungal parasite *Pneumocystis carinii,* seen only in immunocompromised individuals, characterized by interstitial pneumonia and foamy intra-alveolar exudate.

DISEASE ENTITIES; SYNONYMS AND ACRONYMS   PCP, pneumocystosis; plasma cell pneumonia.

INCIDENCE   Common in immunocompromised patients, especially AIDS; not seen in those with normal immune status.

AGE   Any age, depending on age; follows age distribution of AIDS.

ETIOLOGY, PATHOGENESIS, AND PREDISPOSING FACTORS   Pneumocystis may infect any patient who is immunosuppressed for renal transplantation, by chemotherapy for lymphoma or leukemia, by steroid therapy, by malnutrition, or by AIDS.

SITES INVOLVED   Lungs, within alveoli. Occasionally disseminates throughout body and localizes within another organ (e.g., spleen).

GROSS LESIONS   Diffuse bilateral consolidation of lungs.

MICROSCOPIC LESIONS   Foamy eosinophilic alveolar exudate; interstitial inflammation by lymphocytes and plasma cells; diffuse alveolar damage with hyaline membranes; Type II cell hyperplasia; alveolar fibrosis.

COMPLICATIONS   Respiratory failure.

SIGNS AND SYMPTOMS   Dyspnea, fatigue; fever may not be present; weight loss and other manifestations of underlying immunosuppressive disease.

CLINICAL DIAGNOSIS AND OTHER CLINICAL FEATURES   Pulmonary disease in an immunosuppressed patient is likely to be PCP. Chest x-ray shows patchy bilateral alveolar infiltrates.

LABORATORY DIAGNOSIS   Microscopic examination of silver-stained material from sputum, open or bronchoscopic lung biopsy, or from bronchoalveolar lavage shows diagnostic round or cup-shaped organisms.

PROGNOSIS   Poor, probably progressing to death if untreated; specific treatment is usually effective.

THERAPY   Pentamidine, trimethoprim-sulfamethoxazole.

OTHER INFORMATION   PCP frequently coexists with cytomegalovirus (CMV) pneumonia. Pneumocystis was previously considered a protozoan parasite. (See also pg. 127.)

Pneumonia—Bacterial

DESCRIPTION   Bacterial infection of lung characterized by intra-alveolar exudate of PMNs, fibrin, and fluid; categorized anatomically (bronchopneumonia or lobar pneumonia) or etiologically (specific bacteria).

DISEASE ENTITIES; SYNONYMS AND ACRONYMS   Pneumococcal, Klebsiella, staphylococcal, or gram-negative pneumonia; Legionnaire's disease.

INCIDENCE   Common, particularly in the elderly and during epidemics of viral respiratory infections.

AGE   Bronchopneumonia affects infants and elderly; lobar pneumonia affects middle-aged individuals.

ETIOLOGY, PATHOGENESIS, AND PREDISPOSING FACTORS   *S. pneumoniae* (Pneumococcus) and Klebsiella cause lobar pneumonia, especially in alcoholics. Heart failure, stroke, cystic fibrosis, viral pneumonia, immunosuppression predispose to bronchopneumonia.

SITES INVOLVED   Lung parenchyma. Bronchopneumonia has a patchy peribronchial distribution, often in lower lobes. Lobar pneumonia involves entire lobe(s) diffusely.

GROSS LESIONS   Consolidation (solidification) of lung parenchyma. Stages: congestion and edema; then "red hepatization"; followed by "gray hepatization"; ending with resolution as the lung returns to normal.

MICROSCOPIC LESIONS   Exudation of PMNs filling alveolar air spaces. Early, there is fibrin along with the PMNs; during resolution, the exudate is digested and macrophages are present.

COMPLICATIONS   Sepsis, respiratory failure; empyema, pyothorax, lung abscess, bronchopleural fistula.

SIGNS AND SYMPTOMS   Cough with rusty purulent sputum, chest pain, fever, dyspnea; changes in percussion and auscultation, rales. Elderly patients with bronchopneumonia may remain afebrile.

CLINICAL DIAGNOSIS AND OTHER CLINICAL FEATURES   Presentation and physical examination are essentially diagnostic; chest x-ray is important to assess extent of disease, to follow progress, and to exclude tumor as underlying cause.

LABORATORY DIAGNOSIS   Microbiologic culture of sputum or transtracheal aspirate with testing for antibiotic sensitivity; Gram stain of sputum may give a quick preliminary identification. Blood cultures are often positive.

PROGNOSIS   Good if previously healthy; poor for debilitated patient or virulent organism (e.g., Legionella).

THERAPY   Specific antibiotics, especially penicillin for pneumococcal pneumonia.

OTHER INFORMATION   Legionnaire's disease, caused by gram-negative *L. pneumophila,* causes pneumonia in the elderly and in those with chronic lung disease; it cannot be routinely cultured or Gram-stained.

Pneumonia—Viral

DESCRIPTION Infection of the lung caused by certain viruses, characterized by interstitial inflammation and diffuse alveolar damage.

DISEASE ENTITIES; SYNONYMS AND ACRONYMS Interstitial pneumonia, atypical pneumonia.

INCIDENCE Common but usually not life-threatening except in immunocompromised patients.

AGE Any age; most serious in infants and in the elderly.

ETIOLOGY, PATHOGENESIS, AND PREDISPOSING FACTORS Viruses that primarily affect airways: adenovirus, respiratory syncytial virus, influenza virus; other viruses: cytomegalovirus, measles virus, varicella virus.

SITES INVOLVED Lungs, often bilateral and panlobar; inflammation is confined to septa rather than the intra-alveolar space, in contrast to bacterial pneumonia.

GROSS LESIONS Congestion, edema, and scattered hemorrhages in the lung. Consolidated areas indicate superimposed bacterial pneumonia.

MICROSCOPIC LESIONS Interstitial inflammation with lymphocytes infiltrating alveolar septa; necrosis of Type I pneumocytes; hyaline membranes; hyperplasia of Type II cells; intranuclear inclusions; giant cells (measles).

COMPLICATIONS Respiratory failure; secondary bacterial pneumonia, often staphylococcal; adult respiratory distress syndrome (ARDS); interstitial fibrosis.

SIGNS AND SYMPTOMS Dyspnea, fever, chest pain, cough; rales on auscultation

CLINICAL DIAGNOSIS AND OTHER CLINICAL FEATURES Symptoms and physical examination indicate lung infection. Chest x-ray shows a patchy interstitial infiltrate.

LABORATORY DIAGNOSIS Viral cultures; histologic demonstration of characteristic viral inclusions; elevation of cold agglutinins (adenovirus); bacterial cultures may show a secondary infection.

PROGNOSIS Usually full recovery; more often serious outcome in infants, elderly, and immunocompromised.

THERAPY Amantidine; supportive therapy; treatment of superimposed bacterial infection.

OTHER INFORMATION Viral pneumonia is a major predisposing factor leading to bacterial pneumonia; bacterial pneumonia is the leading cause of death during influenza epidemics; vaccination is recommended for the elderly.

Pneumothorax

DESCRIPTION   Air within the pleural cavity, caused by a defect in the visceral pleura or chest wall, resulting in compression and collapse of the lung.

DISEASE ENTITIES; SYNONYMS AND ACRONYMS   Traumatic pneumothorax, spontaneous pneumothorax; tension pneumothorax, open pneumothorax.

INCIDENCE   Common, especially with trauma or after medical/surgical procedures that puncture the chest wall.

AGE   Any age. Spontaneous pneumothorax typically affects young adults.

ETIOLOGY, PATHOGENESIS, AND PREDISPOSING FACTORS   Trauma, including surgical, with puncture of chest wall or lung; rupture of an emphysematous bleb or bulla; positive pressure mechanical ventilation; bronchopleural fistula.

SITES INVOLVED   Pleura, pleural space, and lung. The causative pleural defect may be in the visceral (lung) pleura or the parietal (chest wall) pleura.

GROSS LESIONS   Pleural space is filled with air and the lung is atelectatic. To demonstrate pneumothorax at autopsy, the chest cavity is opened under water, letting air bubbles escape.

MICROSCOPIC LESIONS   Section of lung shows collapsed alveolar air spaces.

COMPLICATIONS   Respiratory failure, especially with tension pneumothorax in which air accumulates under pressure and causes mediastinal shift, compressing the opposite lung.

SIGNS AND SYMPTOMS   Chest pain and dyspnea developing suddenly in a tall young man at exercise; after chest injury; after a pleural tap or central line placement; or in a patient with COPD and emphysema.

CLINICAL DIAGNOSIS AND OTHER CLINICAL FEATURES   Should be an immediate consideration for patients presenting as described above. Absent breath sounds and chest x-ray showing collapsed lung confirm the diagnosis.

LABORATORY DIAGNOSIS   No specific tests. Blood gas measurements indicate the degree of respiratory impairment.

PROGNOSIS   Good, if recognized and treated promptly.

THERAPY   Repair or closure of pleural defect; evacuation of air from pleural space.

OTHER INFORMATION   Following chest trauma, both air and blood are likely to escape into the pleural space; this is called hemopneumothorax.

Pulmonary Edema

DESCRIPTION Excessive fluid within the lungs, which may accumulate in the interstitium, in the alveoli, or in both; caused by increased intracapillary hydrostatic pressure or increased capillary permeability.

DISEASE ENTITIES; SYNONYMS AND ACRONYMS Pulmonary congestion and edema.

INCIDENCE Common; accompanies most mechanisms of death.

AGE Any age; increasing incidence with age due to heart failure.

ETIOLOGY, PATHOGENESIS, AND PREDISPOSING FACTORS Left ventricular failure, mitral stenosis, ARDS, fluid overload, drowning, aspiration, toxic gas inhalation, viral infection, fat embolism, drug overdose, severe brain injury.

SITES INVOLVED Lung; alveolar spaces and interstitium.

GROSS LESIONS Lungs are heavy and usually dark red due to concurrent congestion; they exude white or pink frothy fluid from their bronchi and from cut surfaces.

MICROSCOPIC LESIONS Interstitium is widened and loose; lymphatics are dilated; pink, smooth acellular material is present within alveoli; the darkness of the pink color correlates with the amount of protein in the fluid.

COMPLICATIONS Hypoxia, respiratory failure; bronchopneumonia.

SIGNS AND SYMPTOMS Dyspnea exaggerated by lying flat and relieved by sitting upright (orthopnea); moist rales first heard at bases of lung; pink or white frothy sputum.

CLINICAL DIAGNOSIS AND OTHER CLINICAL FEATURES Recognition of characteristic presentation. Chest x-ray shows increased vascular pattern, increased opacity of lungs especially at bases, Kerley B lines, and frequently a coexistent pleural effusion.

LABORATORY DIAGNOSIS No specific tests. Blood gas measurements indicate degree of functional impairment. Microbiologic cultures may be needed to exclude a superimposed bronchopneumonia.

PROGNOSIS Depends on underlying condition; often reversible with clinical management.

THERAPY Oxygen, diuretics, fluid restriction; correction of mitral stenosis, positive pressure ventilation.

OTHER INFORMATION Pulmonary edema is a common complication of many disease processes; it is a major predisposing factor in the development of pneumonia that complicates heart failure and ARDS.

Pulmonary Embolism

DESCRIPTION Mass of blood clot that lodges within the pulmonary artery; nearly all pulmonary emboli are thromboemboli arising from deep veins of the legs; air, fat, and foreign material are other types of embolus.

DISEASE ENTITIES; SYNONYMS AND ACRONYMS Embolus, thromboembolus, PE.

INCIDENCE Common. Most common cause of sudden death in hospitalized patients.

AGE Any age, depending on predisposing condition; increased incidence with age due to heart failure.

ETIOLOGY, PATHOGENESIS, AND PREDISPOSING FACTORS Pathogenically: endothelial damage, stasis of blood, hypercoagulability. Clinically: heart failure, trauma, surgery, pregnancy, birth control pills, prolonged bed rest.

SITES INVOLVED Any level of the pulmonary artery, from the main trunk to the distal branches are sites for emboli to lodge. Sites of origin of most thromboemboli are the deep veins of the calf and thigh.

GROSS LESIONS Cylindrical mass of fresh or organizing thrombus. A saddle embolus is large and occludes the main pulmonary artery at its bifurcation. Others are smaller, often multiple, within distal arteries.

MICROSCOPIC LESIONS Alternating bands of red cells, fibrin strands, and leukocytes. Organization is indicated by a rim of fibroblasts at the periphery of the thrombus.

COMPLICATIONS Sudden death, pulmonary hemorrhage, pulmonary infarct (a wedge-shaped pleural based lesion that is hemorrhagic due to dual blood supply of the lung), bloody pleural effusion, pulmonary hypertension.

SIGNS AND SYMPTOMS Dyspnea, tachypnea, chest pain, tachycardia, hemoptysis, a feeling of impending death, sudden death.

CLINICAL DIAGNOSIS AND OTHER CLINICAL FEATURES High suspicion of sudden onset of chest pain and/or dyspnea in a hospitalized, postsurgical, or trauma patient. Ventilation/perfusion scans and pulmonary angiography are used to confirm diagnosis.

LABORATORY DIAGNOSIS Fibrin split products and fibrinopeptides are measured to detect thrombogenic activity. Coagulation tests are used to monitor therapy. Blood gas measurements indicate degree of respiratory failure.

PROGNOSIS Poor with large or multiple emboli. Small emboli may resolve without serious morbidity.

THERAPY Anticoagulation with heparin; thrombolytic agents; embolectomy; vena cava ligation or umbrella.

OTHER INFORMATION Prevention of PE is an important aspect of patient management. Other pulmonary emboli involve fat (following trauma with bone fractures), air (100–150 ml is fatal), talc (IV drug abuse), tumor.

Pulmonary Hypertension

DESCRIPTION Increased blood pressure within the pulmonary circulation; either primary or secondary to increased flow within the pulmonary vasculature, increased vascular resistance, or left heart failure.

DISEASE ENTITIES; SYNONYMS AND ACRONYMS Primary pulmonary hypertension, secondary pulmonary hypertension.

INCIDENCE The primary form is rare; secondary forms are common, especially with left heart failure.

AGE Primary disease affects women aged 20–30 years; secondary to left heart failure affects the elderly.

ETIOLOGY, PATHOGENESIS, AND PREDISPOSING FACTORS Idiopathic (primary), congenital heart disease, recurrent pulmonary emboli, chronic lung disease, obesity (Pickwickian syndrome), kyphoscoliosis, mitral stenosis, left heart failure, high altitudes.

SITES INVOLVED Pulmonary arteries of all sizes; diseases affecting the left ventricle or the mitral valve cause congestion and hypertension within pulmonary capillaries.

GROSS LESIONS Atherosclerosis of the main pulmonary artery and its major branches; arterial dilatation; plexiform or angiomatoid formations; webs due to organized thromboemboli in arteries; pulmonary hemorrhage.

MICROSCOPIC LESIONS Arterial walls thickened by muscular hyperplasia and intimal fibrosis; increased elastic fibers in media. Lung shows congestion, edema, hemorrhage, and "heart failure cells" (hemosiderin macrophages).

COMPLICATIONS Right heart failure, right ventricular hypertrophy (cor pulmonale), pulmonary congestion and edema, pulmonary hemorrhage, pulmonary embolism.

SIGNS AND SYMPTOMS Dyspnea, cyanosis, signs of right heart failure.

CLINICAL DIAGNOSIS AND OTHER CLINICAL FEATURES Rales due to pulmonary edema in cases of left heart failure; chest x-ray shows increased vascular pattern. Pulmonary artery catheterization with direct pressure measurement is diagnostic.

LABORATORY DIAGNOSIS No specific tests. Blood gas measurements indicate degree of hypoxemia.

PROGNOSIS Poor; patients die of progressive heart failure or pulmonary embolism.

THERAPY Treatment of underlying primary condition; diuretics, nitrites; heart-lung transplantation.

OTHER INFORMATION Examples of dietary and drug-related pulmonary hypertension include: monocrotaline and fulvine in Jamaican bush tea, contaminated rapeseed oil; aminorex, fenfluramine, and phenformin.

Pulmonary Tuberculosis

DESCRIPTION   Infection of lungs with the acid-fast staining *Mycobacterium tuberculosis,* characterized by granulomatous inflammation, caseous necrosis, and spread to lymph nodes and other organs.

DISEASE ENTITIES; SYNONYMS AND ACRONYMS   Primary TB, secondary (reactivation) TB, postprimary TB, miliary TB, cavitary TB; acid fast bacteria (AFB).

INCIDENCE   Uncommon in developed countries except in certain lower economic groups; high in undeveloped areas.

AGE   Primary TB involves children; reactivation TB affects adults, especially in advanced age.

ETIOLOGY, PATHOGENESIS, AND PREDISPOSING FACTORS   *M. tuberculosis* is highly virulent; primary TB affects healthy persons. Reactivation TB is a consequence of immune depression—alcoholism, immunosuppression, silicosis, old age, cancer, etc.

SITES INVOLVED   Primary TB involves subpleural lung and hilar lymph node (Ghon complex); reactivation TB affects apex of upper lung lobes; miliary TB is disseminated throughout all organs including lungs.

GROSS LESIONS   Ghon complex lesions are small granulomas (1 cm) that become fibrous and calcified; secondary TB causes large caseating cavities; multiple small (1–2 mm) caseating granulomas are seen in miliary TB.

MICROSCOPIC LESIONS   Central caseous necrosis rimmed by lymphocytes, epithelioid cells and Langhan's giant cells are seen in all lesions; variables are the confluence of granulomas and fibrous scar tissue formation.

COMPLICATIONS   Progression of disease with cavitary destruction of lung leading to respiratory failure; empyema; TB pneumonia; massive hemoptysis; pleural effusion; spread to other organs.

SIGNS AND SYMPTOMS   Fever, weight loss, night sweats, malaise; cough, hemoptysis; primary TB is usually mild and becomes arrested but occasionally becomes progressive.

CLINICAL DIAGNOSIS AND OTHER CLINICAL FEATURES   Recognition of classical symptoms; chest x-ray evidence of cavities or pleural effusion. Mantoux, Tine, or PPD skin tests may indicate infection but not whether the infection is active.

LABORATORY DIAGNOSIS   Acid fast stain (Ziehl-Neelsen) is rapid but not sensitive; cultures are more sensitive but require weeks. Granulomas and AFB are seen histologically in biopsies from lung or lymph node.

PROGNOSIS   Good for early treated disease; poor for advanced cavitary TB; terrible for miliary TB.

THERAPY   Multidrug antitubercular chemotherapy especially INH; also rifampin, ethambutal, streptomycin.

OTHER INFORMATION   The incidence of TB is increasing because of the AIDS epidemic. In addition, multiple drug-resistant strains are emerging.

Sarcoidosis

DESCRIPTION Idiopathic disease characterized by granulomatous inflammation involving any organ; lung and lymph nodes are involved most commonly.

DISEASE ENTITIES; SYNONYMS AND ACRONYMS Boeck's sarcoid.

INCIDENCE Somewhat common, especially among Southern US blacks and in Scandinavian countries.

AGE Adults, young to middle aged; more common in females.

ETIOLOGY, PATHOGENESIS, AND PREDISPOSING FACTORS Idiopathic; hypersensitivity to an environmental antigen or a viral infection are possible but unlikely etiologies; abnormal activation of T-cells is somehow involved in the pathogenesis.

SITES INVOLVED Any organ: lungs, lymph nodes commonly; spleen, liver, bone marrow, skin, eye, brain, heart. In lung, granulomas are distributed along lymphatics, around blood vessels, bronchi, and interstitium.

GROSS LESIONS Firm nodules, individually usually only a few millimeters in size; these become confluent and give rise to larger nodules and lymphadenopathy.

MICROSCOPIC LESIONS Noncaseating granulomas with fibrotic acellular core surrounded by lymphocytes, epithelioid cells and Langhan's giant cells. Asteroids and Schauman bodies may be seen.

COMPLICATIONS Progressive respiratory failure with obstructive and/or restrictive lung disease; cor pulmonale. Lesions in other organs (heart, brain) may cause arrhythmias or seizures.

SIGNS AND SYMPTOMS Dyspnea, cough; fever, malaise, weight loss; erythema nodosum.

CLINICAL DIAGNOSIS AND OTHER CLINICAL FEATURES Likely diagnosis for a disease showing hilar adenopathy and reticulonodular opacities on chest x-ray. Lytic bone lesions may be seen, particularly in the hand. Kveim skin test is rarely done.

LABORATORY DIAGNOSIS Histology is mandatory; biopsy of lung or lymph node is usual source of tissue. Special stains and microbiologic cultures are required to exclude other granulomatous diseases, particularly TB.

PROGNOSIS Variable, ranging from spontaneous remissions to progressive lung disease with honeycombing.

THERAPY Corticosteroids often obtain a rapid response; some patients require no therapy.

OTHER INFORMATION Patients with sarcoidosis display cutaneous anergy to multiple antigens; T-cells are decreased in the blood but overabundant in the tissues with granulomas.

Pathology Facts, by Richard C.
Harruff, J.B. Lippincott
Company, Philadelphia © 1994.

Chapter 14

Gastrointestinal Tract

Appendicitis—Acute

DESCRIPTION Acute inflammatory condition of the vermiform appendix; different stages may be recognized: suppurative, gangrenous, and ruptured appendicitis.

DISEASE ENTITIES; SYNONYMS AND ACRONYMS Periappendicitis, periappendiceal abscess, phlegmonous appendicitis.

INCIDENCE Common; most common disease of appendix.

AGE Any age; peak incidence in second and third decades.

ETIOLOGY, PATHOGENESIS, AND PREDISPOSING FACTORS Fecalith in lumen causes distention and ischemia in one third of cases; tumor, parasite, foreign body, or lymphoid hyperplasia may also obstruct; in 50%, there is no obstruction and cause is unknown.

SITES INVOLVED Appendix; inflammation starts in mucosa and extends into and through wall.

GROSS LESIONS Early: swollen and hyperemic, covered with fibrinous exudate; later: purulent exudate on serosa; advanced: black coloration of gangrene, perforation of wall; fecalith may be within proximal lumen.

MICROSCOPIC LESIONS Early: luminal purulence, acute exudate in mucosa; later: purulent exudate extending through wall and on surface; advanced: complete necrosis of wall with perforation.

COMPLICATIONS Perforation, particularly in infants under 2 years of age and in adults over 60 because of atypical presentations; periappendiceal abscess; liver abscess; peritonitis and septicemia.

SIGNS AND SYMPTOMS Epigastric or periumbilical pain, shifting to the right lower quadrant; nausea and vomiting; low-grade fever; moderate leukocytosis; atypical presentations are common in infants and elderly.

CLINICAL DIAGNOSIS AND OTHER CLINICAL FEATURES Recognition of typical symptoms and suspicions regarding atypical symptoms, which may be present with a retrocecal appendix or in an elderly patient.

LABORATORY DIAGNOSIS Complete blood count to demonstrate leukocytosis; histologic examination of resected appendix to confirm diagnosis.

PROGNOSIS Good, unless perforation occurs and leads to complications; peritonitis has a poor prognosis.

THERAPY Appendectomy; antibiotics if surgical facilities are not available.

OTHER INFORMATION At least 10% of appropriately resected appendices are normal; similar symptoms are produced by mesenteric lymphadenitis, Meckel's diverticulitis, ovarian follicle rupture, and acute salpingitis.

Carcinoid Tumors

DESCRIPTION   Tumors of the gastrointestinal tract, which may be benign or malignant, arising from argentaffin cells of the neuroendocrine system of the gut.

DISEASE ENTITIES; SYNONYMS AND ACRONYMS   Endocrine tumors of GI tract; neuroectodermal tumor; APUDoma.

INCIDENCE   Constitute less than 1% of all GI tumors but are fairly frequent small intestinal tumors.

AGE   Adults; increasing incidence with age.

ETIOLOGY, PATHOGENESIS, AND PREDISPOSING FACTORS   Neoplasm, unknown etiology; may be part of a multiple endocrine neoplasia (MEN) syndrome; arise from amine precursor uptake and decarboxylating (APUD) cells; carcinoid syndrome is caused by serotonin.

SITES INVOLVED   Any site within the GI tract, by far most commonly in the ileum and appendix; they develop initially within the submucosa.

GROSS LESIONS   Firm, yellowish nodule in the submucosa, covered by mucosa; may be multicentric; enlargement produces a polypoid mass protruding into the lumen, an intramural mass, or an annular neoplasm.

MICROSCOPIC LESIONS   Nests and cords of small round uniform cells in fibrous stroma; regular nuclei; marginal cells in nests have smaller dark nuclei; neurosecretory granules seen by silver stains or electron microscopy.

COMPLICATIONS   Local spread, metastasis; carcinoid syndrome with extensive hepatic metastases, causing diarrhea, episodic flushing, bronchospasm, skin rash, and right-sided valvular heart disease.

SIGNS AND SYMPTOMS   Often asymptomatic until advanced; pain and symptoms of obstruction; carcinoid syndrome is a rare presentation.

CLINICAL DIAGNOSIS AND OTHER CLINICAL FEATURES   X-rays with contrast media (e.g., upper GI series); endoscopy with biopsy.

LABORATORY DIAGNOSIS   Histochemical stains demonstrate substances that can reduce silver (argentaffin, argyrophil); immunohistochemistry demonstrates neuropeptides; electron microscopy shows neurosecretory granules.

PROGNOSIS   Depends on size; for resected small intestinal carcinoids, the 5-year survival is 50%.

THERAPY   Surgical resection.

OTHER INFORMATION   The malignant potential of carcinoid tumors is related to size: tumors less than 1 cm rarely metastasize; between 1 and 2 cm, 50% metastasize; greater than 2 cm, 80% metastasize.

Carcinoma of Colon and Rectum

DESCRIPTION Malignant neoplasm of the colonic or rectal mucosa, almost always an adenocarcinoma.

DISEASE ENTITIES; SYNONYMS AND ACRONYMS Adenocarcinoma of colon or rectum, colorectal carcinoma, colon cancer.

INCIDENCE Second most common cancer causing death in men; third most common in women.

AGE Rapidly increasing incidence with age, starting at age 40 years.

ETIOLOGY, PATHOGENESIS, AND PREDISPOSING FACTORS Low-fiber, high animal-fat diet; adenomatous polyps; ulcerative colitis, Crohn's disease; familial polyposis; high population of anaerobic bacteria in colon; low dietary vitamins A, E, C, and selenium.

SITES INVOLVED Any site in colon; one third in rectum and rectosigmoid colon; one fourth in sigmoid colon; large polypoid tumors are most common in the cecum; annular constricting tumors are more common distally.

GROSS LESIONS Polypoid, ulcerating, or infiltrating tumors; the infiltrating type is often annular and constricting; polypoid tumors protrude into the lumen; all types invade through the wall into serosal fat.

MICROSCOPIC LESIONS Nearly all are adenocarcinomas, well or moderately differentiated; some secrete excessive mucus (mucinous adenocarcinomas); some are composed of signet ring cells.

COMPLICATIONS Intestinal obstruction, perforation, bleeding; anemia; fistulas between other bowel loops, vagina, or skin; ascites; distant metastases to liver most commonly, also to lungs, bones, and brain.

SIGNS AND SYMPTOMS Rectal bleeding, occult or obvious; iron-deficiency anemia; change in bowel habits, gaseousness, abdominal pain, tenesmus.

CLINICAL DIAGNOSIS AND OTHER CLINICAL FEATURES Rectal examination, proctoscopy, sigmoidoscopy, colonoscopy with biopsy of lesion; barium enema x-rays.

LABORATORY DIAGNOSIS Histologic examination of resected or biopsied tumor; screening tests for occult fecal blood; carcinoembryonic antigen (CEA) detection in serum as a tumor marker to help manage postoperative course.

PROGNOSIS 5-year survival according to Duke's stage: A—95%; B—60%; C—35%; D—poor.

THERAPY Surgical resection may be curative; chemotherapy or radiotherapy is adjunctive or palliative.

OTHER INFORMATION Dukes staging scheme: A—confined to the mucosa and submucosa; B—into and possibly through the muscle wall but no lymph node metastases; C—regional lymph node metastases; D—distant metastases.

Carcinoma of Esophagus

DESCRIPTION Malignant tumor of the esophagus, most often squamous cell carcinoma, which may be polypoid, infiltrating, or ulcerating; has a poor prognosis due to invasion of surrounding mediastinal structures.

DISEASE ENTITIES; SYNONYMS AND ACRONYMS Squamous cell carcinoma of esophagus, esophageal cancer.

INCIDENCE Constitutes 7% of all GI cancers; male:female = 3:1; more common in US blacks and in urban groups.

AGE Middle aged to elderly.

ETIOLOGY, PATHOGENESIS, AND PREDISPOSING FACTORS Chronic esophageal disease (rings, webs, diverticula, stricture from lye ingestion, achalasia, chronic esophagitis); excessive alcohol consumption; cigarette smoking; nitrosamines; aniline dyes; diet.

SITES INVOLVED Middle third of esophagus in about half of cases; upper third in 15%; lower third in 35%.

GROSS LESIONS Polypoid: exophytic growth projecting into the lumen; infiltrating: growth is within the wall, thickening the wall and narrowing the lumen; ulcerating: growth extends through the wall with ulceration.

MICROSCOPIC LESIONS Most are squamous carcinomas: well, moderately, or poorly differentiated. About 5% are adenocarcinomas arising in Barrett's epithelium.

COMPLICATIONS Esophageal obstruction with malnutrition, cachexia; tracheoesophageal fistula with pneumonia; mediastinal extension; metastasis to lymph nodes, liver, and lung as well as other organs.

SIGNS AND SYMPTOMS Dysphagia with pain during swallowing or continuously, anorexia, weight loss; hoarseness due to compression of laryngeal nerve; cough due to tracheoesophageal fistula.

CLINICAL DIAGNOSIS AND OTHER CLINICAL FEATURES Recognition of clinical presentation; x-rays with radiopaque media (barium swallow); endoscopy; CT and MRI scans visualize extent of invasion into mediastinal structures.

LABORATORY DIAGNOSIS Histology of endoscopic biopsy or cytology of brushings are usually accurate; biopsy of necrotic slough from the surface or ulcer cavity may produce false negatives.

PROGNOSIS Dismal; overall 4% 5-year survival; symptomatic tumors are usually unresectable at presentation.

THERAPY Surgery and radiotherapy, usually only for palliation; only 40% of surgical cases are resectable.

OTHER INFORMATION Palliative procedures include endoscopic laser fulguration; placement of a gastrostomy or jejunostomy feeding tube or a polyvinyl esophageal prosthesis.

Carcinoma of Stomach

DESCRIPTION Malignant neoplasm arising from the gastric mucosa, most often an adenocarcinoma showing one of three growth patterns: polypoid or fungating, ulcerating, diffuse or infiltrating (linitis plastica).

DISEASE ENTITIES; SYNONYMS AND ACRONYMS Adenocarcinoma; advanced gastric cancer; early gastric cancer; superficial spreading carcinoma; linitis plastica.

INCIDENCE Sixth most common cancer causing death; male predominance; more common in low socioeconomic groups.

AGE Incidence increases sharply after age 50.

ETIOLOGY, PATHOGENESIS, AND PREDISPOSING FACTORS Atrophic gastritis, pernicious anemia, subtotal gastrectomy, gastric polyps; dietary factors, e.g., smoked fish and meat containing benzpyrene; nitrosamines produced endogenously in chronic gastritis.

SITES INVOLVED Stomach, usually the distal portion, on the lesser curvature of the antrum and prepyloric region. Often arises in a site of intestinal metaplasia in chronic gastritis.

GROSS LESIONS Polypoid: raised fungating mass projecting into the lumen; ulcerating: shallow ulcer with firm raised nodular edges and ragged base; infiltrating: diffuse wall thickening with no exophytic tumor.

MICROSCOPIC LESIONS Most are adenocarcinomas, ranging from a well-differentiated pattern (often seen in the polypoid type) to an anaplastic growth with signet ring cells (common in linitis plastica).

COMPLICATIONS Gastric obstruction leading to malnutrition and cachexia; bleeding, usually low grade and causing anemia; metastasis to regional lymph nodes and to liver, lung, brain, or ovary (Krukenberg tumor).

SIGNS AND SYMPTOMS Weight loss, anorexia, nausea; epigastric or back pain possibly relieved by antacids; dysphagia, dyspepsia; melena or anemia; lympadenopathy, especially supraclavicular (Virchow's or sentinel node).

CLINICAL DIAGNOSIS AND OTHER CLINICAL FEATURES Often found during evaluation of a patient suspected of having peptic ulcer disease; endoscopy; radiography with contrast media. Metastases at presentation are common.

LABORATORY DIAGNOSIS Histology of endoscopic biopsy; false negatives are not infrequent, especially with linitis plastica; carcinoembryonic antigen (CEA) is a tumor marker to monitor recurrences or metastases.

PROGNOSIS Poor; most have metastasized at presentation; of those surgically resectable, 20% survive 10 years.

THERAPY Surgery, radiotherapy, chemotherapy; usually for palliation only.

OTHER INFORMATION Early gastric cancer, common in Japan, is usually limited to the mucosa and submucosa, although polypoid and ulcerative types occur. Its prognosis is much better than for advanced gastric cancer.

Celiac Disease

DESCRIPTION   Disease of the small intestine related to gluten sensitivity, characterized by atrophy of the small intestine mucosal villi and generalized malabsorption.

DISEASE ENTITIES; SYNONYMS AND ACRONYMS   Celiac sprue, gluten-sensitive enteropathy, nontropical sprue.

INCIDENCE   Highly variable; 1 in 300 population in Ireland, 1 in 3000 in other countries; female:male = 1.3:1.

AGE   Most are diagnosed in childhood, after first feedings of cereals; few cases appear much later.

ETIOLOGY, PATHOGENESIS, AND PREDISPOSING FACTORS   Sensitivity to water-insoluble gluten and its alcoholic extract, gliadin, contained in wheat, barley, and rye flours; may involve altered immunologic responses to gluten; linked to HLA-B8 and DW3.

SITES INVOLVED   Small intestine mucosal villi, particularly in the distal duodenum and proximal jejunum.

GROSS LESIONS   The mucosal surface may appear smoother than normal; the lesion is best recognized microscopically.

MICROSCOPIC LESIONS   Flat mucosal surface with blunting or total loss of villi; flattening and basophilia of absorptive cells with loss of nuclear polarity; increased lymphocytes and plasma cells in the lamina propria.

COMPLICATIONS   Malnutrition most immediately; later, malignant lymphoma of small intestine; ulcerative jejunitis.

SIGNS AND SYMPTOMS   Failure to thrive in an infant growing normally until cereals are started; other signs of malabsorption may or may not be present; vesicular skin lesions (dermatitis herpetiformis).

CLINICAL DIAGNOSIS AND OTHER CLINICAL FEATURES   Recognition of the clinical presentation, followed by a rapid response to a gluten-free diet. Diagnosis in an adult is similar but recognition of the disease is usually delayed.

LABORATORY DIAGNOSIS   Histology of small bowel biopsy shows characteristic changes; other tests are those suggested for evaluating malabsorption.

PROGNOSIS   There is almost always a good response to a gluten-free diet.

THERAPY   Avoidance of gluten.

OTHER INFORMATION   Dermatitis herpetiformis, the associated skin disease, is related to circulating antigluten IgA antibodies that are deposited in skin.

Crohn's Disease

DESCRIPTION An inflammatory bowel disease that may affect any part of the gastrointestinal tract, characterized by transmural granulomatous inflammation with ulcers, strictures, fissures, and fistulas.

DISEASE ENTITIES; SYNONYMS AND ACRONYMS Regional enteritis, terminal ileitis, granulomatous colitis; inflammatory bowel disease, IBD.

INCIDENCE 0.5–5/100,000 per year; female:male = 1.6:1; more common in people of European ancestry and Jews.

AGE Usually appears in adolescents and young adults.

ETIOLOGY, PATHOGENESIS, AND PREDISPOSING FACTORS Idiopathic despite much speculation regarding bacterial or viral infections, disordered cell-mediated immunity, dietary or emotional factors; there is a positive family history of IBD in 40% of cases.

SITES INVOLVED Ileum and cecum in 30%; small bowel only, 15%; colon only, 20%; anorectal region, 15%; duodenum and stomach occasionally; rare in esophagus and oral cavity; female genitalia with anorectal disease.

GROSS LESIONS Discontinuous involvement; thickened bowel wall; edema and fibrosis; narrowed lumen; serpinginous mucosal ulcers; cobblestone appearance of mucosal surface; fissures into wall; fistulas; adhesions.

MICROSCOPIC LESIONS Chronic inflammation in all layers of the intestine (transmural); fibrosis; granulomatous inflammation; granulomas usually in the submucosa; fissures lined by granulation tissue.

COMPLICATIONS Intestinal obstruction; fistulas (bladder, uterus, vagina, skin, perianal region); malabsorption; episcleritis; uveitis; arthritis; erythema nodosum; colon cancer; liver disease; amyloidosis.

SIGNS AND SYMPTOMS Abdominal pain and diarrhea; fever; occasionally presents like appendicitis; right lower quadrant pain, tenderness, and possible mass; anorectal fistulas.

CLINICAL DIAGNOSIS AND OTHER CLINICAL FEATURES X-ray studies with contrast (barium enema or small bowel series); sigmoidoscopy, colonoscopy; differential: ulcerative colitis, infection (TB, Yersinia, Campylobacter), parasites, lymphoma.

LABORATORY DIAGNOSIS Stool cultures for bacteria; fecal examinations for ameba and other parasites; TB cultures; histology of mucosal biopsy tissue or resected bowel.

PROGNOSIS Chronic debilitating illness with no cure; anti-inflammatory therapy may provide some relief.

THERAPY Anti-inflammatory steroids; sulfasalazine; 6-mercaptopurine; metronidazole; surgical resections.

OTHER INFORMATION IBD includes Crohn's disease and ulcerative colitis; many cases (10%) show overlapping features and cannot be distinguished; see entry for ulcerative colitis, which lists differentiating criteria.

Diverticular Disease

DESCRIPTION Condition of the colon in which the mucosa and submucosa herniate through the muscular layers of the colon to form outpouchings containing feces.

DISEASE ENTITIES; SYNONYMS AND ACRONYMS Diverticulosis coli, diverticulosis (uncomplicated disease), diverticulitis (complicated by inflammation), "tics."

INCIDENCE Common; diverticula may be demonstrated in as many as one half of elderly persons.

AGE Increasing incidence with age, starting after age 40.

ETIOLOGY, PATHOGENESIS, AND PREDISPOSING FACTORS Current hypothesis: low-fiber diet results in increased intraluminal pressure that pushes the mucosa through connective tissue sheathes that surround nutrient blood vessels penetrating the muscularis.

SITES INVOLVED Any segment of the colon may be involved; sigmoid colon is involved in 95% of cases.

GROSS LESIONS External outpouchings containing feces along the colon between the taenia coli up to 1 cm in diameter; from the lumen, small mouths open through the mucosa into the pouches.

MICROSCOPIC LESIONS A diverticulum sectioned along its axis shows mucosa invested with connective tissue herniating through a defect in the internal circular layer of muscularis.

COMPLICATIONS Inflammation resulting in progressive fibrosis, stricture and obstruction; bleeding leading to hypovolemia or iron-deficiency anemia; perforation with pericolonic abscess or peritonitis.

SIGNS AND SYMPTOMS Usually asymptomatic unless complicated by diverticulitis; episodic or constant abdominal pain; constipation alternating with diarrhea; fever; sudden onset of painless rectal bleeding; anemia.

CLINICAL DIAGNOSIS AND OTHER CLINICAL FEATURES Investigation of abdominal pain, gastrointestinal bleeding, bowel dysfunction, or iron deficiency; barium enema x-rays show the characteristic configuration of diverticula; colonoscopy, sigmoidoscopy.

LABORATORY DIAGNOSIS No specific tests; fecal examination for occult blood may be positive; iron-deficiency anemia may be present; stool cultures and examinations exclude bacterial or parasitic infections.

PROGNOSIS Usually good; complications are occasionally serious (e.g., severe bleeding, peritonitis).

THERAPY High-fiber diet; antibiotics for diverticulitis; surgical resection of severely involved segments.

OTHER INFORMATION Colonic diverticula are pseudodiverticula because they do not contain all layers of the intestinal wall.

Enterocolitis (Diarrheal Diseases)

DESCRIPTION Infections of predominantly small intestine, characterized by watery feces due to excessive secretions; caused by adhesive, toxigenic, or invasive bacteria, preformed bacterial toxins, or viruses.

DISEASE ENTITIES; SYNONYMS AND ACRONYMS Infectious diarrhea, cholera, dysentery, typhoid fever, shigellosis, salmonellosis, food poisoning, traveler's diarrhea.

INCIDENCE Very common; most common cause of infant mortality in undeveloped countries.

AGE Any age; most serious in infants and elderly.

ETIOLOGY, PATHOGENESIS, AND PREDISPOSING FACTORS Toxigenic bacteria: *V. cholera, E. coli;* invasive bacteria: Shigella, Salmonella, Yersinia, Campylobacter; food poisoning: *S. aureus, Clostridium perfringens;* virus: Rotaviruses, Norwalk viruses.

SITES INVOLVED Usually small intestine; shigellosis affects the colon; salmonella (typhoid fever) attacks the Peyer's patches in the distal ileum: Yersinia causes granulomatous lymphadenitis in mesenteric nodes.

GROSS LESIONS Only the invasive bacteria show lesions; shigellosis: mucosal hyperemia, multiple serpinginous ulcers; typhoid fever: necrosis and ulceration of lymphoid follicles and overlying mucosa.

MICROSCOPIC LESIONS Toxigenic bacteria and food poisoning: minimal or no lesions; viruses: blunting of villi; invasive bacteria: fibrin, acute inflammation and granulation tissue in mucosal ulcers.

COMPLICATIONS Dehydration, shock (especially cholera or any diarrhea in infants); hemorrhage, perforation (typhoid fever); sepsis; bacteremia (salmonellosis); salmonella osteomyelitis in sickle cell disease.

SIGNS AND SYMPTOMS Abundant watery stools with variable abdominal pain, worse pain accompanied by fever with invasive bacteria; erythema nodosum or multiforme may follow Yersinia enterocolitis.

CLINICAL DIAGNOSIS AND OTHER CLINICAL FEATURES Presence of diarrhea; history of travel is important; blood in stools or fever indicates an invasive strain; symptoms occurring after eating improperly stored food indicates food poisoning.

LABORATORY DIAGNOSIS Stool cultures are fairly successful in isolating an etiologic bacteria; presence of leukocytes in the feces indicates an invasive bacteria; blood cultures may be positive in salmonella infections.

PROGNOSIS Good in developed countries; high mortality in infants in undeveloped regions.

THERAPY Fluid and electrolyte replacement, oral or intravenous; specific antibiotics when indicated.

OTHER INFORMATION See Section II: Infectious Diseases for discussion of specific organisms. Amebic dysentery is also considered a diarrheal disease.

Esophagitis

DESCRIPTION   Inflammation of the esophagus due to reflux of gastric juices, infections, chemical irritants, involvement by systemic diseases, or physical agents (including radiation).

DISEASE ENTITIES; SYNONYMS AND ACRONYMS   Reflux esophagitis, peptic esophagitis; candidal or herpetic esophagitis; chemical esophagitis; pemphigoid esophagitis.

INCIDENCE   Reflux esophagitis is the most common type; infectious esophagitis occurs with immunosuppression.

AGE   Increasing incidence with age.

ETIOLOGY, PATHOGENESIS, AND PREDISPOSING FACTORS   Reflux: incompetent cardiac sphincter, hiatal hernia, certain foods or drugs; infectious: immunosuppression; chemical: caustic chemicals, acid or alkali; physical agents: nasogastric tube, radiation.

SITES INVOLVED   Esophagus, particularly the distal portion in reflux esophagitis; diffuse involvement with esophagitis due to corrosives; multifocal or diffuse involvement with infectious esophagitis.

GROSS LESIONS   Reflux: erythema, linear mucosal ulcers (erosions) of distal esophagus; infectious: scattered round ulcers throughout the mucosa; chemical: extensive diffuse erythema and mucosal sloughing.

MICROSCOPIC LESIONS   Acute and possibly also chronic inflammation; mucosal ulcers with granulation tissue; multinucleated cells and intranuclear inclusions with herpetic infection; fungal hyphae with candidal.

COMPLICATIONS   Ulceration with hematemesis; perforation causing pleuritis or mediastinitis; glandular metaplasia of squamous mucosa (Barrett's epithelium); esophageal stricture due to scarring of deep ulcers.

SIGNS AND SYMPTOMS   Heartburn, regurgitation, dysphagia, painful swallowing.

CLINICAL DIAGNOSIS AND OTHER CLINICAL FEATURES   Recognition of typical symptoms, which must be differentiated from cardiac pain; symptoms are reproduced by dripping dilute acid into the esophagus via a nasogastric tube; endoscopy with biopsy.

LABORATORY DIAGNOSIS   No specific test for the reflux type; for the infectious type, histologic examination of biopsy to document hyphae or intranuclear inclusions.

PROGNOSIS   Good for reflux esophagitis; often poor for infectious; variable for the chemical type.

THERAPY   Elevation of head of bed; antacids or H2 blockers; surgery for hiatal hernia; nystatin for candida.

OTHER INFORMATION   Barrett's epithelium predisposes to adenocarcinoma of the lower esophagus.

Gastritis—Acute

DESCRIPTION   Acute inflammation with focal necrosis of the gastric mucosa, leading to hemorrhage and possibly ulcers.

DISEASE ENTITIES; SYNONYMS AND ACRONYMS   Erosive gastritis, stress ulcers, Curling's ulcers, Cushing's ulcers.

INCIDENCE   Common, especially following trauma, with corticosteroid therapy, and in alcoholism.

AGE   Any age depending on predisposing factors; increasing incidence with age.

ETIOLOGY, PATHOGENESIS, AND PREDISPOSING FACTORS   Ingestion of corrosive substances; steroids; aspirin and other nonsteroidal anti-inflammatory drugs; stress in the form of trauma, particularly burns, CNS injury, shock, sepsis, and incapacitation.

SITES INVOLVED   Gastric mucosa at any site in the stomach; inflammation and erosions may also involve the esophagus and duodenum.

GROSS LESIONS   Petechial hemorrhages or confluent hemorrhages in the mucosa with small mucosal erosions (few millimeters) or punched-out ulcers (1–2 cm) that may extend into the submucosa or deeper.

MICROSCOPIC LESIONS   Focal necrosis of the mucosa with acute inflammation and erosion or ulceration.

COMPLICATIONS   Progression to gastric ulcer; deep gastric ulcers can perforate and cause peritonitis; gastrointestinal hemorrhage, sometimes severe enough to cause exsanguination.

SIGNS AND SYMPTOMS   Epigastric pain; gastrointestinal hemorrhage in a trauma victim or patient treated with steroids, aspirin, or other nonsteroidal anti-inflammatory agent.

CLINICAL DIAGNOSIS AND OTHER CLINICAL FEATURES   Suspicion regarding epigastric pain; endoscopy. Alcoholics, trauma victims, and any patient treated with steroids or anti-inflammatory drugs are predisposed to GI hemorrhage due to gastritis.

LABORATORY DIAGNOSIS   Histology of endoscopic biopsy material; occult fecal blood tests to detect GI bleeding.

PROGNOSIS   Usually good with removal of predisposing factor; significant mortality is due to hemorrhage.

THERAPY   Antacids; H2 blocking agents that reduce gastric acid secretion; removal of predisposing condition.

OTHER INFORMATION   Pathogenic mechanisms involve decreased mucus secretion, hypersecretion of acid, microcirculatory changes producing mucosal ischemia, local prostaglandin deficiency, and decreased intramucosal pH.

Gastritis—Chronic

DESCRIPTION   Chronic inflammation of the gastric mucosa, divided into fundic and antral gastritis, ranging in severity from mild superficial gastritis to gastric atrophy.

DISEASE ENTITIES; SYNONYMS AND ACRONYMS   Nonerosive gastritis, atrophic gastritis, achlorhydria, pernicious anemia.

INCIDENCE   Common. Antral gastritis is considerably more common than the fundal type.

AGE   Increasing incidence with age, particularly after age 40.

ETIOLOGY, PATHOGENESIS, AND PREDISPOSING FACTORS   Aging is the most important factor; autoantibodies are present in the fundal type; genetic factors may be important; partial gastrectomy results in chronic gastritis in the remaining stomach.

SITES INVOLVED   Fundal gastritis: gastric mucosa of fundus and body; antral gastritis: mucosa of antrum.

GROSS LESIONS   Superficial gastritis may show no gross changes; with atrophic gastritis, there is thinning of the mucosa and flattening of the gastric rugal folds.

MICROSCOPIC LESIONS   Lymphocyte and plasma cell infiltrates in the lamina propria; germinal centers may be present; decreased number of glands and thinning of mucosa; intestinal metaplasia or pseudopyloric metaplasia.

COMPLICATIONS   Achlorhydria due to loss of parietal cells; pernicious anemia due to loss of intrinsic factor; gastric ulcer; carcinoma of stomach.

SIGNS AND SYMPTOMS   Few if any symptoms; dyspepsia and indigestion are not constant; pallor and neurologic signs due to pernicious anemia.

CLINICAL DIAGNOSIS AND OTHER CLINICAL FEATURES   Endoscopy with biopsy to assess inflammation and intestinal metaplasia; many cases are clinically insignificant; possible complications of ulcer and carcinoma need to be excluded.

LABORATORY DIAGNOSIS   Histologic examination of biopsy material; decreased gastric acid and pepsin secretion; macrocytic/megaloblastic anemia; demonstration of autoantibodies to parietal cells.

PROGNOSIS   Fairly good unless gastric carcinoma develops.

THERAPY   No specific therapy other than treating the complications.

OTHER INFORMATION   Chronic gastritis with loss of intrinsic factor, due to destruction of parietal cells, causes malabsorption of vitamin B_{12} leading to megaloblastic anemia (pernicious anemia).

Hemorrhoids

DESCRIPTION   Dilated venous channels of the hemorrhoidal plexus; internal hemorrhoids arise above the pectinate line and external hemorrhoids below the line.

DISEASE ENTITIES; SYNONYMS AND ACRONYMS   Piles.

INCIDENCE   Very common, affecting as many as 50% of the population over 50 years of age.

AGE   Middle-aged persons; young women during or after pregnancy.

ETIOLOGY, PATHOGENESIS, AND PREDISPOSING FACTORS   Increased abdominal pressure due to pregnancy; low-fiber diet; association with portal hypertension is debatable.

SITES INVOLVED   Superior hemorrhoidal plexus (internal hemorrhoids); inferior hemorrhoidal plexus (external hemorrhoids).

GROSS LESIONS   Purplish-red nodular masses protruding from anal canal; possible thrombosis or ulceration with bleeding; fibrous polyps of anal canal and anal tags represent old hemorrhoids with organized thrombus.

MICROSCOPIC LESIONS   Dilated vascular channels containing blood and possibly fresh or organizing thrombus; smooth muscle hyperplasia in walls; variable amount of inflammation; covered with squamous or columnar epithelium.

COMPLICATIONS   Rectal bleeding with potential iron-deficiency anemia; rectal prolapse; strangulation of hemorrhoids; thrombosis.

SIGNS AND SYMPTOMS   Anal discomfort ranging to severe pain with thrombosed hemorrhoids; bright red rectal bleeding, especially after bowel movement; sensation of incomplete evacuation.

CLINICAL DIAGNOSIS AND OTHER CLINICAL FEATURES   Rectal examination; proctoscopy; occasionally a rectal carcinoma may present with hemorrhoids.

LABORATORY DIAGNOSIS   No specific tests; histologic examination confirms clinical diagnosis.

PROGNOSIS   Usually good.

THERAPY   Local topical therapy; surgical excision (hemorrhoidectomy); high-fiber diet.

OTHER INFORMATION   Chronic hemorrhoids predispose to carcinoma of the anus.

Hiatal Hernia

DESCRIPTION   Herniation of the stomach through an enlarged esophageal hiatus in the diaphragm, subclassified as sliding (axial) or paraesophageal.

DISEASE ENTITIES; SYNONYMS AND ACRONYMS   Hiatus hernia; sliding hiatal hernia, paraesophageal hiatal hernia.

INCIDENCE   Common; the sliding type is present in 10% of the population on routine barium swallow.

AGE   Adult; increasing incidence with age.

ETIOLOGY, PATHOGENESIS, AND PREDISPOSING FACTORS   Unknown etiology; acquired condition.

SITES INVOLVED   Lower esophagus and cardia of stomach.

GROSS LESIONS   With a sliding hernia, the cardia moves upward into the thorax through the dilated hiatus. In the paraesophageal type, a portion of the fundus protrudes through the hiatus adjacent to the esophagus.

MICROSCOPIC LESIONS   Variable degrees of inflammation, both acute and chronic, due to associated reflux esophagitis; ulceration or columnar metaplasia (Barrett's epithelium) may be present.

COMPLICATIONS   Esophagitis, bleeding. Large paraesophageal herniations may compress lung or strangulate and become infarcted.

SIGNS AND SYMPTOMS   Heartburn, regurgitation, exacerbated when lying down; dysphagia, painful swalllowing. Most persons with radiographic evidence of hiatal hernia are asymptomatic.

CLINICAL DIAGNOSIS AND OTHER CLINICAL FEATURES   Suspected on the basis of history; must be differentiated from peptic ulcer pain and angina pectoris; radiographic studies with barium swallow; esophagoscopy with biopsy.

LABORATORY DIAGNOSIS   No specific tests; histologic examination of biopsy shows variable inflammation.

PROGNOSIS   Overall good, but recurrences are expected.

THERAPY   Elevation of head of bed; antacids or H2 blocking agents; surgical correction.

OTHER INFORMATION   Hiatal hernia and reflux esophagitis are not necessarily related, and each can occur independently; surgery for sliding hernia is indicated only if symptoms are not controllable by other means.

Hirschsprung's Disease

DESCRIPTION   Congenital absence of ganglion cells in the rectum and possibly higher segments of the colon, causing dilatation of the colon proximal to the aganglionic segment.

DISEASE ENTITIES; SYNONYMS AND ACRONYMS   Congenital megacolon; aganglionosis of the colon.

INCIDENCE   Uncommon; occurs in 2% of Down's syndrome; 10 times more common in Down's syndrome than normal.

AGE   Usually presents within a few days after birth; others may present in early childhood.

ETIOLOGY, PATHOGENESIS, AND PREDISPOSING FACTORS   Arrest of embryonic caudal migration of neural crest cells that become intramural ganglion cells; the aganglionic segment remains contracted; the proximal segment dilates secondary to the obstruction.

SITES INVOLVED   Rectum is always involved; in one fourth of cases, more proximal portions of the colon are deficient in ganglion cells; in rare cases, the lesion extends to the small bowel.

GROSS LESIONS   Marked dilatation of the proximal segment of colon that narrows rapidly into the distal aganglionic segment; hypertrophy of dilated segment.

MICROSCOPIC LESIONS   Absence of ganglion cells in the distal segment; increase in nonmyelinated fibers in the submucosa and between layers of muscularis; hypertrophic smooth muscle in dilated segment.

COMPLICATIONS   Fecal impaction; colitis with mucosal ulceration and necrosis in the proximal dilated segment; toxic megacolon; perforation of colon leading to peritonitis.

SIGNS AND SYMPTOMS   Delayed passage of meconium with vomiting starting 2–3 days after birth; chronic constipation, abdominal distention, recurrent fecal impaction.

CLINICAL DIAGNOSIS AND OTHER CLINICAL FEATURES   Recognition of typical presentation; barium enema.

LABORATORY DIAGNOSIS   Transmural rectal biopsy that demonstrates absence of ganglion cells.

PROGNOSIS   Usually good with therapy; complication of ulcerating colitis is serious and may be fatal.

THERAPY   Surgical resection of the aganglionic segment with reanastomosis at the distal rectum.

OTHER INFORMATION   Acquired megacolon occurs when there is mechanical obstruction of the colon (e.g., carcinoma, inflammatory bowel disease) or dysfunctional motility.

Ischemic Bowel Disease

DESCRIPTION   A group of intestinal diseases characterized by ischemia of small or large bowel, caused either by intrinsic vascular disease or by extrinsic compression of intestinal blood vessels.

DISEASE ENTITIES; SYNONYMS AND ACRONYMS   Intestinal infarct, gangrene of bowel, ischemic colitis; volvulus, intussusception, incarcerated hernia.

INCIDENCE   Common as a complication of atherosclerosis; volvulus is less common.

AGE   Any age depending on cause; increasing incidence with age, due to incidence of atherosclerosis.

ETIOLOGY, PATHOGENESIS, AND PREDISPOSING FACTORS   Atherosclerosis of celiac axis and mesenteric artery with superimposed thrombus; embolus to mesenteric artery; arteritis; venous thrombus; shock; volvulus; intussusception; incarcerated hernia.

SITES INVOLVED   Occlusion of the superior mesenteric artery (SMA) in half the cases; inferior mesenteric artery occlusion, venous thrombus, or arteritis are found in a quarter; in many cases, no occlusion is found.

GROSS LESIONS   Hemorrhagic infarction of intestine, extent depending on artery occluded; proximal SMA occlusion causes infarction of the entire small bowel and cecum; wall is purple, then green-black with gangrene.

MICROSCOPIC LESIONS   Hemorrhage, necrosis, and acute inflammation of the intestinal wall, first involving mucosa and submucosa and later becoming transmural.

COMPLICATIONS   Intestinal perforation, peritonitis, overwhelming sepsis; bowel gangrene is fatal; chronic ischemia and necrosis that involves less than the entire wall thickness produce fibrosis and strictures.

SIGNS AND SYMPTOMS   Abrupt onset of abdominal pain, bloody diarrhea, hematochezia, shock; chronic ischemic bowel disease is characterized by abdominal (intestinal) angina, which commences shortly after eating.

CLINICAL DIAGNOSIS AND OTHER CLINICAL FEATURES   Prompt recognition of presenting signs and symptoms; arteriography revealing vascular obstruction; laparotomy for acute abdomen quickly reveals necrotic bowel.

LABORATORY DIAGNOSIS   No specific tests; histologic examination confirms the necrosis and may reveal the etiology for the vascular occlusion.

PROGNOSIS   Poor, especially if gangrene develops.

THERAPY   Surgical resection of necrotic bowel; reduction of volvulus, hernia, or intussusception.

OTHER INFORMATION   Certain cases of ischemic colitis, in which only the colonic mucosa suffers ischemic damage, are clinically similar to inflammatory bowel disease; biopsy may be required to establish the diagnosis.

Malabsorption Syndromes

DESCRIPTION Conditions with inadequate absorption of nutrients from the intestine; categorized as generalized malabsorption or as specific (isolated) malabsorption, if only a particular nutrient is involved.

DISEASE ENTITIES; SYNONYMS AND ACRONYMS Celiac disease, chronic pancreatitis, cystic fibrosis, Crohn's disease; abetalipoproteinemia, pernicious anemia.

INCIDENCE Somewhat common, depending on particular condition and nutrient involved.

AGE Any age, depending on condition; cystic fibrosis presents in childhood.

ETIOLOGY, PATHOGENESIS, AND PREDISPOSING FACTORS Gastrectomy; biliary or pancreatic disease (pancreatitis, cystic fibrosis); bacterial overgrowth in small bowel; absent or diseased ileum (Crohn's disease); small intestinal disease (celiac disease).

SITES INVOLVED Primary disease may involve: stomach (intrinsic factor); pancreas (enzymes, especially lipase); biliary system (bile salts); intestinal mucosa (disaccharidase, absorptive area); lymphatics (transport).

GROSS LESIONS See specific primary condition.

MICROSCOPIC LESIONS See specific primary condition.

COMPLICATIONS Malnutrition, cachexia, failure to thrive; macrocytic anemia due to B_{12} deficiency; bleeding diathesis (vitamin K deficiency); tetany, osteomalacia, rickets (vitamin D and calcium deficiency).

SIGNS AND SYMPTOMS Bulky malodorous stools with excessive fat (steatorrhea); diarrhea; signs of specific deficiencies (e.g., anemia, rickets, bleeding tendency, glossitis).

CLINICAL DIAGNOSIS AND OTHER CLINICAL FEATURES Steatorrhea indicates generalized malabsorption; explosive diarrhea: disaccharidase deficiency; chronic diarrhea and macrocytic anemia: disease of ileum (Crohn's disease).

LABORATORY DIAGNOSIS Fecal fat analysis; lactose tolerance test; Schilling test; d-xylose absorption; breath test for radioactive CO_2; sweat chloride test; histology of small bowel biopsy; hypoalbuminemia, hypocalcemia.

PROGNOSIS Often good if the underlying defect can be corrected.

THERAPY Depends on underlying condition, e.g., replacement of pancreatic enzymes, avoidance of gluten.

OTHER INFORMATION Small intestinal disease produces the most severe forms of malabsorption; pancreatic insufficiency usually does not cause malabsorption of fat soluble vitamins, B_{12} or folate.

Malignant Lymphoma of Small Intestine

DESCRIPTION   Primary malignant neoplasm of lymphoid tissue in the small intestine, separated into two major categories: Western type and Mediterranean type; another category affects patients with sprue.

DISEASE ENTITIES; SYNONYMS AND ACRONYMS   Immunoproliferative small intestinal disease, IPSID, heavy-chain disease, alpha-chain disease.

INCIDENCE   Uncommon; accounts for 15% of small bowel cancers in US and two thirds in undeveloped countries.

AGE   Western type: adults over 40 years, children under 10; Mediterranean: men under 40 years.

ETIOLOGY, PATHOGENESIS, AND PREDISPOSING FACTORS   Associated with chronic inflammatory intestinal conditions, such as celiac disease and parasitism, especially with the Mediterranean type; sustained lymphocytic stimulation may induce the neoplasm.

SITES INVOLVED   Western type: usually in ileum; Mediterranean type: predominantly duodenum and proximal jejunum.

GROSS LESIONS   Western: fungating mass projecting into the lumen, with or without ulceration, diffuse thickening of wall, mucosal nodules; Mediterranean: diffuse thickening of long segments of mucosa and submucosa.

MICROSCOPIC LESIONS   Western: any type of non-Hodgkin's malignant lymphoma may be seen (large or small cell, nodular or diffuse); Mediterranean: neoplasm is composed of plasma cells and plasmacytoid lymphocytes.

COMPLICATIONS   Malabsorption, especially with the Mediterranean type; intestinal obstruction; intestinal hemorrhage; intussusception; perforation with peritonitis; extraintestinal spread.

SIGNS AND SYMPTOMS   Chronic abdominal pain, diarrhea, clubbing of fingers, weight loss; signs of malabsorption.

CLINICAL DIAGNOSIS AND OTHER CLINICAL FEATURES   Radiographic studies of small intestine; CT or MRI scans; lesion is usually inaccessible to endoscopy; laparotomy is often required for diagnosis.

LABORATORY DIAGNOSIS   Histology of resected or biopsied lesion; alpha-heavy chains may be detected in serum by immunoelectrophoresis in Mediterranean type lymphoma.

PROGNOSIS   Poor; better for Mediterranean type; with extraintestinal spread, 5-year survival is less than 10%

THERAPY   Surgical resection; radiation therapy; chemotherapy.

OTHER INFORMATION   In the US, primary lymphoma is more common in the stomach than in small intestine; gastric lymphoma must be differentiated from undifferentiated carcinoma because the lymphoma is more treatable.

Meckel's Diverticulum

DESCRIPTION   A true diverticulum of the small intestine caused by persistence of the vitelline duct.

DISEASE ENTITIES; SYNONYMS AND ACRONYMS   True or congenital diverticulum of small intestine.

INCIDENCE   Most common congenital anomaly of the small intestine.

AGE   Any age; found incidentally in adults; presents with symptoms in children under 2 years.

ETIOLOGY, PATHOGENESIS, AND PREDISPOSING FACTORS   Congenital anomaly due to persistence of vitelline duct (omphalomesenteric duct), which is the embryonic communication between the midgut and the yolk sac.

SITES INVOLVED   Ileum of small intestine, 60–100 cm from ileocecal valve, on the antimesenteric border.

GROSS LESIONS   A tubular outpouching of the small intestine, usually about 5 cm in length, containing all layers of the intestinal wall.

MICROSCOPIC LESIONS   Serosa, muscularis, submucosa and normal mucosa are present; occasionally there is ectopic gastric, duodenal, biliary or pancreatic tissue.

COMPLICATIONS   Peptic ulceration with gastrointestinal hemorrhage or perforation with peritonitis; intussusception or volvulus with intestinal obstruction or infarction; diverticulitis.

SIGNS AND SYMPTOMS   Abdominal pain with nausea and vomiting; melena; gastrointestinal bleeding from an occult site. Most cases are asymptomatic.

CLINICAL DIAGNOSIS AND OTHER CLINICAL FEATURES   Often discovered incidentally at autopsy or during laparotomy for unrelated conditions. May be visualized in radiographic examinations of the small bowel using contrast media.

LABORATORY DIAGNOSIS   No specific tests. Histology may confirm the origin and cause of ulceration and bleeding, e.g., from ectopic gastric mucosa.

PROGNOSIS   Good except in the rare cases that cause infarction or peritonitis.

THERAPY   Surgical resection.

OTHER INFORMATION   Ectopic gastric mucosa in a Meckel's diverticulum can be detected by nuclear imaging using radioactive pertechnetate.

Meconium Ileus

DESCRIPTION A characteristic complication of cystic fibrosis where there is intestinal obstruction in the neonate produced by accumulation of thick, viscous, inspissated meconium.

DISEASE ENTITIES; SYNONYMS AND ACRONYMS Meconium ileus of cystic fibrosis.

INCIDENCE Common only in cystic fibrosis patients.

AGE Neonatal period.

ETIOLOGY, PATHOGENESIS, AND PREDISPOSING FACTORS The secretory defect characteristic of cystic fibrosis results in highly viscous, small intestinal mucus that becomes inspissated and fails to pass normally.

SITES INVOLVED Usually the point of obstruction is the midileum. Similar but less serious obstructions occur in the distal colon, which eventually pass without intervention.

GROSS LESIONS Sticky, thick green mucus plug within lumen; distal to the obstruction, the ileum is contracted and proximally it is dilated.

MICROSCOPIC LESIONS No specific features; mucus within the lumen of normal small intestine.

COMPLICATIONS Occur in about half of cases: volvulus, perforation with meconium peritonitis, intestinal atresia.

SIGNS AND SYMPTOMS Failure to pass meconium after birth; abdominal distention.

CLINICAL DIAGNOSIS AND OTHER CLINICAL FEATURES Recognition of clinical presentation.

LABORATORY DIAGNOSIS No specific tests for the obstruction; sweat chloride test may confirm cystic fibrosis.

PROGNOSIS High mortality if complications develop.

THERAPY Detergent hypertonic enema for uncomplicated cases; surgery if complications develop.

OTHER INFORMATION Delayed passage of meconium may be the first indication of cystic fibrosis, which later causes malabsorption and recurrent pulmonary infections.

Peptic Ulcer Disease

DESCRIPTION Ulceration produced by gastric acid, involving mucosa and often deeper layers of stomach or small intestine, due to hypersecretion of gastric acid and/or abnormalities of the mucosa.

DISEASE ENTITIES; SYNONYMS AND ACRONYMS Gastric ulcer, pyloric ulcer, duodenal ulcer; Zollinger-Ellison syndrome; PUD.

INCIDENCE Up to 10% of population at some time during their life; duodenal ulcers affect males predominately.

AGE Duodenal ulcers: 30–60 years; gastric: older age groups, middle aged and elderly.

ETIOLOGY, PATHOGENESIS, AND PREDISPOSING FACTORS Peptic acid and gastrin hypersecretion; gastritis; gastrinoma; accelerated gastric emptying; *Helicobacter pylori;* cirrhosis; chronic renal failure; chronic lung disease; blood group O nonsecretors.

SITES INVOLVED Lesser curvature, antrum or prepyloric region of stomach; first part of the duodenum. In the Zollinger-Ellison syndrome, jejunum may be involved.

GROSS LESIONS Circumscribed ulcer in the mucosa that may extend part or all the way through the wall; gastric ulcers are larger and solitary; duodenal ulcers are smaller and may occur as two (kissing) ulcers.

MICROSCOPIC LESIONS Base of ulcer is covered with fibrinopurulent exudate and necrotic tissue; deeper there is granulation tissue and fibrous scar tissue with chronic and acute inflammation.

COMPLICATIONS Hemorrhage, which may be slow, causing iron-deficiency anemia, or fast, causing shock; perforation leading to peritonitis; pyloric obstruction due to scarring; malignant transformation (a rare event).

SIGNS AND SYMPTOMS Burning epigastric pain starting 1–3 hours after eating or awakening the patient at night, relieved by food or antacids; dyspepsia, i.e., fatty food intolerance, bloating, belching.

CLINICAL DIAGNOSIS AND OTHER CLINICAL FEATURES Recognition of symptoms; radiographic studies; endoscopy. Black tarry stools and coffee ground emesis indicate massive bleeding; pneumoperitoneum (air under the diaphragm) indicates perforation.

LABORATORY DIAGNOSIS Histology of endoscopic biopsy, useful primarily to exclude neoplasia; detection of occult fecal blood; culture or histologic detection of *Helicobacter pylori.*

PROGNOSIS Usually good; massive hemorrhage or perforation carries high mortality.

THERAPY Antacids, H_2-receptor antagonists; surgical partial gastrectomy, antrectomy, vagotomy.

OTHER INFORMATION Gastric ulcers differ from those in the duodenum by their association with decreased acid secretion, reflux of bile into the antrum, and chronic atrophic gastritis.

Peritonitis—Bacterial

DESCRIPTION   Acute inflammatory disease of the peritoneum which may be localized or generalized, caused by bacterial infection introduced most commonly by perforation of a viscus.

DISEASE ENTITIES; SYNONYMS AND ACRONYMS   Generalized or localized peritonitis; spontaneous peritonitis; pelvic peritonitis, pelvic inflammatory disease, PID.

INCIDENCE   Fairly common.

AGE   Any age.

ETIOLOGY, PATHOGENESIS, AND PREDISPOSING FACTORS   Perforated appendix, ulcer, diverticulum; bowel infarct; peritoneal dialysis; nephrotic syndrome; urinary infection; ascites; organisms: *E. coli*, Bacteroides, Staphylococcus, Streptococcus, pneumococcus, gonococcus.

SITES INVOLVED   Peritoneum, entire surface (generalized) or restricted sites (localized); pelvic peritonitis (pelvic inflammatory disease) results from gonococcal or other types of salpingitis.

GROSS LESIONS   Fibrinopurulent exudate covering peritoneal surface, between loops of bowel, and often collecting in the pouch of Douglas; exudate becomes organized and fibrotic, leading to adhesions.

MICROSCOPIC LESIONS   PMNs and fibrin covering serosal surface with various stages of organization indicated by the presence of granulation tissue and fibrosis.

COMPLICATIONS   Septic shock; peritoneal abscess; obstruction or volvulus caused by fibrous adhesions.

SIGNS AND SYMPTOMS   Diffuse abdominal pain and tenderness; rebound tenderness; high fever; paralytic ileus; septic shock.

CLINICAL DIAGNOSIS AND OTHER CLINICAL FEATURES   Recognition of signs and symptoms that indicate an acute abdomen, which requires surgical intervention; diagnosis is confirmed by laparotomy at which time the cause is usually determined.

LABORATORY DIAGNOSIS   Microbiologic cultures.

PROGNOSIS   50% mortality with generalized peritonitis; PID is usually successfully treated.

THERAPY   Antibiotics, supportive measures; surgical drainage, repair of perforation or resection of infarct.

OTHER INFORMATION   Chemical peritonitis is a noninfectious inflammation caused by bile leakage from a perforated gallbladder, by pancreatitis, or by other substances such as talc, gastric acid, blood, foreign material.

Polyps of Colon—Adenomatous

DESCRIPTION   Benign neoplastic mass of colonic epithelium protruding from the mucosal surface; classified as sessile or pedunculated and as villous, tubular, or tubulovillous.

DISEASE ENTITIES; SYNONYMS AND ACRONYMS   Colonic polyps; tubular adenomas, villous adenomas, tubulovillous adenomas.

INCIDENCE   Very common; two thirds of population over 65 may have at least one polyp; male:female = 1.4:1.

AGE   Increasing incidence with age in adults.

ETIOLOGY, PATHOGENESIS, AND PREDISPOSING FACTORS   Low-fiber, high animal-fat diet; autosomal dominant genetic diseases, familial polyposis coli and Gardner's syndrome, develop numerous polyps; rare Turcot's syndrome is polyposis with CNS tumors.

SITES INVOLVED   Any part of colon, particularly the rectosigmoid region. Lesions involve mucosa only.

GROSS LESIONS   Tubular: smooth spherical pedunculated mass usually less than 2 cm in diameter; villous: flat sessile shaggy masses, often greater than 2 cm; tubulovillous: similar to the tubular type, only larger.

MICROSCOPIC LESIONS   Tubular: round or elongated glands on fibrovascular stalk lined by colonic epithelium: villous: long finger-like projections arising from the colonic surface; tubulovillous: features of both.

COMPLICATIONS   Adenocarcinoma, particularly with villous adenoma; intestinal bleeding leading to anemia; profuse diarrhea, hypokalemia, and intussusception with large villous adenomas.

SIGNS AND SYMPTOMS   Often asymptomatic and discovered during rectal or colonic examination; bleeding, either obvious or occult; anemia; abdominal pain; diarrhea.

CLINICAL DIAGNOSIS AND OTHER CLINICAL FEATURES   Rectal examination, proctoscopy, sigmoidoscopy, colonoscopy; x-rays with barium enema.

LABORATORY DIAGNOSIS   Histologic examination of resected polyp is important to exclude invasive carcinoma, particularly if the invasion involves the stalk or goes beyond the muscularis mucosae.

PROGNOSIS   Good, if resected before invasive carcinoma extending beyond the muscularis mucosae develops.

THERAPY   Polypectomy through sigmoidoscope or colonoscope; a large villous adenoma may require laparotomy.

OTHER INFORMATION   Carcinoma, in situ or invasive, may be found in any adenoma; the chance increases with size and if the polyp is villous. Up to 50% of villous adenomas greater than 2 cm contain invasive carcinoma.

Polyps of Colon—Nonneoplastic

DESCRIPTION Raised lesions protruding from the surface of the colonic mucosa, derived from hyperplasia of epithelium or lymphoid tissue, hamartomatous proliferation, or inflammation.

DISEASE ENTITIES; SYNONYMS AND ACRONYMS Hyperplastic (metaplastic) polyps, juvenile (retention) polyps, inflammatory polyps, lymphoid polyps.

INCIDENCE Common; the most common in this group is the hyperplastic polyp.

AGE Hyperplastic: adults; juvenile: usually children; inflammatory: usually adults; lymphoid: any age.

ETIOLOGY, PATHOGENESIS, AND PREDISPOSING FACTORS Hyperplastic: epithelial maturation defect; juvenile: hamartomatous overgrowth of mucosa; inflammatory: regeneration of epithelium plus granulation tissue; lymphoid: hyperplasia of lymphoid tissue.

SITES INVOLVED Hyperplastic: any site, particularly rectum, especially around cancers or adenomas; juvenile: usually rectum; inflammatory: any site; lymphoid: any site, most prominently rectum.

GROSS LESIONS Hyperplastic: sessile raised lesions less than 0.5 cm; juvenile: pedunculated nodules up to 2 cm; inflammatory: mucosal masses surrounded by ulcer; lymphoid: small sessile nodules, rarely up to 5 cm.

MICROSCOPIC LESIONS Hyperplastic: elongated crypts, sawtooth surface; juvenile: dilated, cystic tubules in fibrous stroma; inflammatory: inflamed mucosa, granulation tissue; lymphoid: hyperplastic lymphoid follicles.

COMPLICATIONS Associated problems are usually insignificant; lesions should not be confused with neoplasms, preneoplastic conditions, or cancers; juvenile polyps may cause rectal bleeding.

SIGNS AND SYMPTOMS Hyperplastic: asymptomatic; juvenile: rectal bleeding, prolapse into rectum; inflammatory: symptoms of underlying inflammatory bowel disease; lymphoid: usually asymptomatic.

CLINICAL DIAGNOSIS AND OTHER CLINICAL FEATURES Rectal examination, proctoscopy, sigmoidoscopy, colonoscopy; x-rays with barium enema.

LABORATORY DIAGNOSIS Histologic examination of biopsied or resected specimen.

PROGNOSIS Good.

THERAPY Usually none; juvenile polyps may be removed through the proctoscope.

OTHER INFORMATION Inflammatory polyps are often associated with ulcerative colitis or Crohn's disease; hyperplastic polyps are not preneoplastic, although they are often seen near carcinomas and adenomas.

Pseudomembranous Enterocolitis

DESCRIPTION   Inflammatory disease of the colon, characterized by an edematous congested mucosa superficially covered by plaques of pseudomembrane containing mucus, fibrin, PMNs, and necrotic cellular debris.

DISEASE ENTITIES; SYNONYMS AND ACRONYMS   Pseudomembranous enteritis or colitis, antibiotic enterocolitis, staphylococcal enterocolitis (outdated and incorrect).

INCIDENCE   Fairly common in hospitalized patients on antibiotics.

AGE   Any age.

ETIOLOGY, PATHOGENESIS, AND PREDISPOSING FACTORS   Toxins of *Clostridium difficile*; antibiotic therapy, particularly clindamycin and lincomycin; also ampicillin and cephalosporins; gastrointestinal surgery; other intestinal and systemic diseases.

SITES INVOLVED   Large intestine mucosa, particularly in the rectosigmoid colon; small intestine may also be involved, either alone or in combination with the colon.

GROSS LESIONS   Mucosa is swollen and red; pseudomembranes appear as raised yellow plaques adherent to the mucosa, ranging in size from 2 cm to extensive involvement of the mucosa.

MICROSCOPIC LESIONS   Superficial epithelium is denuded and necrotic; disrupted crypts are filled with mucus and PMNs; adherent plaques and pseudomembranes contain PMNs, fibrin, mucus, and necrotic debris.

COMPLICATIONS   Fluid loss, electrolyte imbalance; dehydration, shock; sepsis.

SIGNS AND SYMPTOMS   Watery diarrhea containing pus, mucus, and sometimes blood; fever, leukocytosis, abdominal cramps.

CLINICAL DIAGNOSIS AND OTHER CLINICAL FEATURES   Suspicion regarding the onset of diarrhea in a patient treated with antibiotics or otherwise predisposed by GI surgery or intestinal disease; sigmoidoscopy reveals the presence of pseudomembranes.

LABORATORY DIAGNOSIS   Stool culture; detection of toxin in the feces; histology of colonic biopsy shows the characteristic features and serves to exclude other causes for the colitis.

PROGNOSIS   Mortality is high with severe cases; early recognition and therapy improves recovery rate.

THERAPY   Withdrawal of agent; vancomycin, metronidazole, or bacitracin; fluid and electrolyte replacement.

OTHER INFORMATION   Diarrhea develops in up to 20% of patients treated with clindamycin; 10% of these progress to pseudomembranous enterocolitis.

Pyloric Stenosis—Congenital

DESCRIPTION   Obstruction of the outlet of the stomach due to congenital hypertrophy of smooth muscle of the pyloric sphincter.

DISEASE ENTITIES; SYNONYMS AND ACRONYMS   Hypertrophic pyloric stenosis.

INCIDENCE   One in 250–300 births; rare in blacks and Asians; male:female = 4:1; mostly affects first-borns.

AGE   Becomes apparent within the first month of life.

ETIOLOGY, PATHOGENESIS, AND PREDISPOSING FACTORS   Unknown; may be genetic; occasionally associated with other congenital anomalies, maternal rubella, or thalidomide; gastrin administered to pregnant dogs causes pyloric stenosis in their litters.

SITES INVOLVED   Smooth muscle of pylorus.

GROSS LESIONS   Concentric enlargement of the pylorus with narrowing of the pyloric canal and distention of the stomach.

MICROSCOPIC LESIONS   Hypertrophy of the pyloric smooth muscle.

COMPLICATIONS   Gastric outlet obstruction leading to malnutrition and fluid and electrolyte abnormalities.

SIGNS AND SYMPTOMS   Projectile vomiting starting in the first month of life; after vomiting, the infant is hungry and feeds actively; pyloric tumor and active peristalsis are apparent in the epigastrium.

CLINICAL DIAGNOSIS AND OTHER CLINICAL FEATURES   Recognition of the clinical presentation; palpation of the epigastric tumor; observation of the hyperactive peristalsis. X-rays with contrast media in the stomach show the stenosis and obstruction.

LABORATORY DIAGNOSIS   There may be electrolyte abnormalities (hypochloremic alkalosis) due to prolonged vomiting.

PROGNOSIS   Good, with surgery.

THERAPY   Surgical pyloromyotomy.

OTHER INFORMATION   Pyloric stenosis in adults is usually caused by scarring from peptic ulcer disease; other causes may be mild congenital stenosis or pyloric stenosis due to pyloric spasm with an ulcer.

Smooth Muscle Tumors

DESCRIPTION   Benign or malignant neoplasms of smooth muscle origin, located and arising within the wall of the esophagus, stomach, or intestine.

DISEASE ENTITIES; SYNONYMS AND ACRONYMS   Leiomyoma; leiomyoblastoma (epithelioid leiomyoma); leiomyosarcoma.

INCIDENCE   Leiomyomas are the most common tumor of stomach; small intestinal leiomyomas are fairly common.

AGE   Increasing incidence with age.

ETIOLOGY, PATHOGENESIS, AND PREDISPOSING FACTORS   Neoplastic disease of unknown etiology.

SITES INVOLVED   Wall of esophagus, stomach or small intestine, usually the jejunum; leiomyoblastoma (epithelioid leiomyoma) is a variant peculiar to the stomach.

GROSS LESIONS   Leiomyoma: firm, circumscribed nodular mass within the wall, a few millimeters to 20 cm in size, covered by mucosa; leiomyosarcoma: similar shape, usually larger, necrosis and invasive margins may be present.

MICROSCOPIC LESIONS   Whorling interlaced bundles of spindle-shaped cells; cellularity, hyperchromasia and pleomorphism are variable; leiomyosarcoma has more mitoses than leiomyoma; leiomyoblastoma has polygonal cells.

COMPLICATIONS   Mucosal ulceration, gastrointestinal bleeding, pain; intestinal obstruction, volvulus; local spread or metastasis to lungs and other sites with the malignant tumors.

SIGNS AND SYMPTOMS   Substernal or epigastric pain that may mimic peptic ulcer; dysphagia, difficulty swallowing; chronic blood loss anemia; the smaller tumors are often asymptomatic.

CLINICAL DIAGNOSIS AND OTHER CLINICAL FEATURES   X-rays with contrast in the lumen (barium swallow, upper GI series); by endoscopy, recognition of a mass covered by mucosa. Most gastric leiomyomas are small and clinically insignificant.

LABORATORY DIAGNOSIS   Histologic examination of biopsied or resected tumor. Endoscopic biopsy must be sufficiently deep to sample the submucosal mass.

PROGNOSIS   Excellent for leiomyoma; poor for leiomyosarcoma (25–50% 5-year survival rate).

THERAPY   Surgical excision.

OTHER INFORMATION   It may be difficult to differentiate a leiomyosarcoma from a leiomyoma; the most reliable criterion is the mitotic count. These tumors are unpredictable; seemingly benign tumors may metastasize.

Tracheoesophageal Fistula

DESCRIPTION   Congenital esophageal anomaly in which there is an abnormal communication between the lower portion of the esophagus and the trachea, often combined with some form of esophageal atresia.

DISEASE ENTITIES; SYNONYMS AND ACRONYMS   T-E fistula; VATER syndrome.

INCIDENCE   The most common esophageal anomaly and one of the most common congenital defects.

AGE   Recognized in the neonatal period.

ETIOLOGY, PATHOGENESIS, AND PREDISPOSING FACTORS   Congenital disease; etiology unknown.

SITES INVOLVED   Esophagus and trachea.

GROSS LESIONS   In 90% the esophagus ends in a blind pouch; the distal portion communicates with the trachea. Less often, the proximal esophagus communicates with the trachea or the esophagus is continuous (H-type).

MICROSCOPIC LESIONS   Section through the fistula may show transition between respiratory columnar and squamous mucosa.

COMPLICATIONS   Aspiration pneumonia, especially if the proximal esophagus communicates with the trachea or if there is an H-type fistula.

SIGNS AND SYMPTOMS   Aspiration of milk during initial feeding with coughing, asphyxia, choking; development of pneumonia. Rarely a small lesion escapes detection until adulthood, causing repeated pulmonary infections.

CLINICAL DIAGNOSIS AND OTHER CLINICAL FEATURES   Suspected on the basis of characteristic clinical presentation; confirmed by radiographic studies using contrast media introduced into the esophagus.

LABORATORY DIAGNOSIS   No specific laboratory tests.

PROGNOSIS   Good if recognized early to avoid feedings causing aspiration.

THERAPY   Surgical anastomosis of proximal with distal esophagus and ablation of fistula.

OTHER INFORMATION   The VATER syndrome is a complex of anomalies with vertebral defects, anal atresia, tracheal-esophageal fistula, and renal dysplasia.

Ulcerative Colitis

DESCRIPTION   Inflammatory bowel disease characterized by recurrent episodes of colonic and rectal mucosal ulceration with rectal bleeding, bloody stools, abdominal pain, fever, and occasionally massive bleeding.

DISEASE ENTITIES; SYNONYMS AND ACRONYMS   Ulcerative proctitis, pancolitis, inflammatory bowel disease, UC, IBD.

INCIDENCE   4–7/100,000; females and males equally; US whites more than blacks.

AGE   Usually begins in early adult life; peak incidence in 30s.

ETIOLOGY, PATHOGENESIS, AND PREDISPOSING FACTORS   Unknown; there are various speculations regarding viral or bacterial agents (especially *C. difficile*), psychosomatic factors, and immune cross-reactions between shared bacterial and mucosal antigens.

SITES INVOLVED   Involvement starts at the most distal part of the rectum and extends continuously for a variable distance proximally, depending on the severity of the disease, as far as the ileocecal junction.

GROSS LESIONS   Early disease: mucosa is hyperemic, granular, edematous; advanced disease: crater-like ulcers surround islands of mucosa, forming pseudopolyps; long-standing disease: mucosa is flat and atrophic.

MICROSCOPIC LESIONS   Congestion, edema, diffuse inflammation of mucosa; crypt abscesses; ulcers through part or all of the mucosa; inflammatory polyps; granulation tissue in base of ulcers; focal epithelial dysplasia.

COMPLICATIONS   Massive intestinal hemorrhage with shock and sepsis; anemia; toxic megacolon with perforation; colon cancer; uveitis; erythema nodosum, pyoderma gangrenosum; liver disease; deep leg vein thrombosis.

SIGNS AND SYMPTOMS   Severity ranges from mild to fulminant: intermittent rectal bleeding; recurrent bloody stools with abdominal cramps and fever; massive bloody diarrhea with hypovolemic and septic shock.

CLINICAL DIAGNOSIS AND OTHER CLINICAL FEATURES   Barium enema x-rays; sigmoidoscopy, colonoscopy; differential: Crohn's disease, bacterial or amebic dysentery, opportunistic infections due to AIDS, ischemic colitis.

LABORATORY DIAGNOSIS   Stool culture, fecal examination for ameba and other parasites (to exclude other diseases); histology of colonic mucosal biopsy or resected colon.

PROGNOSIS   10% of patients with UC have fulminant disease: 15% of those with fulminant UC die of complications.

THERAPY   Steroids, other anti-inflammatory drugs; colectomy for toxic megacolon or for prevention of cancer.

OTHER INFORMATION   Differentiation of UC from Crohn's: diffuse disease (UC), patchy (Crohn's); mucosal inflammation (UC), transmural (Crohn's); colon only (UC), small bowel also (Crohn's); granulomas (Crohn's).

Pathology Facts, by Richard C.
Harruff, J.B. Lippincott
Company, Philadelphia © 1994.

Chapter 15

Liver, Biliary Tract, and Pancreas

Alcoholic Liver Disease

DESCRIPTION   Liver diseases produced by excessive consumption of ethanol, including fatty liver, alcoholic hepatitis, and cirrhosis.

DISEASE ENTITIES; SYNONYMS AND ACRONYMS   Fatty liver, steatosis; alcoholic hepatitis; Laennec's cirrhosis, micronodular cirrhosis, alcoholic cirrhosis.

INCIDENCE   Common; about 15% of alcoholics develop cirrhosis. Alcoholism causes 70% of cases of cirrhosis.

AGE   Middle-aged adults, usually males.

ETIOLOGY, PATHOGENESIS, AND PREDISPOSING FACTORS   Ethyl alcohol: a pint of whiskey (approximately 80 grams of ethanol) per day for 10–15 years is considered a threshold for development of cirrhosis.

SITES INVOLVED   Liver, hepatocytes.

GROSS LESIONS   Fatty liver: enlarged, yellow, and greasy; hepatitis may also show fatty enlargement; cirrhosis is micronodular.

MICROSCOPIC LESIONS   Fatty liver: hepatocytes distended with fat, displacing nucleus to side; hepatitis: hepatocellular necrosis, acute inflammation, alcoholic hyaline (Mallory bodies); cirrhosis: micronodular pattern.

COMPLICATIONS   Fatty liver: reversible with abstinence, associated with sudden death; alcoholic hepatitis: hepatic failure; cirrhosis: portal hypertension, ascites and esophageal varices, progressive liver failure.

SIGNS AND SYMPTOMS   Fatty liver: hepatic enlargement; hepatitis: anorexia, malaise, fever, right upper abdominal pain, jaundice; cirrhosis: ascites, GI bleeding, liver failure, palmar erythema, spider angiomas.

CLINICAL DIAGNOSIS AND OTHER CLINICAL FEATURES   Recognition of signs and symptoms in an alcoholic; amount of alcohol consumption may be denied by patient.

LABORATORY DIAGNOSIS   Hyperbilirubinemia, elevated aminotransferases and alkaline phosphatase indicate hepatitis; tests may be normal with fatty liver; laboratory values in cirrhosis are variable.

PROGNOSIS   Depends on abstinence; poor for cirrhosis; fatty liver and alcoholic hepatitis may recover fully.

THERAPY   Abstinence; treatment of complications of cirrhosis; liver transplantation.

OTHER INFORMATION   Uncontrolled diabetes mellitus, kwashiorkor, pregnancy, obesity, and prolonged steroid therapy are other causes of fatty liver.

Bacterial Infections of Liver

DESCRIPTION Bacterial infection of liver characterized by suppuration, often caused by spread from intra-abdominal infection, from biliary obstruction with secondary infection, or complicating sepsis.

DISEASE ENTITIES; SYNONYMS AND ACRONYMS Pyogenic liver abscess, pylephlebic abscess; ascending cholangitis, cholangitic abscess.

INCIDENCE Uncommon in US; often regarded as complications of other diseases.

AGE Any age depending on etiology; most likely in adults.

ETIOLOGY, PATHOGENESIS, AND PREDISPOSING FACTORS Gram-negative and anaerobic organisms; spread via portal vein from appendicitis, peritonitis, or diverticulitis; via arterial blood in sepsis; via biliary tract in obstruction; 50% are cryptogenic.

SITES INVOLVED Liver, portal vein, extra- and intrahepatic biliary system.

GROSS LESIONS Abscess: single or multiple foci of suppuration with central liquefaction, usually in the right lobe; may be up to several centimeters in diameter and is often multiloculated.

MICROSCOPIC LESIONS Cholangitis: acute inflammatory cells within portal bile ducts, edema of the portal triad; suppuration may rupture through the bile ducts and produce pericholangitis and abscesses.

COMPLICATIONS Rupture and spread of infection leading to pleuropulmonary fistula, empyema, or peritonitis; septicemia and metastatic abscesses in other parts of body.

SIGNS AND SYMPTOMS Right upper quadrant pain, hepatomegaly, high spiking fever; jaundice with cholangitis, less often with abscess; abdominal pain may be absent in half of cases of abscess.

CLINICAL DIAGNOSIS AND OTHER CLINICAL FEATURES Recognition of localizing signs, especially in a patient with abdominal sepsis or biliary obstruction; radiographic imaging (ultrasound, MRI, CT scans) readily detect an abscess.

LABORATORY DIAGNOSIS Elevated bilirubin (in 25% of cases); elevated liver enzymes, particularly alkaline phosphatase; leukocytosis; liver biopsy showing ascending cholangitis; blood cultures may be positive.

PROGNOSIS High mortality, 40–80%; may be lower with early diagnosis and aggressive therapy.

THERAPY Surgical drainage, which is often percutaneous; antibiotics.

OTHER INFORMATION Most abscesses involve enteric bacteria; two thirds are polymicrobial and one third contain anaerobes; *S. aureus* sometimes causes abscesses in septicemia.

Carcinoma of Pancreas

DESCRIPTION   Primary malignant tumor of pancreas, usually adenocarcinoma arising from pancreatic ducts.

DISEASE ENTITIES; SYNONYMS AND ACRONYMS   Adenocarcinoma of pancreas, pancreatic cancer.

INCIDENCE   Fourth most common cause of cancer death; highest in men, blacks, Native Americans, Polynesians.

AGE   Highest incidence in ages over 60 years.

ETIOLOGY, PATHOGENESIS, AND PREDISPOSING FACTORS   Chronic gallbladder disease, diabetes mellitus, chronic hereditary pancreatitis; cigarette smoking; diets high in meat and fat; occupational exposure to carcinogens (e.g., beta-naphthylamine).

SITES INVOLVED   Head of pancreas, 60% of cases; body, 13%; tail, 5%; in 22% the entire pancreas is diffusely involved.

GROSS LESIONS   Hard nodular mass with ill-defined borders invading pancreatic parenchyma; tumors in the head are usually smaller than those in other locations; extensive spread throughout peritoneum is common.

MICROSCOPIC LESIONS   Most (75%) are well-differentiated adenocarcinomas secreting mucin; a dense collagenous desmoplastic stroma is common.

COMPLICATIONS   Obstructive jaundice especially with tumors of the head; widespread metastasis, commonly to liver, lung, and peritoneum; intestinal obstruction; migratory thrombophlebitis (Trousseau's sign); cachexia.

SIGNS AND SYMPTOMS   Anorexia, weight loss; epigastric pain radiating to back; jaundice with acute painless dilatation of gallbladder (Courvoisier's sign); carcinomas of the head are detected early due to jaundice.

CLINICAL DIAGNOSIS AND OTHER CLINICAL FEATURES   Except for those in the head presenting early with jaundice, many are silent and are advanced when first discovered; ultrasonography, CT or MRI scans localize the tumor; laparotomy confirms diagnosis.

LABORATORY DIAGNOSIS   Histologic examination of pancreatic biopsy from laparotomy or laparoscopy; needle biopsy of liver or other metastatic site; fine needle aspiration cytology performed under CT or ultrasound guidance.

PROGNOSIS   Dismal; 2% 5-year survival; slightly better survival with cancers involving the head.

THERAPY   Surgical pancreatoduodenectomy (Whipple procedure); chemotherapy, support, and palliation.

OTHER INFORMATION   One of the earliest symptoms, pain, is due to extrapancreatic spread; thus, most cancers with this symptom are unresectable.

Cholecystitis—Acute

DESCRIPTION   Acute inflammatory condition of the gallbladder with secondary bacterial infection. Most cases are associated with gallstones; less than 5–10% are acalculous.

DISEASE ENTITIES; SYNONYMS AND ACRONYMS   Empyema of the gallbladder; gangrenous cholecystitis.

INCIDENCE   Develops in less than 20% of cases of cholelithiasis.

AGE   As with cholelithiasis, incidence increases with age.

ETIOLOGY, PATHOGENESIS, AND PREDISPOSING FACTORS   Obstruction of cystic duct by gallstone leads to stasis and degradation of bile components into toxic and irritating products; bacterial infection is secondary to the obstruction, not a primary event.

SITES INVOLVED   Gallbladder, cystic duct.

GROSS LESIONS   Distended gallbladder with congested wall covered with fibrinous exudate; wall is thickened with edema; mucosa is ulcerated; contents may be purulent (empyema); gangrene or perforation may develop.

MICROSCOPIC LESIONS   Acute inflammatory cellular reaction, starting in the ulcerated mucosa, with edema and congestion throughout the wall; transmural necrosis is seen in gangrenous cholecystitis.

COMPLICATIONS   Gangrene of gallbladder, bacterial sepsis; perforation, peritonitis; pericholecystic abscess; cholecystenteric fistula; emphysematous cholecystitis with gas-forming bacteria.

SIGNS AND SYMPTOMS   Nausea, vomiting, fever, abdominal pain, tender right upper quadrant; gallbladder may be palpable; biliary colic refers to intense pain.

CLINICAL DIAGNOSIS AND OTHER CLINICAL FEATURES   Clinical presentation; cholescintigraphy, ultrasonography, abdominal x-rays; gallbladder usually will not visualize with oral cystogram.

LABORATORY DIAGNOSIS   Leukocytosis; hyperbilirubinemia, elevated amylase; microbiologic culture from resected specimen.

PROGNOSIS   Usually good with acute attacks resolving spontaneously; complications are often quite serious.

THERAPY   Antibiotics and medical support; cholecystectomy after acute inflammation subsides.

OTHER INFORMATION   Differential includes peptic ulcer, acute appendicitis, acute pyelonephritis, acute pancreatitis, myocardial infarction, and acute hepatitis.

Cholelithiasis

DESCRIPTION Gallstones in the lumen of the gallbladder or extrahepatic biliary system. Most stones are composed predominantly of cholesterol; the less common pigment stones are composed of bilirubin salts.

DISEASE ENTITIES; SYNONYMS AND ACRONYMS Gallstones; cholesterol stones or calculi; pigment stones; mixed stones; gallbladder disease; chronic cholecystitis.

INCIDENCE Common; female:male = 3:1; particularly common in Native American Indians (Pima Indians).

AGE Increasing incidence with age; 20% of men and 35% of women over 75 years have gallstones at autopsy.

ETIOLOGY, PATHOGENESIS, AND PREDISPOSING FACTORS High bile cholesterol (hyperlipidemia, obesity, diabetes); low bile salts (hydroxylase deficiency, malabsorption); estrogens (pregnancy, oral contraceptives); hemolytic anemia (pigment stones).

SITES INVOLVED Gallbladder lumen, cystic duct; common bile duct (choledocholithiasis), usually at the juncture with the ampulla of Vater.

GROSS LESIONS Cholesterol stones are pale yellow to green, round or multifaceted, with a radial crystalline cut surface; pigment stones are green-black and amorphous in composition.

MICROSCOPIC LESIONS Collections of lipid-laden foamy macrophages may be present in the gallbladder mucosa, a condition called cholesterolosis; chronic cholecystitis is frequently present.

COMPLICATIONS Obstruction of cystic duct or common bile duct; biliary colic, acute cholecystitis, chronic cholecystitis; obstructive jaundice, ascending cholangitis, pancreatitis; hydrops (mucocele) of gallbladder.

SIGNS AND SYMPTOMS Most gallstones remain asymptomatic (silent); approximately only 20% develop serious complications; one third have symptoms of biliary colic or chronic cholecystitis with right upper quadrant pain.

CLINICAL DIAGNOSIS AND OTHER CLINICAL FEATURES Investigation of abdominal pain; few gallstones are radiopaque (15%, usually pigment stones containing calcium); cholecystogram with contrast agent and ultrasonography may visualize the others.

LABORATORY DIAGNOSIS Bilirubin and alkaline phosphatase may be elevated with stones impacted in the common bile duct.

PROGNOSIS Usually good unless complications of bacterial infection develop in a compromised patient.

THERAPY Cholecystectomy; oral administration of bile acids; percutaneous cholesterol solvent; lithotripsy.

OTHER INFORMATION Chronic cholecystitis usually accompanies cholelithiasis; the gallbladder is thickened, fibrotic, rigid, and may calcify (porcelain gallbladder).

Chronic Hepatitis

DESCRIPTION Persistent inflammation with necrosis of the liver lasting for more than 6 months, caused by viral infections, hepatotoxic drugs, autoimmune disease, or unknown etiology.

DISEASE ENTITIES; SYNONYMS AND ACRONYMS Chronic persistent hepatitis, chronic active (aggressive) hepatitis, lupoid hepatitis, autoimmune hepatitis.

INCIDENCE Common chronic liver disease; complicates 5–10% of hepatitis B, at least 20% of hepatitis C (NANB).

AGE Any age; more common in adults.

ETIOLOGY, PATHOGENESIS, AND PREDISPOSING FACTORS Previous viral hepatitis (B, C, or NANB); autoimmune disease, commonly with HLA-B8; isoniazid, methyldopa; Wilson's disease, alpha-1-antitrypsin deficiency; most cases are idiopathic.

SITES INVOLVED Liver; portal tracts, and surrounding hepatocytes.

GROSS LESIONS Liver may be grossly normal or enlarged; macronodular cirrhosis or hepatocellular carcinoma may be present.

MICROSCOPIC LESIONS Chronic persistent: lymphocytic inflammation limited to portal tracts; chronic active: portal inflammation plus "piece-meal" periportal necrosis along with focal lobular necrosis and inflammation.

COMPLICATIONS Cirrhosis with portal hypertension; hepatocellular carcinoma, especially if etiologically related to HBV; hepatic failure with coma and coagulopathy.

SIGNS AND SYMPTOMS Anorexia, malaise; jaundice, hepatomegaly; signs of portal hypertension as cirrhosis develops.

CLINICAL DIAGNOSIS AND OTHER CLINICAL FEATURES Suspicion regarding presenting signs and symptoms, confirmed by laboratory tests and liver biopsy; follow-up of cases of acute hepatitis for 6 months to a year.

LABORATORY DIAGNOSIS Persistent elevation of serum aminotransferases; alkaline phosphatase mildly elevated; hyperbilirubinemia. After hepatitis B: HBeAg in serum, HBsAb absent. Autoimmune type: antinuclear antibodies.

PROGNOSIS Chronic active hepatitis progresses to cirrhosis; chronic persistent does not progress.

THERAPY Supportive; some cases, especially lupoid hepatitis, respond to steroid therapy.

OTHER INFORMATION Most cases with known etiology (10–20%) are positive for HBsAg, and most of these lack HBsAb; if HBsAb is present, it has the wrong subtype specificity.

Cirrhosis

DESCRIPTION   End-stage liver disease in which the normal hepatic architecture is destroyed and replaced by bands of fibrous scar tissue encircling nodules of regenerating hepatocytes.

DISEASE ENTITIES; SYNONYMS AND ACRONYMS   Micronodular cirrhosis: alcoholic, Laennec's cirrhosis; macronodular cirrhosis: posthepatitic, postnecrotic cirrhosis.

INCIDENCE   Most common chronic liver disease; 70% of cases are caused by alcoholism.

AGE   Usually adults; occasionally children, depending on the etiology of the liver disease.

ETIOLOGY, PATHOGENESIS, AND PREDISPOSING FACTORS   Alcoholism, viral or chronic active hepatitis, primary biliary cirrhosis, extrahepatic biliary obstruction, hemochromatosis, cystic fibrosis, alpha-1-antitrypsin deficiency, Wilson's disease, others.

SITES INVOLVED   Liver, both parenchyma and connective tissue stroma. Obliteration and disorganization of the normal vascular architecture causes portal hypertension.

GROSS LESIONS   Diffuse nodularity replacing normal liver; micronodular: nodules predominantly 3 mm or smaller; macronodular: nodules greater than 3 mm; mixed: nodules in both size ranges.

MICROSCOPIC LESIONS   Regenerating nodules of hepatocytes lacking normal organization, surrounded by bands of fibrous tissue where there is variable inflammation and proliferation of bile ductules.

COMPLICATIONS   Portal hypertension with ascites and esophageal varices; gastrointestinal bleeding from ruptured varices; hepatic failure with coma and coagulopathy.

SIGNS AND SYMPTOMS   Ascites, splenomegaly, gynecomastia in males, jaundice, other signs of liver failure; sudden onset of upper GI bleeding; many cases are silent until complications develop.

CLINICAL DIAGNOSIS AND OTHER CLINICAL FEATURES   Investigation of chronic liver disease, often confirmed by liver biopsy. Splenomegaly indicates portal hypertension.

LABORATORY DIAGNOSIS   Bilirubin and liver enzymes may be elevated, depending on the etiology and stage of disease; liver biopsy is the most specific diagnostic test.

PROGNOSIS   Poor, although survival may be prolonged.

THERAPY   Supportive with treatment of complications; portasystemic shunts; liver transplantation.

OTHER INFORMATION   Micronodular cirrhosis is associated with alcoholic hepatitis, antitrypsin deficiency, and hemochromatosis; macronodular follows viral hepatitis; micronodular cirrhosis progresses to macronodular.

Hemochromatosis

DESCRIPTION Accumulation of excess iron within all cells of the body, due to excessive intake or unregulated intestinal absorption, causing cirrhosis, pancreatic fibrosis with diabetes, and cardiac dysfunction.

DISEASE ENTITIES; SYNONYMS AND ACRONYMS Primary hemochromatosis; secondary hemochromatosis; hemosiderosis, siderosis; bronze diabetes.

INCIDENCE Gene frequency is .056; homozygous, 1 per 200–400; male:female > 5:1; clinical disease is less common.

AGE Increasing incidence with age due to the long time required to accumulate the iron; 40–60 years.

ETIOLOGY, PATHOGENESIS, AND PREDISPOSING FACTORS Primary: autosomal recessive defect in regulation of intestinal iron absorption; secondary: excessive iron consumption in food or alcoholic beverages, refractory anemias, multiple blood transfusions.

SITES INVOLVED Parenchymal cells of liver, pancreas, heart, skin (especially sweat glands), and pituitary gland; macrophages in bone marrow and throughout body; gene is on chromosome 6, linked to HLA-A3.

GROSS LESIONS Rusty discoloration of affected organs, especially liver, pancreas, and heart. Liver shows micronodular cirrhosis; pancreas is fibrotic. Skin coloration is due to melanin hyperpigmentation.

MICROSCOPIC LESIONS Brownish intracellular hemosiderin pigment that stains with Prussian blue; deposition is largely parenchymal in the primary form, within macrophages in the secondary forms. Cirrhosis is micronodular.

COMPLICATIONS Complications of cirrhosis (varices, GI bleeding, ascites); diabetes mellitus; cardiac failure; arthropathy; testicular atrophy; hepatocellular carcinoma in 10–20% of cases.

SIGNS AND SYMPTOMS Skin pigmentation and diabetes (bronze diabetes); signs of cirrhosis or hepatic failure; heart failure.

CLINICAL DIAGNOSIS AND OTHER CLINICAL FEATURES Suspicion of presenting signs, confirmed by laboratory tests.

LABORATORY DIAGNOSIS Elevated serum iron, transferrin, and especially ferritin; liver biopsy shows cirrhosis with hemosiderin in hepatocytes and macrophages, parenchymal distribution more prominent in the primary disease.

PROGNOSIS 10-year survival: untreated, 6%; treated, at least 30%.

THERAPY Repeated phlebotomy; iron chelation therapy.

OTHER INFORMATION Finding hemosiderin prominently within parenchymal cells helps differentiate primary hemochromatosis from secondary hemosiderosis coexisting with cirrhosis due to other causes.

Hepatic Failure

DESCRIPTION   Clinical syndrome that results when there is significant loss of liver cell mass or when hepatocyte function is impaired, as in cirrhosis.

DISEASE ENTITIES; SYNONYMS AND ACRONYMS   Liver failure, hepatic encephalopathy, hepatic coma, massive hepatic necrosis, fulminant hepatitis, cirrhosis.

INCIDENCE   Common, especially with end-stage cirrhosis.

AGE   Any age; more common in adults due to cirrhosis.

ETIOLOGY, PATHOGENESIS, AND PREDISPOSING FACTORS   Cirrhosis is the most common cause; viral or toxic hepatitis with massive hepatic necrosis; Budd-Chiari syndrome; veno-occlusive disease.

SITES INVOLVED   Liver. In cirrhosis, the vascular disorganization impairs the function of a potentially adequate mass of hepatocytes. Secondary changes are seen in other organs.

GROSS LESIONS   Depends on the morphology of the underlying liver disease. Cerebral edema is a feature of hepatic encephalopathy; ascites, splenomegaly, and esophageal varices occur with cirrhosis.

MICROSCOPIC LESIONS   Depends on the morphology of the underlying liver disease (necrosis, cirrhosis, fatty change). Alzheimer Type II astrocytes are seen in the brain; bile staining of renal tubule cells in the kidneys.

COMPLICATIONS   Hepatic encephalopathy due to elevated ammonia and other neurotoxic amines; renal failure (hepatorenal syndrome); coagulopathy; hypoalbuminemia; feminization, hypogonadism; portal hypertension.

SIGNS AND SYMPTOMS   Depends on the underlying liver disease (cirrhosis, fulminant hepatitis, fatty liver). Jaundice, coma, and bleeding diathesis from coagulopathy are strong indicators.

CLINICAL DIAGNOSIS AND OTHER CLINICAL FEATURES   Recognition of signs; malodorous breath (fetor hepatis); presence of asterixis (liver flap); liver may be enlarged and tender, or shrunken.

LABORATORY DIAGNOSIS   Hyperammonemia, hyperbilirubinemia, elevated aminotransferases and other enzymes, prolonged prothrombin time, hypoalbuminemia; presence of viral antigens with viral hepatitis.

PROGNOSIS   Poor, at least 80% mortality; liver transplantation may offer the only hope.

THERAPY   Treatment of complications; low-protein diet to reduce ammonia; liver transplantation.

OTHER INFORMATION   Both indirect and direct bilirubin are elevated; direct bilirubin predominates because secretion from the hepatocyte is the rate-limiting step in bile metabolism.

Hepatitis A

DESCRIPTION   Infectious disease involving liver, characterized by hepatocellular necrosis and jaundice, caused by an RNA enterovirus transmitted by the fecal-oral route.

DISEASE ENTITIES; SYNONYMS AND ACRONYMS   Infectious hepatitis, epidemic hepatitis, epidemic jaundice, acute viral hepatitis, HAV.

INCIDENCE   Causes 10–25% of hospitalized cases of viral hepatitis in US; hyperendemic in undeveloped countries.

AGE   May infect any age; childhood infections in hyperendemic areas reduce frequency of adult infections.

ETIOLOGY, PATHOGENESIS, AND PREDISPOSING FACTORS   RNA enterovirus transferred by fecal-oral route; overcrowding, poverty, unsanitary conditions, shellfish from contaminated water, mental institutions, and male homosexuals.

SITES INVOLVED   Liver, hepatocytes.

GROSS LESIONS   Often normal; may show congestion, enlargement, and greenish discoloration; rarely there is acute yellow atrophy evident by a flabby shrunken liver with wrinkled capsule.

MICROSCOPIC LESIONS   Multifocal hepatocellular necrosis with acidophilic (Councilman) bodies; balloon cells; predominantly lymphocytic infiltrates around necrotic foci and in portal tracts; lobular disarray.

COMPLICATIONS   Fulminant hepatitis with submassive or massive hepatic necrosis is rare with hepatitis A; chronic hepatitis does not occur.

SIGNS AND SYMPTOMS   Fever, malaise, and anorexia start after an incubation period of 3–6 weeks; jaundice may or may not develop; liver may be enlarged and painful; dark urine, light stools; itching, rash, joint pains.

CLINICAL DIAGNOSIS AND OTHER CLINICAL FEATURES   Recognition of the signs and symptoms in a predisposed person or one who has just traveled to an endemic region. Vague signs and symptoms require laboratory studies.

LABORATORY DIAGNOSIS   Only IgM anti-HAV indicates acute infection; IgG antibody persists for life after infection; hyperbilirubinemia; elevated aminotransferases; prolonged prothrombin time; hypergammaglobulinemia.

PROGNOSIS   Good; never causes chronic hepatitis; rarely causes fulminant hepatitis.

THERAPY   Nonspecific supportive care; isolation to prevent transmission to others.

OTHER INFORMATION   Pooled gammaglobulin is commonly recommended for prophylaxis of close contact to an infected patient in homes, day care centers, hospitals, and of exposure in restaurants to an infected food handler.

Hepatitis B

DESCRIPTION   Infectious disease producing liver inflammation and necrosis transmitted by a DNA virus; the severity varies from an asymptomatic carrier state to fulminant hepatitis; chronic hepatitis is common.

DISEASE ENTITIES; SYNONYMS AND ACRONYMS   Serum hepatitis, HBV; acute viral hepatitis.

INCIDENCE   Depends on population; carrier rate in US is 0.3%; in less developed areas, the rate approaches 20%.

AGE   Any age; in highly endemic areas, vertical transmission affects neonates.

ETIOLOGY, PATHOGENESIS, AND PREDISPOSING FACTORS   Virus is transmitted by blood, saliva, or semen via defects in skin or mucosa; blood transfusion was a major problem in the past; sexual and transplacental transmission are important routes.

SITES INVOLVED   Liver; hepatocytes.

GROSS LESIONS   Liver may be enlarged, congested, or jaundiced. In fulminant hepatitis with massive hepatic necrosis, the liver is yellow, shrunken, and flabby and its capsule is wrinkled (acute yellow atrophy).

MICROSCOPIC LESIONS   Hydropic swelling; hepatocellular necrosis with acidophil (Councilman) bodies, lobular disarray; predominantly mononuclear (lymphocytic) infiltrates within lobules associated with foci of necrosis.

COMPLICATIONS   Hepatic failure; chronic hepatitis progressing to macronodular cirrhosis; hepatocellular carcinoma; aplastic anemia; immune complex diseases: polyarteritis, glomerulonephritis, cryoglobulinemia.

SIGNS AND SYMPTOMS   Fever, malaise, anorexia, and jaundice developing 2–3 months after exposure (6 weeks to 6 months); light-colored stools, dark urine; liver is often enlarged and tender.

CLINICAL DIAGNOSIS AND OTHER CLINICAL FEATURES   Recognition of clinical signs; suspicion is confirmed by laboratory studies.

LABORATORY DIAGNOSIS   Antigens HBs, HBc, and HBe and their corresponding antibodies may be detected, depending on the course and stage of disease; aminotransferases and bilirubin are elevated.

PROGNOSIS   Usually recovery; fulminant hepatitis causes hepatic failure; chronic hepatitis in 5% of cases.

THERAPY   Supportive care in acute illness; vaccination with HBsAg is effective for prevention.

OTHER INFORMATION   Hepatitis B immune globulin plus hepatitis B vaccine are recommended for parenteral or mucosal exposures to infected patients' blood and for newborns of HBsAg-positive mothers.

Hepatocellular Carcinoma

DESCRIPTION   Malignant primary neoplasm of liver, usually arising in cirrhosis and frequently associated with hepatitis B virus (HBV) infection.

DISEASE ENTITIES; SYNONYMS AND ACRONYMS   Hepatoma.

INCIDENCE   Uncommon in developed countries; common in Asia and Africa, depending on prevalence of HBV.

AGE   Usually in adults; increasing incidence with age; more common in elderly men.

ETIOLOGY, PATHOGENESIS, AND PREDISPOSING FACTORS   Chronic HBV infection; alcoholic cirrhosis; cirrhosis with hemochromatosis and alpha-1-antitrypsin deficiency; with HBV infection, viral genome is incorporated into tumor cells and hepatocytes.

SITES INVOLVED   Liver; other sites depending on metastasis.

GROSS LESIONS   Single tumor mass or multiple simultaneous nodules, tan, sometimes greenish from bile production; hemorrhage and necrosis within tumor; often spreads into portal vein, hepatic vein, and vena cava.

MICROSCOPIC LESIONS   Pleomorphic tumor cells resembling hepatocytes arranged in trabeculae or pseudoglandular structures; occasional intracellular bile production.

COMPLICATIONS   Cachexia; tumor rupture with hemoperitoneum; thrombosis of portal or hepatic vein; tumor embolism; portal hypertension with esophageal varices, ascites; hepatic failure; widespread metastases.

SIGNS AND SYMPTOMS   Painful enlarging mass in liver. Paraneoplastic syndromes due to ectopic hormone: polycythemia, hypoglycemia, hypercalcemia.

CLINICAL DIAGNOSIS AND OTHER CLINICAL FEATURES   Right upper quadrant mass may be palpable; ultrasound, CT, and MRI scans; angiography; background of cirrhosis and absence of an extrahepatic cancer should establish the primary site as liver.

LABORATORY DIAGNOSIS   Levels of alpha-fetoprotein are often very high but are not absolutely diagnostic; liver biopsy is often diagnostic.

PROGNOSIS   Poor , 5-year survival rate with therapy is 12–30%.

THERAPY   Lobectomy; hepatectomy with liver transplantation; chemotherapy is not effective.

OTHER INFORMATION   Noncirrhotic causes of hepatocellular carcinoma include aflatoxin poisoning (from *Aspergillus flavus* in mold-contaminated food) and steroids (oral contraceptives, androgens).

Islet Cell Tumors

DESCRIPTION   Tumors arising from specialized cells of pancreatic islets, named for and characterized by their hormonal secretions that produce distinctive clinical syndromes; most are benign, some are malignant.

DISEASE ENTITIES; SYNONYMS AND ACRONYMS   Insulinoma, gastrinoma (ulcerogenic islet cell tumor), glucagonoma, VIPoma, somatostatinoma; carcinoid, APUDoma.

INCIDENCE   Altogether uncommon; insulinoma, then gastrinoma are the most frequent islet cell tumors.

AGE   Adults.

ETIOLOGY, PATHOGENESIS, AND PREDISPOSING FACTORS   Neoplasms of unknown etiology; clinical syndromes are due to hormone secretions: insulinoma, hypoglycemia; gastrinoma, peptic ulcers (Zollinger-Ellison syndrome); VIPoma, profuse watery diarrhea.

SITES INVOLVED   Tumors usually arise within pancreatic parenchyma; a few gastrinomas are primary in the duodenum; malignant variants metastasize to regional lymph nodes and liver.

GROSS LESIONS   Commonly small (few millimeters to few centimeters) solitary demarcated nodules; malignant variants have invasive margins and are larger; gastrinomas are usually malignant or multiple.

MICROSCOPIC LESIONS   Proliferation of small uniform cells with regular round or oval nuclei; cytoplasm may stain with special silver stains (argyrophilia); immunoperoxidase stains demonstrate specific peptide secretions.

COMPLICATIONS   Depends on particular hormone secretion: insulinoma, hypoglycemic coma; gastrinoma, intractable ulcers with hemorrhage, perforation; VIPoma, fluid, and electrolyte abnormalities.

SIGNS AND SYMPTOMS   Depends on specific hormonal secretion: sweating, nervousness, hunger, lethargy, confusion, coma (insulin); peptic ulcer symptoms (gastrin); explosive, profuse watery diarrhea (VIP).

CLINICAL DIAGNOSIS AND OTHER CLINICAL FEATURES   Recognition of clinical syndromes and finding of elevated peptide hormones; tumor may be discovered during laparotomy for ulcers.

LABORATORY DIAGNOSIS   Radioimmunoassay of peptide hormones; histology of biopsied or resected pancreas; immunohistochemical techniques allow direct visualization of cells producing specific hormones.

PROGNOSIS   Good if tumor is benign and resectable; gastrinomas produce intractable disease and debilitation.

THERAPY   Surgical resection.

OTHER INFORMATION   These tumors are derived from amine precursor uptake and decarboxylating (APUD) cells and are related to intestinal carcinoid tumors; they may be seen in multiple endocrine neoplasia (MEN) syndromes.

Jaundice

DESCRIPTION   A condition characterized by yellow discoloration of skin, sclera, and tissues caused by various defects in bile excretion that produce elevation of bilirubin and other components of bile in the blood.

DISEASE ENTITIES; SYNONYMS AND ACRONYMS   Icterus, hyperbilirubinemia, cholestasis, intrahepatic cholestasis, obstructive jaundice, kernicterus.

INCIDENCE   Common; a leading manifestation of liver disease of any etiology; also produced by hemolytic anemia.

AGE   Any age, depending on etiology.

ETIOLOGY, PATHOGENESIS, AND PREDISPOSING FACTORS   Hemolytic anemia, erythroblastosis fetalis; prematurity; familial defects in bile metabolism; drugs (e.g., chlorpromazine, ethinyl estradiol); hepatitis, cirrhosis; extrahepatic biliary obstruction.

SITES INVOLVED   Liver, hepatocytes, intrahepatic or extrahepatic bile ducts; skin, sclera, and all tissues are yellow; bile casts in renal tubules; basal ganglia of brain in kernicterus.

GROSS LESIONS   Organs and tissues show yellow or green pigmentation, liver is often dark green with other features depending on primary disease process (e.g., cirrhosis).

MICROSCOPIC LESIONS   In liver: centrilobular bile pigment initially, later throughout lobule; bile plugs in canaliculi, bile pigment in hepatocytes and macrophages; cellular degeneration, bile infarcts, portal fibrosis.

COMPLICATIONS   Depends largely on the underlying disease; extrahepatic biliary obstruction results in portal fibrosis; high bilirubin in the neonate causes neurologic damage (kernicterus).

SIGNS AND SYMPTOMS   Jaundice becomes obvious with bilirubin levels exceeding 2.0–2.5 mg/dl; pruritis is common; specific features depend on underlying disease.

CLINICAL DIAGNOSIS AND OTHER CLINICAL FEATURES   Jaundice, when present, is most apparent in the sclera under good lighting; diagnostic workup is directed at determining the cause.

LABORATORY DIAGNOSIS   Unconjugated/conjugated bilirubin ratio to differentiate hemolysis, obstructive, or intrahepatic causes; alkaline phosphatase, aminotransferases to differentiate hepatic necrosis vs. biliary disease.

PROGNOSIS   Depends on underlying disease.

THERAPY   Surgery for obstructive jaundice; medical management; withdrawal of cholestatic drug.

OTHER INFORMATION   In jaundice caused by hemolysis, indirect (unconjugated) bilirubin is elevated; with obstruction, direct (conjugated) bilirubin is elevated; in hepatocellular necrosis, both are elevated.

Pancreatitis—Acute

DESCRIPTION Destruction of pancreatic acinar tissue with release of activated digestive enzymes, resulting in acute inflammation, fat necrosis, and hemorrhage; associated with alcoholism and biliary disease.

DISEASE ENTITIES; SYNONYMS AND ACRONYMS Acute hemorrhagic pancreatitis, interstitial pancreatitis, edematous pancreatitis.

INCIDENCE Limited to alcoholics and cholelithiasis; more common in men due to higher incidence of alcoholism.

AGE Middle age; peak incidence at 60 years.

ETIOLOGY, PATHOGENESIS, AND PREDISPOSING FACTORS Alcoholism and biliary disease account for most cases; less commonly: direct trauma to the pancreas, mumps virus, ischemia, certain drugs, hypercalcemia, and hypertriglyceridemia.

SITES INVOLVED Pancreatic acinar tissue is first involved; as the autodigestion progresses, the surrounding mesenteric fat becomes saponified and hemorrhagic; pseudocysts may impinge on adjacent duodenum or spleen.

GROSS LESIONS In mild cases, there is edema and hyperemia; with progression, pasty yellow-white foci of fat necrosis develop and expand to form pseudocysts; hemorrhage and cystic cavitation mark the worst cases.

MICROSCOPIC LESIONS Edema of connective tissue, infiltrates of PMNs, hemorrhage, necrosis of pancreatic acini; fat necrosis appears as pale-blue amorphous foci where adipocyte membranes are dissolved.

COMPLICATIONS Shock, ARDS, acute renal failure; hypercalcemia; fat necrosis at extrapancreatic sites due to liberated lipase; pancreatic pseudocyst, abscess; chemical or septic peritonitis.

SIGNS AND SYMPTOMS Severe epigastric pain, radiating to back; nausea and vomiting; rapid development of shock; often preceded by a heavy meal or excessive alcohol consumption.

CLINICAL DIAGNOSIS AND OTHER CLINICAL FEATURES Recognition of clinical presentation, confirmed by laboratory tests; abdominal ultrasound or CT scans may demonstrate pseudocyst.

LABORATORY DIAGNOSIS Elevation of serum lipase and amylase in blood and ascitic fluid; hypocalcemia may be present.

PROGNOSIS Depends on severity; complications of shock and ARDS are associated with high mortality.

THERAPY Supportive with fluid and electrolytes; cessation of oral intake reduces pancreatic secretions.

OTHER INFORMATION Alcohol causes acinar injury and sphincter of Oddi spasm; gallstones may impact in the distal common duct; activation of lytic enzymes (trypsin) initiates autodigestion and formation of lysolecithin.

Pancreatitis—Chronic

DESCRIPTION   Chronic destruction of the pancreatic acinar tissue with fibrosis, atrophy, fatty replacement, and calcification; associated with alcoholism, biliary tract disease, and cystic fibrosis.

DISEASE ENTITIES; SYNONYMS AND ACRONYMS   Chronic calcifying pancreatitis, pancreatic insufficiency, pancreatic malabsorption; cystic fibrosis.

INCIDENCE   Occurs mainly in chronic alcoholics and in cystic fibrosis; more common in men due to alcoholism.

AGE   Childhood in cystic fibrosis; middle aged due to alcoholism.

ETIOLOGY, PATHOGENESIS, AND PREDISPOSING FACTORS   Inspissated pancreatic secretions causing chronic duct obstruction in cystic fibrosis; recurrent episodes of acute pancreatitis in alcoholism; congenital pancreas divisum.

SITES INVOLVED   Pancreatic acini are destroyed and replaced first; obliteration of islets usually occurs later or not at all.

GROSS LESIONS   Pancreatic tissue is reduced in mass and replaced with fibrosis and/or fat; foci of calcification and dilatation of ducts are common, especially with alcoholic etiology; pseudocyst may be present.

MICROSCOPIC LESIONS   Acini replaced with fat or fibrosis; islets conspicuously preserved; chronic inflammation; focal calcification; dilated ducts filled with proteinaceous material is a feature of alcoholic pancreatitis.

COMPLICATIONS   Pancreatic insufficiency with malabsorption and steatorrhea; diabetes mellitus; pancreatic pseudocyst.

SIGNS AND SYMPTOMS   Malabsorption with weight loss, malnutrition, and steatorrhea; glucose intolerance, diabetes mellitus; chronic abdominal pain.

CLINICAL DIAGNOSIS AND OTHER CLINICAL FEATURES   Recognition of malabsorption in a patient with predisposing conditions; diabetes mellitus is an uncommon presentation.

LABORATORY DIAGNOSIS   Demonstration of malabsorption; decreased pancreatic enzymes in stool or intestinal aspirate.

PROGNOSIS   Variable, depending on other disease processes; in cystic fibrosis lung infections cause mortality.

THERAPY   Oral supplements of pancreatic enzymes; insulin therapy.

OTHER INFORMATION   Risk factors are similar to acute pancreatitis; in half of cases, risk factors are absent and there may be no preceding episodes of acute pancreatitis.

Portal Hypertension

DESCRIPTION Elevation of portal venous pressure due to obstruction of the portal blood flow, either within the hepatic lobule (intrahepatic), in the hepatic vein (posthepatic), or in the portal vein (prehepatic).

DISEASE ENTITIES; SYNONYMS AND ACRONYMS Cirrhosis, portal vein thrombosis, Budd-Chiari syndrome, hepatic veno-occlusive disease.

INCIDENCE Common, particularly with cirrhosis.

AGE Any age, depending on cause; most cases affect adults due to alcoholic cirrhosis.

ETIOLOGY, PATHOGENESIS, AND PREDISPOSING FACTORS Prehepatic: portal vein thrombosis; intrahepatic: cirrhosis from any cause, schistosomiasis; posthepatic: hepatic vein thrombosis (Budd-Chiari syndrome, hepatic veno-occlusive disease).

SITES INVOLVED Prehepatic: portal vein; intrahepatic: liver sinusoids, intrahepatic veins; posthepatic: extrahepatic hepatic veins.

GROSS LESIONS Depends on particular lesion; cirrhosis is described elsewhere; thrombi in portal or hepatic veins may be completely organized; liver in Budd-Chiari syndrome is markedly congested and swollen.

MICROSCOPIC LESIONS Depends on cause; in veno-occlusive disease, small intrahepatic veins are occluded, central zones congested and necrotic, fibrous bands join central zones forming nodules with portal tracts centrally.

COMPLICATIONS Bleeding from ruptured esophageal varices; splenomegaly, splenic consumption of blood cells; ascites, possibly complicated by peritonitis; portasystemic encephalopathy; hepatic failure.

SIGNS AND SYMPTOMS Splenomegaly, ascites, and esophageal varices are important signs; hepatic vein thrombosis presents acutely with abdominal pain, liver enlargement, ascites, and jaundice.

CLINICAL DIAGNOSIS AND OTHER CLINICAL FEATURES Detection of ascites by physical examination, x-ray, and paracentesis; splenomegaly by palpation or imaging techniques; varices by endoscopy; workup is directed at determining the cause.

LABORATORY DIAGNOSIS Abnormalities in liver function tests are likely, depending on underlying disease; liver biopsy may be needed to determine the etiology.

PROGNOSIS Poor; patients commonly die of bleeding varices or hepatic failure.

THERAPY Treatment of complications; portasystemic shunt to reduce portal pressure; liver transplantation.

OTHER INFORMATION Portasystemic shunt surgery carries high mortality but may be required to control variceal bleeding; peritoneovenous shunt is preferred to control ascites.

Primary Biliary Cirrhosis

DESCRIPTION   Chronic liver disease of probable autoimmune etiology occurring mostly in women, characterized by nonsuppurative obliterative cholangitis that progresses to cirrhosis.

DISEASE ENTITIES; SYNONYMS AND ACRONYMS   PBC.

INCIDENCE   Not common; accounts for up to 2% of deaths from cirrhosis. Women are involved in 90–95% of cases.

AGE   Usually between 30 and 65 years; peak age 55.

ETIOLOGY, PATHOGENESIS, AND PREDISPOSING FACTORS   Presumed autoimmune disease; associated with another autoimmune disease in 85%; initial lesion involves attack on bile duct epithelium by cytotoxic T-cells; autoantibodies are also present.

SITES INVOLVED   Liver; intrahepatic bile ducts are involved in Stage I; in Stage II, there is scarring and chronic inflammation of the portal region; in Stage III lesions, the entire liver is involved with cirrhosis.

GROSS LESIONS   There may be no gross alteration until the terminal stage, which is a dark-green cirrhotic liver.

MICROSCOPIC LESIONS   Stage I: lymphocytes, mononuclear cells, eosinophils, and epithelioid granulomas around altered bile ducts; Stage II: disappearance of small bile ducts, scarring of larger ducts; Stage III: cirrhosis.

COMPLICATIONS   Cirrhosis and its complications, particularly portal hypertension; malabsorption with steatorrhea; osteoporosis, osteomalacia due to malabsorption of vitamin D and calcium.

SIGNS AND SYMPTOMS   Initially fatigue and pruritis, with or without jaundice; complications develop within several years of progression; xanthomas may appear secondary to hyperlipidemia.

CLINICAL DIAGNOSIS AND OTHER CLINICAL FEATURES   Recognition of the early sign of pruritis; investigation of jaundice or fatigue. Chronic thyroiditis, rheumatoid arthritis, scleroderma, or Sjogren's syndrome may coexist.

LABORATORY DIAGNOSIS   Elevated alkaline phosphatase, bilirubin rises later; moderate aminotransferase elevation; hypercholesterolemia with lipoprotein-X; antimitochondrial antibodies and other autoantibodies.

PROGNOSIS   Usually progressive indolent course with survival of 10–15 years.

THERAPY   Cholestyramine resin to control pruritis; immunosuppression; liver transplantation.

OTHER INFORMATION   The target of cytotoxic T lymphocytes in PBC, bile duct epithelial cells, express large amounts of Class I HLA antigens and Class II HLA-DR antigens, which are not expressed by normal bile duct cells.

Toxic Liver Injury

DESCRIPTION Broad spectrum of hepatic changes caused by drug or chemical injury; may be either predictable or unpredictable (idiosyncratic) and is usually reversible upon withdrawal of the offending agent.

DISEASE ENTITIES; SYNONYMS AND ACRONYMS Micro- or macrovesicular fatty change (steatosis), cholestasis, toxic hepatitis, veno-occlusive disease, adenoma.

INCIDENCE Common; may occur with industrial or agricultural exposures and with common therapeutic agents.

AGE Any age depending on exposure; e.g., Reye's syndrome in children may be related to aspirin toxicity.

ETIOLOGY, PATHOGENESIS, AND PREDISPOSING FACTORS Predictable hepatotoxin injury is dose dependent and often due to toxic metabolites; unpredictable injury may be related to immunologic reactions or atypical metabolic pathways in sensitive persons.

SITES INVOLVED Usually the hepatocyte; vascular lesions may be seen with estrogens or anabolic steroids; malignant tumors of bile ducts and blood vessels are associated with Thorotrast, arsenic, and vinyl chloride.

GROSS LESIONS Fatty liver: enlarged, pale yellow, greasy texture; cholestasis: greenish speckling; fulminant hepatitis: soft shrunken liver, wrinkled capsule, yellow or greenish parenchyma; cirrhosis: macronodular.

MICROSCOPIC LESIONS Fatty change: micro- or macrovesicular; cholestasis: usually centrilobular bile plugs, mild inflammation; necrosis: zonal, often centrilobular, may be massive; cirrhosis: bands of fibrosis, nodules.

COMPLICATIONS Acute: hepatic failure with coma. Chronic, usually due to continued exposure: cirrhosis with portal hypertension; malignant neoplasms (hepatocellular carcinoma, cholangiocarcinoma, angiosarcoma).

SIGNS AND SYMPTOMS Jaundice, signs of hepatic failure; anorexia, nausea, vomiting, malaise.

CLINICAL DIAGNOSIS AND OTHER CLINICAL FEATURES Should be suspected in a patient with liver disease exposed to known hepatotoxin or taking virtually any therapeutic agent; following viral illness in a child treated with aspirin.

LABORATORY DIAGNOSIS Elevation of bilirubin and liver enzymes; elevation of ammonia and prolongation of coagulation tests indicate severe injury; liver biopsy may reveal a distinctive injury pattern.

PROGNOSIS Usually good if toxin is withdrawn; halothane hepatitis is often fatal due to massive necrosis.

THERAPY Removal of agent; supportive therapy until recovery.

OTHER INFORMATION The inflammatory pattern in toxic liver injury can mimic patterns associated with viral infection (focal hepatitis, chronic hepatitis); Amanita mushroom poisoning causes massive hepatic necrosis.

Pathology Facts, by Richard C.
Harruff, J.B. Lippincott
Company, Philadelphia © 1994.

Chapter 16

Urinary System

(cont'd)

Acute Glomerulonephritis

DESCRIPTION Acute inflammatory glomerular disease with hematuria and oliguria following a streptococcal or other infection, caused by immune complex deposition leading to proliferative glomerulonephritis.

DISEASE ENTITIES; SYNONYMS AND ACRONYMS Acute proliferative glomerulonephritis, poststreptococcal glomerulonephritis, postinfectious glomerulonephritis.

INCIDENCE One of the more common renal diseases in childhood.

AGE Usually children; adults are less often affected.

ETIOLOGY, PATHOGENESIS, AND PREDISPOSING FACTORS Glomerular deposition of immune complexes following infection of pharynx (usually) or skin with a nephritogenic strain of group A streptococci; other bacterial or viral infections may produce disease.

SITES INVOLVED Kidney, renal glomerulus, basement membrane.

GROSS LESIONS Usually no gross lesions; on close inspection, glomeruli may appear prominent by their hyperemia.

MICROSCOPIC LESIONS LM: proliferation of mesangial and endothelial cells, exudation of PMNs; EM: electron-dense deposits appearing as subepithelial "humps"; IM: granular deposition of IgG and C3 along basement membrane.

COMPLICATIONS A minor proportion of patients may develop rapidly progressive glomerulonephritis leading to renal failure; this is more likely to occur in adults.

SIGNS AND SYMPTOMS Nephritis with oliguria, hematuria, facial edema, and hypertension; resolution usually occurs within 8 weeks; exacerbation after infection by another nephritogenic organism may occur.

CLINICAL DIAGNOSIS AND OTHER CLINICAL FEATURES Recognition of nephritis with facial (periorbital) edema and hypertension; renal biopsy to confirm diagnosis.

LABORATORY DIAGNOSIS Hematuria with red cell casts; depression of complement C3; characteristic changes in renal biopsy; elevation of antibodies to streptococci, e.g., the antistreptolysin O (ASO) titer.

PROGNOSIS 95% of children recover completely; adults are more likely to develop chronic renal insufficiency.

THERAPY Rarely requires any therapy.

OTHER INFORMATION Crescents in the renal biopsy indicate the complication of rapidly progressive glomerulonephritis and a poor prognosis.

Acute Tubular Necrosis

DESCRIPTION   Acute tubular damage resulting in acute renal failure caused either by shock or by nephrotoxic drugs or chemicals; characterized by necrosis of tubular cells.

DISEASE ENTITIES; SYNONYMS AND ACRONYMS   ATN, ischemic or tubulorrhectic ATN, nephrotoxic ATN, lower nephron nephrosis, shock kidneys.

INCIDENCE   The most frequent cause of acute renal failure.

AGE   Any age; young adults are more commonly involved because of their higher incidence of trauma.

ETIOLOGY, PATHOGENESIS, AND PREDISPOSING FACTORS   Tubular ischemia due to hypovolemic or endotoxic shock, trauma, hemorrhage, burns, dehydration, sepsis; nephrotoxicity due to mercuric chloride, antibiotics, chemotherapy agents, ethylene glycol.

SITES INVOLVED   Renal tubular epithelial cells, particularly the proximal tubules and the ascending limb of Henle's loop.

GROSS LESIONS   Initially, pallor and edema of kidneys; later the medulla is congested relative to the cortex.

MICROSCOPIC LESIONS   Necrosis of tubular epithelial cells that slough into the tubular lumen forming casts; the tubular framework is retained; later there is cellular regeneration with mitotic figures.

COMPLICATIONS   Acute renal failure with oliguria or anuria; during tubular regeneration there is diuresis with electrolyte abnormalities; vulnerability to infection is another feature of the recovery phase.

SIGNS AND SYMPTOMS   Acute renal failure in a trauma patient who has sustained a period of shock; in nephrotoxic ATN, renal failure develops after ingesting a chemical or drug such as aminoglycoside antibiotic.

CLINICAL DIAGNOSIS AND OTHER CLINICAL FEATURES   Ischemic ATN is usually obvious from the clinical presentation; nephrotoxic ATN may be more subtle, for example after consumption of "moonshine" liquor adulterated with antifreeze (ethylene glycol).

LABORATORY DIAGNOSIS   Azotemia, hyperkalemia in the early phase; hypokalemia in the recovery phase; urinalysis may show tubular cell or granular casts; renal biopsy is rarely needed but shows morphologic features of ATN.

PROGNOSIS   Mortality varies from 10 to 60% or more depending on the initiating condition.

THERAPY   Fluid and electrolyte management with dialysis if needed until recovery of renal function.

OTHER INFORMATION   ATN often occurs with multiple system organ failure complicating shock. Because dialysis adequately controls renal failure, death usually results from nonrenal causes, particularly ARDS.

Amyloidosis

DESCRIPTION   Involvement of the kidney in systemic amyloidosis causing renal failure, characterized by accumulation of amyloid within glomeruli and around blood vessels.

DISEASE ENTITIES; SYNONYMS AND ACRONYMS   Renal amyloidosis; renal involvement with systemic amyloidosis; primary (AL) amyloidosis, secondary (AA) amyloidosis.

INCIDENCE   Renal disease is a common complication of amyloidosis; however, amyloidosis is uncommon.

AGE   Usually adults, middle aged and older.

ETIOLOGY, PATHOGENESIS, AND PREDISPOSING FACTORS   Either primary amyloidosis with immunocyte dyscrasia or secondary amyloidosis with a chronic inflammatory condition may cause renal amyloidosis; amyloid deposits in glomeruli interfere with function.

SITES INVOLVED   Renal glomeruli, walls of arterioles, surrounding tubules.

GROSS LESIONS   Kidney may appear waxy; with an iodine-sulfuric acid stain for starch, glomeruli containing amyloid stain brownish-purple, hence the name "amyloid."

MICROSCOPIC LESIONS   Amyloid accumulates as acellular eosinophilic masses within the glomerular mesangium, progressively compressing and obliterating the glomerulus.

COMPLICATIONS   Progresses to end-stage renal failure; other complications of amyloidosis involve other organs, particularly the heart causing heart failure.

SIGNS AND SYMPTOMS   Proteinuria with nephrotic syndrome in more than half of cases; renal insufficiency; renal disease is often the first manifestation of amyloidosis.

CLINICAL DIAGNOSIS AND OTHER CLINICAL FEATURES   Suspected if proteinuria or azotemia develops in a patient with known amyloidosis or in a condition commonly associated with amyloidosis; confirmed by renal biopsy.

LABORATORY DIAGNOSIS   Morphologic changes in renal biopsy; greenish birefringence in polarized light with Congo-red–stained tissue; fibrillary structure of amyloid by electron microscopy.

PROGNOSIS   Poor; renal failure; heart failure, or other organ failure.

THERAPY   Treatment of any underlying condition; dialysis; renal transplantation may not be warranted.

OTHER INFORMATION   AL amyloid is composed of immunoglobulin light chains; AA amyloid is derived from serum amyloid A (SAA), an acute phase reactant protein.

Analgesic Abuse Nephropathy

DESCRIPTION Chronic tubulointerstitial disease caused by prolonged excessive consumption of analgesic agents, particularly phenacetin, resulting in renal failure; characterized by papillary necrosis.

DISEASE ENTITIES; SYNONYMS AND ACRONYMS Renal papillary necrosis; analgesic nephritis.

INCIDENCE Uncommon in US compared with Europe and Australia where phenacetin is more popular.

AGE Usually in a middle-aged woman with chronic headaches.

ETIOLOGY, PATHOGENESIS, AND PREDISPOSING FACTORS At least 2–3 kg of phenacetin consumed over 3 years; aspirin and acetaminophen also cause the lesion; the drug or metabolite may be directly nephrotoxic or may induce local ischemic damage.

SITES INVOLVED Renal papillae.

GROSS LESIONS The involved papilla shows a well-demarcated zone of pallor and necrosis; the necrotic part may slough into the pelvis, causing ureteropelvic obstruction, or may remain attached and calcify.

MICROSCOPIC LESIONS Coagulation necrosis of the papillary tip with an inflammatory cell reaction in the viable tissue lining the necrosis.

COMPLICATIONS Progressive renal failure; acute obstruction of one kidney by a sloughed papillary tip.

SIGNS AND SYMPTOMS Renal insufficiency in a patient with chronic headaches or other chronic pain who habitually consumes excessive analgesic compounds; premature aging and brown skin discoloration are sometimes apparent.

CLINICAL DIAGNOSIS AND OTHER CLINICAL FEATURES History is suggestive; intravenous or retrograde pyelogram shows destruction of papillary tip.

LABORATORY DIAGNOSIS Azotemia; inability to concentrate urine and metabolic acidosis indicating tubular dysfunction; anemia.

PROGNOSIS Often results in chronic renal failure.

THERAPY Discontinuation of the analgesic; dialysis; renal transplantation.

OTHER INFORMATION Renal papillary necrosis also occurs in acute pyelonephritis, especially in diabetics, and in sickle cell disease.

Crescentic Glomerulonephritis

DESCRIPTION   Inflammatory glomerular disease with nephritis and rapid progression to renal failure; characterized by crescents of proliferating cells within Bowman's space and subsequent obliteration of glomeruli.

DISEASE ENTITIES; SYNONYMS AND ACRONYMS   Rapidly progressive glomerulonephritis, RPGN, Goodpasture's syndrome, glomerulonephritis with vasculitis; many others.

INCIDENCE   Fairly common complication of several forms of glomerulonephritis that lead to renal failure.

AGE   Any age; adults are more likely than children to develop RPGN after acute glomerulonephritis.

ETIOLOGY, PATHOGENESIS, AND PREDISPOSING FACTORS   This is a morphologic lesion that may be present in different types of glomerulonephritis; leaking of fibrin and fibrinogen into Bowman's space is possibly the stimulus for crescent formation.

SITES INVOLVED   Glomerulus, particularly the cells lining Bowman's capsule.

GROSS LESIONS   No specific gross lesion.

MICROSCOPIC LESIONS   Epithelial cells, PMNs, and macrophages accumulate in Bowman's capsule compressing glomerulus; in older lesions, there are fibroblasts, collagen, and segmentally or globally scarred glomeruli.

COMPLICATIONS   Crescentic glomerulonephritis is itself a complication of several inflammatory glomerular diseases; most patients with this lesion progress fairly rapidly to irreversible renal failure.

SIGNS AND SYMPTOMS   Nephritis with rapidly progressive azotemia and oliguria or anuria. Hemoptysis with hematuria is a feature of Goodpasture's syndrome.

CLINICAL DIAGNOSIS AND OTHER CLINICAL FEATURES   Should be suspected in a patient with nephritis that shows a rapid decline in renal function; renal biopsy is confirmatory; specific features depend on the primary disease process.

LABORATORY DIAGNOSIS   Examination of renal biopsy; specific EM and IM features depend on the underlying disease; circulating antiglomerular basement membrane antibodies are present in Goodpasture's syndrome.

PROGNOSIS   Usually progresses to chronic renal failure.

THERAPY   Corticosteroid or immunosuppressive therapy; dialysis and renal transplantation for renal failure.

OTHER INFORMATION   Antiglomerular basement membrane antibodies mediate Goodpasture's syndrome; the antibodies cross-react with alveolar basement membrane to produce alveolitis and hemoptysis.

Cystitis

DESCRIPTION   Acute or chronic inflammation of the urinary bladder caused by bacterial infections (usually *E. coli*), indwelling catheters, radiation therapy, or chemotherapy with cyclophosphamide.

DISEASE ENTITIES; SYNONYMS AND ACRONYMS   Polypoid, bullous, eosinophilic, hemorrhagic cystitis; chronic interstitial cystitis (Hunner's ulcer), malakoplakia.

INCIDENCE   Common, especially bacterial infections due to the same factors described with acute pyelonephritis (see below).

AGE   Any age, depending on predisposing condition; most common in females of all ages.

ETIOLOGY, PATHOGENESIS, AND PREDISPOSING FACTORS   Female anatomy; onset of sexual activity (honeymoon cystitis); catheters (polypoid or bullous cystitis); cyclophosphamide (hemorrhagic cystitis); unknown (malakoplakia, chronic interstitial cystitis).

SITES INVOLVED   Urinary bladder mucosa.

GROSS LESIONS   Mucosal hyperemia and edema, polypoid or bullous projections of swollen mucosa; chronic interstitial cystitis: chronic ulcer (Hunner's ulcer); malakoplakia: multiple shaggy yellow plaques.

MICROSCOPIC LESIONS   Acute or chronic inflammation; urothelial hyperplasia and metaplasia (e.g., cystitis cystica); chronic inflammation borders Hunner's ulcer; histiocytes contain Michaelis-Gutmann bodies in malakoplakia.

COMPLICATIONS   Pyelonephritis by ascending infection, urosepsis; chronic interstitial cystitis may be resistant to all therapy; profuse hemorrhage from cyclophosphamide-induced cystitis.

SIGNS AND SYMPTOMS   Suprapubic or abdominal pain, nausea and vomiting, urgency, frequency, and burning on urination, dysuria; hematuria, cloudy or malodorous urine.

CLINICAL DIAGNOSIS AND OTHER CLINICAL FEATURES   Signs and symptoms are usually specific but may be confused with gastroenteritis; urinary tract infection is very common with indwelling catheters; concurrent pyelonephritis should be considered.

LABORATORY DIAGNOSIS   Urinalysis: pyuria, hematuria, bacteriuria; WBC casts indicate pyelonephritis; urine culture: usually positive for gram-negative rods; recurrent *E. coli* infections are a feature of malakoplakia.

PROGNOSIS   Usually good with control of infection; hemorrhagic cystitis and Hunner's ulcer can be intractable.

THERAPY   Antibiotics; methylene blue, bladder irrigation for cyclophosphamide cystitis; cystectomy (rare).

OTHER INFORMATION   Metabolites of the drug are the agents actually causing cyclophosphamide-induced hemorrhagic cystitis; in chronic interstitial cystitis, the urine is usually sterile.

Diabetic Glomerulosclerosis

DESCRIPTION   Glomerular disease of diabetes mellitus causing proteinuria and progressive renal failure; characterized by accumulation of basement membrane material in the capillaries and mesangium.

DISEASE ENTITIES; SYNONYMS AND ACRONYMS   Kimmelstiel-Wilson disease; nodular or diffuse diabetic glomerulosclerosis.

INCIDENCE   Common cause of renal failure in diabetics; one of the most common causes of renal failure.

AGE   Adults; increasing incidence with duration of the diabetes.

ETIOLOGY, PATHOGENESIS, AND PREDISPOSING FACTORS   This is the renal manifestation of diabetic microangiopathy, which causes thickening of vascular basement membranes; appears to be a function of the duration and severity of hyperglycemia.

SITES INVOLVED   Renal glomerulus, capillary basement membrane; in the diffuse form, the capillary basement membrane is thickened; in the nodular type, masses of basement membrane material form nodules in the mesangium.

GROSS LESIONS   With advanced disease, the parenchyma is diffusely contracted and granular; glomeruli may be prominent on close inspection.

MICROSCOPIC LESIONS   Increase of mesangial matrix, thickening of capillary basement membrane alone or combined with acellular eosinophilic nodules in the mesangium; hyaline arteriolosclerosis of both afferent and efferent arterioles.

COMPLICATIONS   Progresses to renal failure within 6 years; often associated with other manifestations of microangiopathy such as retinopathy; control of hyperglycemia may retard development of microangiopathy.

SIGNS AND SYMPTOMS   Initially proteinuria, possibly severe enough to produce the nephrotic syndrome; azotemia progressing to end-stage renal failure.

CLINICAL DIAGNOSIS AND OTHER CLINICAL FEATURES   Common and expected complication of diabetes, manifested by proteinuria and/or azotemia; renal biopsy to confirm diagnosis and exclude other diseases.

LABORATORY DIAGNOSIS   Light microscopic changes as described above; absence of immune complex deposition by electron microscopy and immunofluorescence; elevated BUN, creatinine, and glucose.

PROGNOSIS   End-stage renal failure is expected within several years.

THERAPY   Control of hyperglycemia; dialysis, renal transplantation.

OTHER INFORMATION   Glomerulosclerosis is but one form of diabetic nephropathy; other renal diseases of diabetes include acute and chronic pyelonephritis, papillary necrosis, and arteriolonephrosclerosis.

Focal Glomerulonephritis

DESCRIPTION Inflammatory glomerular diseases of various types characterized morphologically by inflammatory lesions involving only some of the glomeruli.

DISEASE ENTITIES; SYNONYMS AND ACRONYMS IgA nephropathy (Berger's disease); Henoch-Schonlein purpura glomerulonephritis.

INCIDENCE Fairly common; IgA nephropathy causes 3–10% of primary glomerulonephritis in US.

AGE IgA nephropathy: males 15–30 years; Henoch-Schonlein: children.

ETIOLOGY, PATHOGENESIS, AND PREDISPOSING FACTORS IgA immune complexes; IgA nephropathy sometimes occurs in inflammatory mucosal diseases like Crohn's and celiac disease; in Henoch-Schonlein, there is systemic disease with purpura and arthritis.

SITES INVOLVED Renal glomerulus.

GROSS LESIONS No specific gross lesion.

MICROSCOPIC LESIONS LM: variable mesangial proliferation; in worst cases, necrosis and crescents; EM: electron-dense deposits in mesangium; IM: deposits of IgA with lesser amounts of IgM, IgG, and C3.

COMPLICATIONS Nephrotic syndrome; hypertension; acute or chronic renal failure; malignant hypertension; IgA nephropathy recurs in the transplanted kidney.

SIGNS AND SYMPTOMS Proteinuria, hematuria, renal insufficiency. With Henoch-Schonlein, there is skin purpura of the lower extremities, along with arthritis and abdominal pain.

CLINICAL DIAGNOSIS AND OTHER CLINICAL FEATURES May be suspected in a young man presenting with nephritis or a child with nephritis and purpura; confirmed by renal biopsy.

LABORATORY DIAGNOSIS Hematuria with red cell casts; characteristic changes in the renal biopsy; different types of focal glomerulonephritis are differentiated by the EM and IM findings.

PROGNOSIS Usually good, although up to 20% develop chronic renal failure.

THERAPY No specific therapy; dialysis, renal transplantation if renal failure develops.

OTHER INFORMATION Hereditary nephritis (Alport's syndrome), associated with splitting of the basement membrane, also presents with a focal glomerulonephritis.

Focal Segmental Glomerulosclerosis

DESCRIPTION Glomerular disease of adults and children causing the nephrotic syndrome, characterized by collapse, sclerosis, and hyalinosis of focal glomerular segments; progresses to chronic renal failure.

DISEASE ENTITIES; SYNONYMS AND ACRONYMS FSG; focal glomerulosclerosis; primary or idiopathic FSG; FSG associated with other glomerular disease.

INCIDENCE Causes 10% of nephrotic syndrome in children and 20% in adults; males slightly more than females.

AGE Both children and adults.

ETIOLOGY, PATHOGENESIS, AND PREDISPOSING FACTORS Focal segmental sclerosis may be a reaction to chronic proteinuria; other possibilities implicate altered cellular immunity; occurs with intravenous heroin abuse and AIDS.

SITES INVOLVED Glomerulus of kidney.

GROSS LESIONS No gross lesion.

MICROSCOPIC LESIONS LM: segmental collapse, synechiae, sclerosis and hyalinosis; EM: folding and thickening of basement membrane, effacement of foot processes; IM: deposits of IgM and C3 in areas of hyalinosis.

COMPLICATIONS End-stage renal failure develops within 10 years, sometimes much sooner; hypertension; disease recurs in 20–30% of transplanted kidneys.

SIGNS AND SYMPTOMS Onset of nephrotic syndrome with nonselective proteinuria; hypertension; microscopic hematuria.

CLINICAL DIAGNOSIS AND OTHER CLINICAL FEATURES Recognition of nephrotic syndrome; renal biopsy. Many patients have previous diagnosis of minimal change disease.

LABORATORY DIAGNOSIS Findings of nephrotic syndrome; characteristic changes of the renal biopsy; requires adequate sampling of glomeruli to differentiate from minimal change disease which it resembles in early stages.

PROGNOSIS Progresses to chronic renal failure within several years.

THERAPY Steroids, cyclophosphamide, nonsteroidal anti-inflammatory agents; dialysis; renal transplantation.

OTHER INFORMATION Tubular defects are associated with FSG, including renal glycosuria, aminoaciduria, renal tubular acidosis, and phosphate wasting.

Hemolytic-Uremic Syndrome

DESCRIPTION   A clinical syndrome of acute renal insufficiency, microangiopathic hemolytic anemia, and thrombocytopenia; a related and more severe form is thrombotic thrombocytopenic purpura.

DISEASE ENTITIES; SYNONYMS AND ACRONYMS   Hemolytic uremic syndrome, HUS; thrombotic thrombocytopenic purpura, TTP.

INCIDENCE   Uncommon. Females are more commonly affected than males.

AGE   HUS affects mostly infants and children and few adults; TTP affects mostly older adults.

ETIOLOGY, PATHOGENESIS, AND PREDISPOSING FACTORS   Endothelial damage, platelet activation and intravascular coagulation; following a respiratory or GI illness in children; oral contraceptives, pregnancy; sporadic or autosomal dominant forms of HUS.

SITES INVOLVED   Small blood vessels throughout the body; glomerular capillaries are particularly vulnerable in HUS; in TTP many organs are involved with less involvement of the kidneys.

GROSS LESIONS   Skin petechiae and purpura, especially with TTP; petechiae may also be present in the viscera.

MICROSCOPIC LESIONS   Fibrin and platelet thrombi are present in glomerular capillaries with secondary mesangial proliferation and a few PMNs; fibrin thrombi may also be seen in arterioles.

COMPLICATIONS   Renal failure due to the glomerular lesions; bleeding diathesis due to thrombocytopenia; hemolytic anemia due to red cell fragmentation.

SIGNS AND SYMPTOMS   HUS: anemia and renal failure, petechiae, in a child or postpartum woman; TTP: purpura, bleeding from GI or urinary tract, anemia, neurologic symptoms, fever, renal failure.

CLINICAL DIAGNOSIS AND OTHER CLINICAL FEATURES   Recognition of presentation, especially if purpura and bleeding diathesis develop; in a child HUS may follow a respiratory or gastrointestinal illness; renal biopsy for confirmation.

LABORATORY DIAGNOSIS   Azotemia; hematuria; thrombocytopenia; hemolytic anemia with red cell fragments (schistocytes) on peripheral smear; reticulocytosis; fibrin thrombi in glomeruli and arterioles on renal biopsy.

PROGNOSIS   Mortality for childhood HUS is under 5%; for adult and postpartum HUS, 60%; TTP may be fatal.

THERAPY   Plasma infusion, gamma globulin; vincristine; plasmapheresis; dialysis for renal failure.

OTHER INFORMATION   Hemolysis is caused by fragmentation of red cells as they pass through fibrin thrombi in small blood vessels; thrombocytopenia is due to consumption of platelets.

Hypertensive Renal Disease

DESCRIPTION Renal disease caused by hypertensive arteriolosclerosis, ranging from clinically insignificant to renal failure; morphologic changes depend on the severity of the hypertension.

DISEASE ENTITIES; SYNONYMS AND ACRONYMS Arteriolonephrosclerosis; benign nephrosclerosis, malignant nephrosclerosis; hypertension, HTN.

INCIDENCE Hypertension is common, more so in men and in blacks; renal failure due to HTN is less common.

AGE Middle-aged adults; incidence increases with age.

ETIOLOGY, PATHOGENESIS, AND PREDISPOSING FACTORS Arteriolosclerosis causes parenchymal ischemia resulting in atrophy and small foci of fibrosis in benign nephrosclerosis and focal necrosis and hemorrhage in malignant nephrosclerosis.

SITES INVOLVED Kidney; small arteries and arterioles; renal cortex.

GROSS LESIONS Benign: diffuse regular granularity of cortical surface, reduction of kidney size due to loss of cortical thickness; malignant: multiple small hemorrhages on surface giving a "flea-bitten" appearance.

MICROSCOPIC LESIONS Benign: hyaline arteriolosclerosis, multiple small foci of parenchymal fibrosis; malignant: hyperplastic arteriolosclerosis, fibrinoid necrosis of arterioles, focal necrosis of parenchyma.

COMPLICATIONS Benign hypertension for many years causes some degree of renal insufficiency and occasionally renal failure; malignant hypertension is much more likely to lead to acute or chronic renal failure.

SIGNS AND SYMPTOMS Benign hypertension is often asymptomatic; malignant hypertension may cause headaches, mental disturbances, and palpitations.

CLINICAL DIAGNOSIS AND OTHER CLINICAL FEATURES The WHO definition of hypertension is systolic blood pressure greater than 160 mm Hg, diastolic pressure greater than 90 mm Hg, or both. Hypertension may be isolated systolic or systolic-diastolic.

LABORATORY DIAGNOSIS Azotemia; granular or waxy casts in urine; renal biopsy shows arteriolosclerosis, focal obliteration of glomeruli, and possibly fibrinoid arteriolar and glomerular necrosis.

PROGNOSIS Untreated HTN eventuates in heart failure, strokes, and renal failure; treatment reduces mortality.

THERAPY Diuretics and other antihypertensive agents; dialysis and renal transplantation for renal failure.

OTHER INFORMATION Because it complicates many renal diseases, HTN can be either the cause or the effect of a patient's renal disease. Arteriolosclerosis is described in Hypertensive Vascular Disease (pg. 148).

Immune Complex Glomerulonephritis

DESCRIPTION A group of inflammatory glomerular diseases produced by antigen-antibody complexes trapped in the glomerulus from the circulation or formed in situ; the antigen may be endogenous or exogenous.

DISEASE ENTITIES; SYNONYMS AND ACRONYMS GN; circulating immune complex GN; in situ immune complex GN; many specific diseases are included.

INCIDENCE A major mechanism of glomerulonephritis.

AGE Any age; see specific disease.

ETIOLOGY, PATHOGENESIS, AND PREDISPOSING FACTORS Potential antigens: bacterial (streptococcal), viral (hepatitis B), tumor-associated, DNA (lupus nephritis); complexes cause complement activation, cellular proliferation, PMN exudation, and necrosis.

SITES INVOLVED Immune complex deposits may be mesangial, subepithelial, intramembranous, or subendothelial depending on charge and size; mesangial and subendothelial deposits are called intracapillary deposits.

GROSS LESIONS No gross lesion until chronic glomerulonephritis develops; occasionally glomeruli appear prominent by their hyperemia.

MICROSCOPIC LESIONS Most commonly, there is cellular proliferation producing glomerular hypercellularity; other patterns are crescents, exudation of PMNs, and necrosis; may be focal or diffuse, segmental or generalized.

COMPLICATIONS Some diseases are transient; most cause progressive renal failure which is rapidly progressive or develops over many years.

SIGNS AND SYMPTOMS Nephritis (nephritic syndrome) characterized by hematuria is the most likely manifestation; proteinuria and/or the nephrotic syndrome is a less frequent pattern.

CLINICAL DIAGNOSIS AND OTHER CLINICAL FEATURES Suspected in cases of sudden onset of renal insufficiency with hematuria and edema but without signs of urinary tract infection or obstruction; renal biopsy confirms diagnosis.

LABORATORY DIAGNOSIS Hematuria with red cell casts; azotemia; decreased complement; electron microscopy and immunofluorescence microscopy are critical in detecting immune complexes.

PROGNOSIS Depends on specific disease; some spontaneously remit, others progress to renal failure.

THERAPY Corticosteroids; immunosuppressive therapy; dialysis, renal transplantation for end-stage disease.

OTHER INFORMATION Poststreptococcal GN is an example of circulating immune complex GN; in membranous GN, immune complexes form within the basement membrane from separate deposition of free antigen and antibody.

Infarct of Kidney

DESCRIPTION   A region of coagulative necrosis caused by ischemia due to arterial occlusion, which heals by organization and scarring. Less commonly, hemorrhagic infarcts are caused by renal vein thrombosis.

DISEASE ENTITIES; SYNONYMS AND ACRONYMS   Renal infarct, ischemic infarcts, embolic infarcts, atherosclerotic infarcts.

INCIDENCE   Common, particularly in atherosclerosis.

AGE   Middle-aged to elderly.

ETIOLOGY, PATHOGENESIS, AND PREDISPOSING FACTORS   Thrombosis, atherosclerosis; embolization of mural thrombus from heart or aorta, or from vegetation of infective endocarditis; atheroembolus from aortic plaque; vasculitis; sickle cell crisis.

SITES INVOLVED   Branch of renal artery; renal parenchyma.

GROSS LESIONS   Single or multiple wedge-shaped regions of central pallor with hemorrhagic borders; base of wedge is toward capsule, apex toward occluded artery; healed infarct is a depressed scar.

MICROSCOPIC LESIONS   Arterial thrombus in various stages of organization; cholesterol clefts in atheroembolus; coagulation necrosis of parenchyma; suppuration and abscess in septic infarcts.

COMPLICATIONS   Renal failure and hypertension following multiple or recurrent infarcts; acute pyelonephritis and renal abscesses caused by septic emboli from vegetations of infective endocarditis.

SIGNS AND SYMPTOMS   Sharp flank or abdominal pain, hematuria.

CLINICAL DIAGNOSIS AND OTHER CLINICAL FEATURES   Clinical signs and symptoms may provide a presumptive diagnosis difficult to confirm radiographically or by renal biopsy; exclusion of other lesions is important.

LABORATORY DIAGNOSIS   No specific tests, renal function may be unimpaired; urinalysis shows nonspecific hematuria; renal biopsy may show characteristic changes, but the chances of sampling the lesion are small.

PROGNOSIS   Usually good, the size of an infarct being smaller than renal reserve.

THERAPY   Treatment of underlying condition.

OTHER INFORMATION   Scars from renal infarcts may be difficult to distinguish from chronic pyelonephritis; infarcts are V-shaped; pyelonephritis scars are U-shaped; history and severity of atherosclerosis are helpful.

Membranoproliferative Glomerulonephritis

DESCRIPTION   Inflammatory glomerular diseases, Types I and II, presenting with nephritis or nephrosis and progressing to renal failure; characterized by basement membrane thickening and mesangial proliferation.

DISEASE ENTITIES; SYNONYMS AND ACRONYMS   Membranoproliferative glomerulonephritis with subendothelial deposits; dense deposit disease.

INCIDENCE   Less common than poststreptococcal glomerulonephritis.

AGE   Mainly children and young adults.

ETIOLOGY, PATHOGENESIS, AND PREDISPOSING FACTORS   Type I: most are idiopathic, others may be immune complex mediated and associated with hepatitis B; Type II: activation of alternate complement pathway by C3 nephritic factor, an IgG immunoglobulin.

SITES INVOLVED   Renal glomerulus, mesangium and basement membrane.

GROSS LESIONS   No specific gross lesion.

MICROSCOPIC LESIONS   LM: mesangial proliferation, basement membrane thickening with double contour on silver stain; EM: subendothelial deposits (Type I), ribbon-like deposits within the basement membrane (Type II); IM: weak deposition of C3 (Type II).

COMPLICATIONS   End-stage renal failure; Type II disease recurs in transplanted kidney.

SIGNS AND SYMPTOMS   Disease may present as nephritis or nephrotic syndrome and progresses to renal failure.

CLINICAL DIAGNOSIS AND OTHER CLINICAL FEATURES   Often cannot be distinguished from other types of glomerular disease without renal biopsy; persistent depression of complement may suggest the diagnosis.

LABORATORY DIAGNOSIS   Urinalysis findings of hematuria and/or proteinuria; azotemia; characteristic changes in renal biopsy, especially those seen by EM; persistently low levels of complement component C3.

PROGNOSIS   Nearly all cases progress to chronic renal failure.

THERAPY   Dialysis, renal transplantation.

OTHER INFORMATION   A new subtype (Type III membranoproliferative glomerulonephritis) is distinguished from Types I and II by electron dense deposits on both sides of the basement membrane; C3 without Ig is seen by IM.

Membranous Glomerulonephropathy

DESCRIPTION Chronic glomerular disease causing the nephrotic syndrome, characterized by deposition of immune complexes and thickening of basement membrane; progresses to chronic renal failure.

DISEASE ENTITIES; SYNONYMS AND ACRONYMS Membranous glomerulonephritis, membranous nephropathy.

INCIDENCE Most common cause of nephrotic syndrome in adults, causing 30% of cases of nephrotic syndrome.

AGE Usually adults, sometimes children.

ETIOLOGY, PATHOGENESIS, AND PREDISPOSING FACTORS Chronic immune complex disease; most cases are idiopathic; others are secondary to carcinoma, hepatitis B, systemic lupus erythematosus or drug therapy (gold, penicillamine for rheumatoid arthritis).

SITES INVOLVED Glomerulus of kidney, specifically the basement membrane.

GROSS LESIONS No gross lesion.

MICROSCOPIC LESIONS LM: thickened basement membrane with spikes seen with silver stains; EM: subepithelial deposits, later incorporated into thickened basement membrane; IM: granular deposits of IgG and C3 along basement membrane.

COMPLICATIONS Chronic renal failure develops in 10 to 15 years; renal vein thrombosis as a complication of nephrotic syndrome; pulmonary embolism; peritonitis and other infections.

SIGNS AND SYMPTOMS Nephrotic syndrome (edema, hypoalbuminemia, proteinuria); progressive renal failure.

CLINICAL DIAGNOSIS AND OTHER CLINICAL FEATURES Recognition of nephrotic syndrome; renal biopsy.

LABORATORY DIAGNOSIS Characteristic findings in the renal biopsy.

PROGNOSIS Control of the underlying condition, if present, may prevent the otherwise inevitable renal failure.

THERAPY Corticosteroids, cyclophosphamide; dialysis; renal transplantation.

OTHER INFORMATION Membranous nephropathy is similar to the experimental model, Heymann nephritis, in which free antigen and antibody are deposited separately but combine in situ within the basement membrane.

Minimal Change Disease

DESCRIPTION Glomerular disease affecting mostly children, producing the nephrotic syndrome; characterized by near normal glomeruli by light microscopy and loss of foot processes by electron microscopy.

DISEASE ENTITIES; SYNONYMS AND ACRONYMS MCD, epithelial cell disease, lipoid nephrosis, nil disease.

INCIDENCE The most common cause of nephrotic syndrome in children; affects males more than females.

AGE Children under the age of 6 years; also affects adults, causing 18% of nephrotic syndrome in adults.

ETIOLOGY, PATHOGENESIS, AND PREDISPOSING FACTORS Unknown; speculation involves a postallergic reaction, altered T-cell immunity, and circulating immune complexes; several mechanisms may explain defective glomerular filtration function.

SITES INVOLVED Glomerulus of kidney, specifically the epithelial cell foot processes.

GROSS LESIONS No change grossly.

MICROSCOPIC LESIONS LM: minimal glomerular changes, lipid droplets in proximal tubule cells; EM: effacement of epithelial cell foot processes and villous hyperplasia; IM: slight deposition of IgM and C3 within mesangium.

COMPLICATIONS Infections, interstitial nephritis, renal vein thrombosis; altogether, complications are uncommon. Progression to renal failure indicates an incorrect diagnosis.

SIGNS AND SYMPTOMS Nephrotic syndrome in a child; often presents in an atopic child following an allergic episode; edema, hypertension, proteinuria, hypoalbuminemia.

CLINICAL DIAGNOSIS AND OTHER CLINICAL FEATURES Recognition of nephrotic syndrome in a child; renal biopsy.

LABORATORY DIAGNOSIS Urinary and serum findings of nephrotic syndrome. Characteristic renal biopsy changes, particularly EM showing loss of foot processes and LM showing essentially normal glomeruli.

PROGNOSIS Good, with appropriate therapy.

THERAPY Corticosteroid therapy usually produces full remission within several weeks.

OTHER INFORMATION Initially, focal segmental glomerulosclerosis and MCD may be indistinguishable, both clinically and in the renal biopsy; MCD is benign; focal segmental glomerulosclerosis progresses to renal failure.

Myeloma Nephropathy

DESCRIPTION Glomerular and tubular lesions caused by precipitation or deposition of abnormal immunoglobulins or light chains, associated with plasma cell neoplasms that produce monoclonal immunoglobulins.

DISEASE ENTITIES; SYNONYMS AND ACRONYMS Myeloma cast or light chain nephropathy; Waldenstrom's macroglobulinemia, cryoglobulinemia, amyloidosis.

INCIDENCE Common in plasma cell dyscrasias, causing renal disease in more than half of myeloma patients.

AGE Same as myeloma; fifth decade and older.

ETIOLOGY, PATHOGENESIS, AND PREDISPOSING FACTORS Immunoglobulins deposit in glomeruli, occlude capillaries, activate complement and cause proliferative lesions; light chains deposit as amyloid fibrils or filter into tubules and precipitate as casts.

SITES INVOLVED Glomeruli and around blood vessels and tubules in amyloidosis (predominantly lambda light chains); distal and collecting tubules in myeloma cast nephropathy (predominantly kappa light chains).

GROSS LESIONS No specific gross lesion.

MICROSCOPIC LESIONS Thrombi occlude glomerular capillaries in Waldenstrom's and cryoglobulinemia; membranous and proliferative lesions may coexist; tubular casts are surrounded by giant cells in light chain nephropathy.

COMPLICATIONS Progressive renal failure.

SIGNS AND SYMPTOMS Renal insufficiency in a patient with myeloma, macroglobulinemia, or cryoglobulinemia.

CLINICAL DIAGNOSIS AND OTHER CLINICAL FEATURES Paraproteinemia of plasma cell dyscrasia may be already known or is discovered during workup for renal disease; renal biopsy is usually diagnostic.

LABORATORY DIAGNOSIS Hypergammaglobulinemia with monoclonal spike on immunoelectrophoresis; Bence-Jones proteinuria; tubular casts or glomerulopathy in renal biopsy; IM is strongly positive for immunoglobulin.

PROGNOSIS Usually progresses to end-stage renal failure; myeloma itself is fatal.

THERAPY Chemotherapy for underlying neoplasm; renal dialysis; transplantation is unlikely.

OTHER INFORMATION In cryoglobulinemia, the immunoglobulins that precipitate from serum may be monoclonal from an immunocyte neoplasm or polyclonal from a chronic inflammatory or autoimmune disease.

Nephrolithiasis

DESCRIPTION Calculi within the renal pelvis or calyces, produced by a variety of environmental, metabolic, and unknown factors and by infection; causing obstruction, infection, hematuria, and pain.

DISEASE ENTITIES; SYNONYMS AND ACRONYMS Urolithiasis, renal calculi, kidney stones.

INCIDENCE Common; affects men more than women.

AGE Adults in most cases; children with hereditary cystinuria.

ETIOLOGY, PATHOGENESIS, AND PREDISPOSING FACTORS Idiopathic hypercalciuria (calcium oxalate or phosphate stones); infection (magnesium ammonium phosphate, struvite, stones); gout (uric acid stones); cystinuria (cystine stones).

SITES INVOLVED Renal pelvis and calyces, often passing into the ureter.

GROSS LESIONS Calcium-containing calculi are usually hard with sharp edges, pale to dark brown; uric acid stones are smooth; staghorn calculi occur in chronic pyelonephritis; hydronephrosis is often present.

MICROSCOPIC LESIONS Depends on the particular complications or associated renal disease. Acute and chronic pyelonephritis are common; in hydronephrosis, the renal parenchyma is atrophic.

COMPLICATIONS Obstruction of the ureter or ureteropelvic junction; acute or chronic pyelonephritis; hydronephrosis, hydroureter.

SIGNS AND SYMPTOMS Many stones are silent until they pass into the ureter causing renal colic (severe flank pain that radiates to the scrotum); some present with urinary infection.

CLINICAL DIAGNOSIS AND OTHER CLINICAL FEATURES Renal colic is usually obvious; abdominal x-rays may show calcium stones, urate stones are radiolucent; intravenous or retrograde pyelography assesses the site and extent of obstruction.

LABORATORY DIAGNOSIS Urinalysis: hematuria or pyuria; urine culture to detect or exclude infection; chemical analysis of stone and levels of serum calcium, uric acid, and cystine to detect a metabolic disorder.

PROGNOSIS Usually good unless the complications are neglected.

THERAPY Treatment of any metabolic disease, especially gout; surgical lithotomy; ultrasonic lithotripsy.

OTHER INFORMATION Urinary infection may cause renal stones or may complicate renal stones; urolithiasis, urinary obstruction, and urinary infection often constitute a self-perpetuating process.

Polycystic Kidney Disease—Adult Type

DESCRIPTION Autosomal dominant genetic disease in which the renal parenchyma is converted into a mass of fluid-filled cysts, resulting in progressive renal failure that commences in adulthood.

DISEASE ENTITIES; SYNONYMS AND ACRONYMS Adult polycystic disease, autosomal dominant polycystic kidney disease.

INCIDENCE Causes 8–10% of end-stage renal disease.

AGE Presents with renal disease in 30s or 40s; end-stage renal failure age 55–60.

ETIOLOGY, PATHOGENESIS, AND PREDISPOSING FACTORS Autosomal dominant inheritance of gene on chromosome 6; few cases from spontaneous mutation; cysts develop from dilated tubules and Bowman's space and compress surrounding parenchyma.

SITES INVOLVED Kidneys, bilateral. In 30–40% of cases, there are cysts in the liver, lined by biliary epithelium; congenital (berry) aneurysms are present in 10–30%; floppy mitral valve may also be present.

GROSS LESIONS Massive enlargement of kidneys, up to 4500 g; hundreds of cysts measuring up to several centimeters filled with clear yellow fluid replace essentially the entire parenchyma; occasional cyst contains blood.

MICROSCOPIC LESIONS Cysts lined by cuboidal epithelium compress atrophic remnants of renal parenchyma; foci of chronic inflammation and old hemorrhage are present.

COMPLICATIONS Progressive renal failure leading to uremia; hypertension with associated heart disease or intracerebral hemorrhage; subarachnoid hemorrhage from ruptured congenital (berry) aneurysm.

SIGNS AND SYMPTOMS Flank pain, bilateral masses in the flanks; hematuria with blood clots in the urine; hypertension; progressive azotemia.

CLINICAL DIAGNOSIS AND OTHER CLINICAL FEATURES Usually discovered by the fourth decade in work-up for renal insufficiency, hematuria, flank mass or pain, or hypertension; ultrasonography and CT scans are likely to be diagnostic.

LABORATORY DIAGNOSIS No specific tests except to measure renal function by BUN, creatinine, or creatinine clearance; urinalysis confirms hematuria and excludes infection.

PROGNOSIS Progresses to chronic renal failure; fatal if untreated.

THERAPY Dialysis; renal transplantation.

OTHER INFORMATION Autosomal recessive polycystic kidney disease causes progressive renal failure in infancy or early childhood and is associated with hepatic fibrosis.

Pyelonephritis—Acute

DESCRIPTION   Acute bacterial infection of the renal parenchyma affecting predominantly the tubules and interstitium, most often caused by gram-negative organisms ascending from a lower urinary tract infection.

DISEASE ENTITIES; SYNONYMS AND ACRONYMS   Urinary tract infection, UTI.

INCIDENCE   Common, especially in women.

AGE   Women of all ages; elderly men with prostatic enlargement.

ETIOLOGY, PATHOGENESIS, AND PREDISPOSING FACTORS   Female short urethra, moist perineum, absence of prostatic secretions, pregnancy; obstruction by prostate hyperplasia, urolithiasis; diabetes mellitus; catheterization; hematogenous route is uncommon.

SITES INVOLVED   Renal parenchyma, initiating in the papillae and spreading throughout the medulla to the cortex.

GROSS LESIONS   Edema and hyperemia, particularly of the medulla; multiple foci of suppuration (microabscesses) are often apparent in the parenchyma and cortical surface; larger abscesses may form.

MICROSCOPIC LESIONS   Purulent exudate in the tubules and interstitium; glomeruli are often spared; necrosis of underlying parenchyma with abscess formation is common.

COMPLICATIONS   Acute renal failure; chronic renal failure due to chronic pyelonephritis; gram-negative sepsis; renal or perirenal abscess.

SIGNS AND SYMPTOMS   Fever, malaise, lower abdominal pain, flank or costovertebral angle tenderness, dysuria, hematuria.

CLINICAL DIAGNOSIS AND OTHER CLINICAL FEATURES   Signs and symptoms are often diagnostic, although it may be difficult to differentiate a lower from an upper urinary infection; in males especially, obstruction should be suspected.

LABORATORY DIAGNOSIS   Urinalysis: white cells indicate UTI; white cell casts differentiate pyelonephritis from acute cystitis; *E. coli* is most frequently cultured; bacteriuria sometimes occurs without symptoms.

PROGNOSIS   Good, with therapy; however, there is usually some degree of irreversible parenchymal damage.

THERAPY   Antibiotics; bacteriostatic agents; relief of obstruction.

OTHER INFORMATION   In girls, vesicoureteral reflux is likely; many initial cases are associated with sexual activity (honeymoon cystitis); spinal cord defects often cause UTI due to atony (neurogenic bladder).

Pyelonephritis—Chronic

DESCRIPTION Chronic tubulointerstitial disease causing renal failure, characterized by irregular scarring of the kidney; associated with recurrent bacterial infections, obstruction, or vesicoureteral reflux.

DISEASE ENTITIES; SYNONYMS AND ACRONYMS Reflux nephropathy.

INCIDENCE Common cause of renal failure, accounting for 15% of dialysis or renal transplant patients.

AGE Middle-aged adults; more common in women.

ETIOLOGY, PATHOGENESIS, AND PREDISPOSING FACTORS Recurrent episodes of acute pyelonephritis produce accumulation of renal scars; vesicoureteral reflux is an important etiology, as is obstruction due to ureteral strictures or urolithiasis.

SITES INVOLVED Kidney cortex and medulla, particularly the regions overlying the calyces.

GROSS LESIONS Multiple irregular 1–2 cm depressed scars present on the cortical surface with fibrosis and atrophy of the underlying parenchyma; calyces and pelvis may be dilated; renal calculi are common.

MICROSCOPIC LESIONS Dilatation and atrophy of tubules filled with eosinophilic material (thyroidization); interstitial fibrosis; chronic mononuclear inflammatory cell infiltrates; glomeruli may be normal or sclerotic.

COMPLICATIONS End-stage renal failure; hypertension.

SIGNS AND SYMPTOMS Recurrent urinary tract infections; renal insufficiency; episodes of urolithiasis; urinary obstruction due to calculi, prostate enlargement, congenital urethral valves, tumors, etc.

CLINICAL DIAGNOSIS AND OTHER CLINICAL FEATURES Should be considered in the differential of any patient with renal failure; history may indicate recurrent infections; kidneys are shrunken by ultrasonography; renal biopsy to confirm diagnosis.

LABORATORY DIAGNOSIS Azotemia; broad waxy casts on urinalysis; acute pyelonephritis may be superimposed with pyuria and positive urine culture; renal biopsy may support diagnosis or at least exclude other diseases.

PROGNOSIS Usually progresses to chronic renal failure despite treatment of any residual infection.

THERAPY Antibiotics for active infection; treatment of obstruction; dialysis; renal transplantation.

OTHER INFORMATION Xanthogranulomatous pyelonephritis is a type of chronic pyelonephritis with granulomas and accumulation of lipid-laden macrophages caused by chronic bacterial infection.

Renal Cell Carcinoma

DESCRIPTION   Primary malignant neoplasm of the kidney occurring in adults.

DISEASE ENTITIES; SYNONYMS AND ACRONYMS   Hypernephroma, adenocarcinoma of kidney.

INCIDENCE   Constitutes 1–3% of all visceral cancers; male:female = 3:1.

AGE   Most common in the sixth and seventh decade.

ETIOLOGY, PATHOGENESIS, AND PREDISPOSING FACTORS   Neoplastic disease of unknown etiology; more common in tobacco smokers; occurs with high frequency in von Hippel-Lindau syndrome; abnormalities in chromosomes 3, 8, and 11 are seen in inherited cases.

SITES INVOLVED   Kidney, usually one of the poles, most commonly the upper one; usually unilateral; bilateral tumors are seen in the von Hippel-Lindau syndrome.

GROSS LESIONS   Spherical yellowish mass 3–15 cm in diameter, arising within the parenchyma and protruding above the cortex; hemorrhage and necrosis are common; invasion of renal vein or pelvis is likely.

MICROSCOPIC LESIONS   Tumor cells are arranged in solid, papillary, trabecular, or tubular patterns; most common cell is the clear cell, which contains glycogen and lipid; granular or spindle tumor cells are less common.

COMPLICATIONS   Metastases, particularly to lungs and bones. Paraneoplastic syndromes due to hormone secretion: polycythemia (erythropoietin), hypercalcemia (parathormone), hypertension (renin), Cushing's (ACTH).

SIGNS AND SYMPTOMS   Malaise, weakness, weight loss; the classic triad of hematuria, palpable mass, and flank pain are present in less than 10% of cases; 25% present with metastases.

CLINICAL DIAGNOSIS AND OTHER CLINICAL FEATURES   Tumors are frequently silent so that early discovery depends on high suspicion of constitutional symptoms; x-rays, intravenous pyelogram, CT and MRI scans; surgical exploration.

LABORATORY DIAGNOSIS   Histologic examination of resected specimen or of biopsy of primary or metastatic tumor.

PROGNOSIS   Overall 5-year survival, 40%; with spread or renal vein invasion, 15–20%; confined to kidney, 70%.

THERAPY   Nephrectomy.

OTHER INFORMATION   Similar tumors less than 3 cm in diameter are called renal cortical adenomas because they rarely metastasize.

Renovascular Hypertension

DESCRIPTION   Secondary systemic hypertension induced by hypersecretion of renin from an ischemic kidney, caused by renal artery stenosis due to atherosclerosis or fibromuscular dysplasia.

DISEASE ENTITIES; SYNONYMS AND ACRONYMS   Goldblatt kidney, renal artery stenosis, fibromuscular hyperplasia or dysplasia of the renal artery.

INCIDENCE   Constitutes less than 5% of all cases of hypertension; most cases are due to atherosclerosis.

AGE   Atherosclerotic: mostly men, average age 55; fibromuscular dysplasia: mostly women, average age 35.

ETIOLOGY, PATHOGENESIS, AND PREDISPOSING FACTORS   Atherosclerosis or fibromuscular dysplasia produces stenosis of one or both renal arteries; the ischemic kidney is thereby stimulated to secrete excess renin, elevating angiotensin and aldosterone.

SITES INVOLVED   Atheromas of the aorta or proximal renal artery narrows the ostium or lumen of the artery. In fibromuscular dysplasia, usually the distal two thirds of the renal artery are involved.

GROSS LESIONS   In fibromuscular dysplasia, there is segmental thickening of the arterial wall with narrowing of the lumen. The fibrofatty plaque of atherosclerosis is described in Chapter 12: Cardiovascular System (pg. 142).

MICROSCOPIC LESIONS   Fibromuscular dysplasia shows fibrosis and sometimes segmental hyperplasia of the arterial media producing segmental stenosis; some segments are normal, others are severely stenotic.

COMPLICATIONS   Hypertension with cardiac hypertrophy or stroke. The kidney contralateral to the stenosis may develop hypertensive arteriolosclerosis; this reduces the chances for surgical cure of the hypertension.

SIGNS AND SYMPTOMS   Systemic hypertension with its expected manifestations and complications. The degree of hypertension is often more severe and its onset more sudden than with essential hypertension.

CLINICAL DIAGNOSIS AND OTHER CLINICAL FEATURES   Should be suspected in a young woman with hypertension or in an older man who demonstrates sudden elevation of blood pressure; renal artery angiography demonstrates the stenosis.

LABORATORY DIAGNOSIS   Elevated plasma renin; with catheterization of the individual renal veins and measurement of renin levels from each, renin is elevated from the stenotic side and reduced from the contralateral side.

PROGNOSIS   Often good with surgical therapy unless the contralateral kidney is damaged by the hypertension.

THERAPY   Surgical correction of the stenosis or nephrectomy of the ischemic kidney.

OTHER INFORMATION   It is important to recognize this cause of hypertension because of the great potential for surgical cure; delay in recognition risks irreversible damage of the uninvolved kidney.

Systemic Lupus Erythematosus Glomerulonephritis

DESCRIPTION   A spectrum of immune complex diseases of the renal glomeruli, constituting an important part of the manifestations of systemic lupus erythematosus (SLE).

DISEASE ENTITIES; SYNONYMS AND ACRONYMS   SLE; lupus nephritis or nephropathy; WHO classes I–V SLE glomerulonephritis; membranous glomerulonephropathy.

INCIDENCE   Significant renal disease develops in 70% of SLE patients.

AGE   As with SLE, most common in young women.

ETIOLOGY, PATHOGENESIS, AND PREDISPOSING FACTORS   Immune complex glomerulonephritis due to mesangial or basement membrane deposition of endogenous DNA and other nuclear components complexed with autoantibodies (anti-DNA, antinuclear antibodies).

SITES INVOLVED   Renal glomerulus; immune complexes are deposited in the mesangium along the basement membrane; there may be prominent tubulointerstitial inflammation or a necrotizing vasculitis.

GROSS LESIONS   No specific gross lesion; focal hemorrhages may be present due to concomitant vasculitis.

MICROSCOPIC LESIONS   LM: proliferative changes, crescents, BM thickening, wire-loop lesions, necrosis, hematoxylin bodies; IM: IgM,G,A; C3,4,1q deposits; EM: mesangial or subendothelial deposits with fingerprint pattern.

COMPLICATIONS   Nephritis or nephrotic syndrome; renal failure commonly develops and is the cause of death in a third of SLE patients.

SIGNS AND SYMPTOMS   Renal insufficiency; nephritis or nephrotic syndrome in a patient with SLE.

CLINICAL DIAGNOSIS AND OTHER CLINICAL FEATURES   Should be anticipated in any patient with SLE; renal biopsy is indicated to classify the glomerular disease for prognostic purposes.

LABORATORY DIAGNOSIS   Hematuria, red cell casts; variable proteinuria, hypoalbuminemia, azotemia; examination of renal biopsy; antinuclear antibodies, anti-DNA present in serum.

PROGNOSIS   Often poor, depends on WHO class; progression of renal disease is a prognostic indicator for SLE.

THERAPY   Corticosteroids, other immunosuppressive drugs; dialysis; renal transplantation is unlikely in SLE.

OTHER INFORMATION   WHO class I: SLE without glomerular lesion; II: mesangial lesions only; III, IV: inflammatory, proliferative, necrotizing lesions; V: membranous glomerulopathy; classes II and V have best prognosis.

Transitional Cell Carcinoma of Renal Pelvis and Ureter

DESCRIPTION   Primary malignant neoplasm of the renal pelvis or ureter; most often a papillary transitional cell carcinoma (TCC) but may also be squamous carcinoma or rarely adenocarcinoma.

DISEASE ENTITIES; SYNONYMS AND ACRONYMS   Urothelial carcinoma, urothelial neoplasm, transitional cell carcinoma, TCC.

INCIDENCE   Uncommon; 90% are transitional cell type; squamous types constitute most of the remainder.

AGE   Adults, 50–70 years of age; affects predominantly males.

ETIOLOGY, PATHOGENESIS, AND PREDISPOSING FACTORS   Same as for TCC of urinary bladder; urolithiasis may precede the squamous type; multiple separate foci of neoplasm occurring in the pelvis, ureter, and urinary bladder are common with TCC.

SITES INVOLVED   Renal pelvis or ureter; arising from epithelium and either projecting into the lumen or invading the wall and surrounding structures.

GROSS LESIONS   TCC is usually exophytic with papillary projections forming a bulky mass within the lumen; high-grade TCC and squamous carcinoma are more invasive of the pelvic or ureteral wall.

MICROSCOPIC LESIONS   TCC Grade I: well-differentiated cells on papillary fronds; Grade III: poorly differentiated, pleomorphic cells, many mitoses, fusion of papillae, focal squamous change; Grade II is intermediate.

COMPLICATIONS   Urinary obstruction, hydronephrosis, pyelonephritis; invasion of surrounding structures including kidney; metastases; recurrences and neoplasms developing at other sites are common.

SIGNS AND SYMPTOMS   Flank pain; hematuria; fever from secondary pyelonephritis.

CLINICAL DIAGNOSIS AND OTHER CLINICAL FEATURES   Investigation of urinary symptoms; intravenous or retrograde pyelogram. After resection, indefinite close follow-up is required for early detection of TCC developing at other urothelial sites.

LABORATORY DIAGNOSIS   Urine cytology; histologic examination of biopsied or resected lesion; determining depth of invasion (stage) and histologic grading are important for prognosis.

PROGNOSIS   Depends on grade and stage; good for neoplasm limited to mucosa; poor for invasion beyond wall.

THERAPY   Surgical resection which usually involves nephrectomy as well.

OTHER INFORMATION   Carcinoma of the renal pelvis that invades the kidney may be grossly distinguished from a renal cell carcinoma by its site, papillary growth pattern and color.

Transitional Cell Carcinoma of Urinary Bladder

DESCRIPTION Primary malignant neoplasm of the urinary bladder, arising from the urothelium and projecting into the bladder cavity as well as invading into and through the bladder wall.

DISEASE ENTITIES; SYNONYMS AND ACRONYMS Urothelial carcinoma, papillary transitional cell carcinoma, TCC.

INCIDENCE Fairly common; the most common urinary bladder cancer; male:female = 4:1.

AGE Most common from 50 to 80 years.

ETIOLOGY, PATHOGENESIS, AND PREDISPOSING FACTORS Occupational exposure in dye, rubber, paint, chemical industries; beta-naphthylamine and other arylamines are oxidized and conjugated in the liver and excreted as concentrated carcinogens in urine.

SITES INVOLVED Urinary bladder mucosa initially, growing into the lumen and invading the wall and surrounding tissues in advanced neoplasms.

GROSS LESIONS Exophytic papillary mass projecting into the lumen and invading the wall with regions of hemorrhage and necrosis; less exophytic growth, solid, and more invasive lesions indicate higher grade tumors.

MICROSCOPIC LESIONS Range from WHO Grade I well-differentiated papillary tumors to Grade III poorly differentiated neoplasms with cellular pleomorphism, high mitotic count and foci of squamous differentiation.

COMPLICATIONS Invasion of perivesicular tissue; ureteral invasion with urinary obstruction leading to hydronephrosis, pyelonephritis, and renal failure; metastases to lymph nodes, liver, lung, and bone.

SIGNS AND SYMPTOMS Sudden onset of hematuria; associated dysuria is often lacking.

CLINICAL DIAGNOSIS AND OTHER CLINICAL FEATURES Painless hematuria is suspicious; cystograms show mass causing filling defect; cystoscopy permits direct visualization of most lesions except carcinoma-in-situ; biopsy.

LABORATORY DIAGNOSIS Urine cytology; histologic examination of biopsied or resected lesion; depth of invasion and histologic grade determinations are important for prognosis and treatment.

PROGNOSIS Often poor long-term survival due to recurrences; with deep muscle invasion, 1-year median survival.

THERAPY Limited invasion: superficial resection; deep invasion or TCC in situ: cystectomy; chemotherapy.

OTHER INFORMATION Stage 0: limited to mucosa; A: lamina propria invasion; B: muscle invasion, B1-superficial, B2-deep; C: perivesical invasion; D: metastases, D1-local, D2-distant. TCC in situ is an aggressive lesion.

Tubulointerstitial Nephritis
Caused by Drugs

DESCRIPTION   Lesions of tubules and interstitium producing acute renal failure, caused by several drugs, beta-lactam antibiotics particularly, mediated by immunologic mechanisms or direct nephrotoxicity.

DISEASE ENTITIES; SYNONYMS AND ACRONYMS   Allergic interstitial nephritis, methicillin hypersensitivity nephritis; aminoglycoside nephrotoxicity.

INCIDENCE   Fairly common complication of therapy with a number of drugs, including antibiotics.

AGE   Any age; most likely in later adult years due to increased number of therapeutic agents consumed.

ETIOLOGY, PATHOGENESIS, AND PREDISPOSING FACTORS   Hypersensitivity mechanism: methicillin, other antibiotics, diuretics, nonsteroidal anti-inflammatory agents; direct nephrotoxicity: gentamicin, other aminoglycoside antibiotics, amphotericin B.

SITES INVOLVED   Renal tubules and interstitium.

GROSS LESIONS   No specific gross lesions.

MICROSCOPIC LESIONS   In the hypersensitivity type, there is interstitial inflammation with lymphocytes and other mononuclear cells; eosinophils are often prominent; granulomas may be seen.

COMPLICATIONS   Acute renal failure.

SIGNS AND SYMPTOMS   Renal insufficiency developing in a patient treated with methicillin, aminoglycoside antibiotic, or many other therapeutic agents.

CLINICAL DIAGNOSIS AND OTHER CLINICAL FEATURES   Renal insufficiency with indications of tubular defects in a predisposed patient; return of renal function after withdrawal of agent confirms the diagnosis; renal biopsy may be required.

LABORATORY DIAGNOSIS   Defective tubular function is indicated by dilute urine, salt wasting, and metabolic acidosis; renal biopsy shows interstitial nephritis and excludes other causes for the renal failure.

PROGNOSIS   Renal function usually improves after withdrawal of the offending agent.

THERAPY   Avoidance of agent; fluid and electrolyte management; dialysis until renal function recovers.

OTHER INFORMATION   Nephrotoxic damage by aminoglycoside antibiotics produces acute tubular necrosis, the features of which are described separately (pg. 240).

Wilms' Tumor

DESCRIPTION Primary malignant neoplasm of kidney that occurs most often in childhood, originating from the primitive renal blastema.

DISEASE ENTITIES; SYNONYMS AND ACRONYMS Nephroblastoma.

INCIDENCE One of the most common tumors of childhood.

AGE Childhood, peak ages between 2 and 4 years.

ETIOLOGY, PATHOGENESIS, AND PREDISPOSING FACTORS Neoplastic disease of unknown etiology; karyotypic abnormalities, particularly deletions in the short arm of chromosome 11, may be etiologically important.

SITES INVOLVED Kidney; 5–10% are bilateral.

GROSS LESIONS Usually solid tan mass invading and expanding within the kidney, which it often dwarfs; areas of hemorrhage and necrosis may be present.

MICROSCOPIC LESIONS Sheets or nests of small oval cells with scant cytoplasm; primitive glomerular and tubular structures; spindle cell stroma; mesenchymal elements (e.g., cartilage) and sarcomatous patterns are common.

COMPLICATIONS Metastases, commonly to the lung; intestinal obstruction; intra-abdominal hemorrhage; hypertension.

SIGNS AND SYMPTOMS Abdominal mass usually discovered by the mother.

CLINICAL DIAGNOSIS AND OTHER CLINICAL FEATURES Assessment of the abdominal mass by x-rays, intravenous pyelograms, CT and MRI scans; laparotomy with biopsy.

LABORATORY DIAGNOSIS Histologic examination of resected or biopsied mass; anaplasia of the stroma is related to prognosis; urine vanillylmandelic acid assay to exclude neuroblastoma.

PROGNOSIS Long-term survival rates of 90% are expected with aggressive therapy.

THERAPY Surgical resection; chemotherapy; radiation therapy.

OTHER INFORMATION Wilms' tumor must be differentiated from neuroblastoma and malignant lymphoma, which are other small-cell tumors of childhood.

Pathology Facts, by Richard C.
Harruff, J.B. Lippincott
Company, Philadelphia © 1994.

Chapter 17

Male Genital System

Carcinoma of Penis

DESCRIPTION Primary malignant neoplasm of the penis originating from squamous epithelium of the glans or inner surface of the foreskin and progressively invading the shaft of the penis.

DISEASE ENTITIES; SYNONYMS AND ACRONYMS Squamous cell carcinoma of penis; epidermoid carcinoma of penis; cancer of penis; verrucous carcinoma.

INCIDENCE Uncommon in US, constituting about 1% of all cancers; much more common in Asia and Africa.

AGE Average 60 years; range 40–70 years.

ETIOLOGY, PATHOGENESIS, AND PREDISPOSING FACTORS Very rare in males circumcised at birth; collection of smegma under the foreskin is presumed to be carcinogenic; other speculations regard the human papilloma virus as etiologic.

SITES INVOLVED Initially the glans or the inner surface of the foreskin; later there is deep invasion of the shaft.

GROSS LESIONS Early lesions appear as a thickened whitish plaque (leukoplakia); later there is ulceration with ragged heaped up margins and induration; some may show a more exophytic and papillary growth pattern.

MICROSCOPIC LESIONS Most are well-differentiated squamous carcinomas with foci of keratinization, appearing the same as any other squamous carcinoma of skin.

COMPLICATIONS Metastases to inguinal lymph nodes then iliac nodes and distant organs; secondary infection of the ulcerated tumor; occasional destruction of the urethral meatus.

SIGNS AND SYMPTOMS Early nonulcerated lesions are nonpainful and often are undiscovered or ignored; most tumors have been present for at least a year, at which time there is ulceration, infection, exudation, and pain.

CLINICAL DIAGNOSIS AND OTHER CLINICAL FEATURES The typically advanced lesions are quite apparent on inspection; they are differentiated from simple ulcers by the growth at the margins; variants may appear similar to large condylomas.

LABORATORY DIAGNOSIS Histology of biopsy; if biopsy is taken too superficially, only nondiagnostic necrotic tissue is obtained; inguinal lymph node biopsy differentiates metastases from reactive changes due to infection.

PROGNOSIS Depends on extent of invasion; with penile shaft invasion, the prognosis is poor.

THERAPY Partial or complete penectomy.

OTHER INFORMATION Giant condyloma of Buschke-Lowenstein, also called verrucous carcinoma, is associated with human papilloma virus infection; it is invasive and tends to recur after excision but does not metastasize.

Carcinoma of Prostate

DESCRIPTION   Primary malignant neoplasm of prostate, arising from peripheral glands, invading periprostatic tissues, and metastasizing to bone and other tissues.

DISEASE ENTITIES; SYNONYMS AND ACRONYMS   Adenocarcinoma of prostate; prostate cancer.

INCIDENCE   Most common male cancer; third most common cause of male cancer death; highest rates in US blacks.

AGE   Increasing incidence with age; 75% of cases are in ages 60–79 years; uncommon under 50 years.

ETIOLOGY, PATHOGENESIS, AND PREDISPOSING FACTORS   Age-dependent alterations in estrogens and androgens, particularly the latter; hormonal effects may interact with a carcinogen.

SITES INVOLVED   Early adenocarcinoma originates in the periphery of the prostate and then invades throughout the prostate and into periprostatic tissue.

GROSS LESIONS   Early: firm yellowish foci at the peripheral prostate; later: irregular invasion throughout prostate; differs from nodular hyperplasia by its yellowish induration and lack of diffuse nodularity.

MICROSCOPIC LESIONS   Small glandular structures composed of a single layer of uniform neoplastic cells arranged haphazardly within a desmoplastic stroma; appearance depends on grade; perineural invasion is common.

COMPLICATIONS   Urinary obstruction; metastases to lymph nodes, bones (especially vertebra), lung and liver; termination in carcinomatosis with cachexia, sepsis, and pneumonia.

SIGNS AND SYMPTOMS   Most present with urinary symptoms, indicating an advanced stage; earlier stages are asymptomatic and neoplasm is discovered on rectal examination; perineal pain; bone pain from metastases.

CLINICAL DIAGNOSIS AND OTHER CLINICAL FEATURES   Peripheral firm nodules on rectal exam with early disease; enlargement and induration with advanced tumor; lymphangiography, x-rays, bone and CT scans for staging; bone metastases are sclerotic.

LABORATORY DIAGNOSIS   Histology of transrectal biopsy; elevated serum acid phosphatase and prostate-specific antigen; clinically insignificant foci of carcinoma are often found in prostatic tissue resected for hyperplasia.

PROGNOSIS   Depends on stage and grade; 10-year survival of 50–80% for Stages A or B.

THERAPY   Surgical resection; radiotherapy; hormonal manipulation (orchiectomy or estrogen therapy).

OTHER INFORMATION   Stage A: microscopic foci in clinically benign prostate; B: palpable tumor but confined to prostate; C: invasion outside the prostate; D: local or distant metastases.

Epididymitis

DESCRIPTION Inflammatory disease of the epididymis caused in younger men most often by *Neisseria gonorrhoeae* and *Chlamydia trachomatis* from sexually transmitted disease and in older men by *Escherichia coli.*

DISEASE ENTITIES; SYNONYMS AND ACRONYMS Gonorrhea; gonococcal, chlamydial, bacterial, tuberculous epididymitis; granulomatous epididymitis; spermatic granuloma.

INCIDENCE Common as a consequence of sexually transmitted disease (STD) or urinary tract infection (UTI).

AGE Younger than 35 years: *N. gonorrhoeae* or *C. trachomatis* from STD; older men: *E. coli* from UTI.

ETIOLOGY, PATHOGENESIS, AND PREDISPOSING FACTORS STD- and UTI-associated infections: spread from urethritis and prostatitis; tuberculous: spread from lung or kidney infection; spermatic granuloma: a reaction to sperm following trauma or infection.

SITES INVOLVED Epididymis; infection may also involve the testis (orchitis).

GROSS LESIONS Bacterial infections: early suppuration and abscesses, later scarring and contraction; tuberculous: caseous material filling the epididymis; spermatic granuloma: induration of the epididymis.

MICROSCOPIC LESIONS Bacterial infections: early purulence, later chronic inflammation, fibrous obliteration of lumen; tuberculous: caseous granulomas; spermatic granuloma: sperm fragments surrounded by granulomas.

COMPLICATIONS Destructive orchitis; infertility.

SIGNS AND SYMPTOMS Swelling and pain of the epididymis; dysuria indicating urethritis; prostatic enlargement in older men; tuberculous infection is characterized by beading along the epididymis.

CLINICAL DIAGNOSIS AND OTHER CLINICAL FEATURES Obvious in many cases from history and associated signs of STD or UTI; with tuberculous infection, positive skin tests; radiologic studies may disclose the primary site in lung and/or kidney.

LABORATORY DIAGNOSIS Microscopic examination and culture of urine, urethral discharge, and prostatic secretions; histologic examination of biopsied or resected tissue.

PROGNOSIS Minimal residual damage if infection is treated early; neglected infections result in scarring.

THERAPY Specific antibiotic or antitubercular therapy.

OTHER INFORMATION Epididymitis in a young homosexual man is more likely to be caused by enteric gram-negative bacteria than by gonococcus or Chlamydia.

Germ Cell Neoplasms of Testis

DESCRIPTION Primary malignant neoplasms originating from germ cells of the seminiferous tubules; subtypes are categorized by their differentiation and maturation of the primitive elements.

DISEASE ENTITIES; SYNONYMS AND ACRONYMS Germ cell tumor, GCT, seminoma, embryonal carcinoma, yolk sac tumor, choriocarcinoma, teratoma, mixed germ cell tumor.

INCIDENCE Fairly common; highest rates in US whites compared with US blacks and Asians.

AGE Infants/children: yolk sac tumor, teratoma; adults, age 20s: embryonal carcinoma; 30s: seminoma.

ETIOLOGY, PATHOGENESIS, AND PREDISPOSING FACTORS Largely unknown; GCT is 35 times more common in cryptorchidism; one GCT increases the risk of a second GCT in the other testis.

SITES INVOLVED Testis; anaplastic germ cells develop within the seminiferous tumors and then invade throughout the testis; later there is invasion into the epididymis and tunica.

GROSS LESIONS Bulging mass within testis; seminoma: solid white; embryonal carcinoma: variegated with necrosis and hemorrhage; choriocarcinoma: often quite small and completely hemorrhagic; teratoma: cystic mass.

MICROSCOPIC LESIONS Seminoma: sheets of germ cells with lymphocytes; embryonal carcinoma: primitive acinar and papillary structures; yolk sac tumor: Schiller-Duval bodies; teratoma: admixture of mature tissue elements.

COMPLICATIONS Metastatic spread to retroperitoneal lymph nodes, lungs, liver, and mediastinal lymph nodes.

SIGNS AND SYMPTOMS Testicular swelling, palpable mass, and occasionally pain.

CLINICAL DIAGNOSIS AND OTHER CLINICAL FEATURES Painless enlargement of the testis is highly suspicious; any testicular swelling should be considered a neoplasm until disproved; CT scans of chest and abdomen to detect metastases.

LABORATORY DIAGNOSIS Histologic examination of resected testis; serum human chorionic gonadotropin is elevated with choriocarcinoma; alpha-fetoprotein is elevated with yolk sac tumor; both may be elevated with mixed GCT.

PROGNOSIS Depends on subtype and stage; best for seminoma; less favorable for nonseminomatous GCT (< 50%).

THERAPY Orchiectomy; retroperitoneal lymph node dissection; chemotherapy with cisplatin; radiation therapy.

OTHER INFORMATION An uncommon variant, spermatocytic seminoma, is seen in men over 65; teratomas in the infant are benign; in the adult, teratomas are considered malignant. Pure choriocarcinoma is highly malignant.

Nodular Hyperplasia of Prostate

DESCRIPTION Benign enlargement of the prostate due to hyperplastic nodules of stroma and glands distorting the prostate, compressing the urethra and causing urinary obstruction.

DISEASE ENTITIES; SYNONYMS AND ACRONYMS Benign prostatic hyperplasia (hypertrophy is also used but inappropriately), BPH; prostatism.

INCIDENCE Very common.

AGE Increasing incidence with age starting at 40 years; affects up to 75% of men by age 80 years.

ETIOLOGY, PATHOGENESIS, AND PREDISPOSING FACTORS Age-dependent changes of estrogens and androgens are believed to cause prostatic hyperplasia, but the mechanism is not understood.

SITES INVOLVED Earliest nodules develop in the submucosal zone of the proximal urethra; subsequent nodule growth compresses the prostate outward toward its capsule.

GROSS LESIONS Prostate is enlarged with well-demarcated nodules ranging up to 1 cm in diameter; nodules often compress the urethra and bladder neck.

MICROSCOPIC LESIONS Both stroma and glands show hyperplasia; the most common variant is fibromyoadenomatous hyperplasia in which proliferating glands are surrounded by proliferating smooth muscle cells and fibroblasts.

COMPLICATIONS Urethral or bladder neck obstruction with urinary stasis and infection; prostatitis, pyelonephritis; trabeculation of the bladder; hydronephrosis; infarction of nodules may cause acute obstruction.

SIGNS AND SYMPTOMS Multiple urinary problems caused by partial obstruction: frequency, difficulty starting or stopping the stream, nocturia, overflow dribbling, dysuria; signs of urinary tract infection are likely.

CLINICAL DIAGNOSIS AND OTHER CLINICAL FEATURES Prostatic enlargement is suggested by the history; workup is directed at confirming nodular hyperplasia rather than cancer or infection; nodules are usually palpable on rectal examination.

LABORATORY DIAGNOSIS Histologic examination of transrectal prostate biopsy or cytology of fine needle aspiration differentiates hyperplasia from carcinoma; culture of urine or prostate secretions may reveal infection.

PROGNOSIS Usually good with therapy; neglected obstruction may cause chronic pyelonephritis and renal failure.

THERAPY Catheterization for acute obstruction; transurethral or suprapubic resection of prostate.

OTHER INFORMATION Although focal carcinoma may be found in up to 10% of prostatic resections for hyperplasia, nodular hyperplasia of the prostate is not considered premalignant.

Orchitis

DESCRIPTION   Acute or chronic inflammatory disease of testis, often caused by gram-negative organisms complicating urinary tract infection; also seen in cases of mumps and in other infections.

DISEASE ENTITIES; SYNONYMS AND ACRONYMS   Acute orchitis, testicular abscess; mumps, syphilitic, tuberculous orchitis; granulomatous orchitis; malakoplakia.

INCIDENCE   Bacterial orchitis is uncommon; testicular involvement occurs in 20% of adult cases of mumps.

AGE   Any age, mostly in older men due to higher incidence of urinary infections.

ETIOLOGY, PATHOGENESIS, AND PREDISPOSING FACTORS   Gram-negative bacteria, particularly *E. coli;* mumps virus, *Mycobacterium tuberculosis, Treponema pallidum;* etiology is unknown in granulomatous orchitis and malakoplakia.

SITES INVOLVED   Testis; in bacterial orchitis, the epididymis is usually also involved.

GROSS LESIONS   Bacterial infection: suppuration and abscesses; syphilitic orchitis: gummas which produce contracted scars; mumps: edema; tuberculous orchitis: caseous necrosis.

MICROSCOPIC LESIONS   Bacterial: PMNs and liquefactive necrosis; syphilitic: epithelioid cells and central coagulation necrosis; tuberculous: caseous granulomas; granulomatous orchitis: granulomas without central necrosis.

COMPLICATIONS   Infertility if bilateral; rarely a source of gram-negative sepsis.

SIGNS AND SYMPTOMS   Scrotal pain, swelling and redness; testicular swelling and induration; fever.

CLINICAL DIAGNOSIS AND OTHER CLINICAL FEATURES   Acute bacterial infection may be inferred from the suppuration and its response to antibiotics; less acutely inflamed testicular swellings need to be differentiated from neoplasm.

LABORATORY DIAGNOSIS   CBC showing leukocytosis; bacterial culture of urine, prostatic fluid or needle aspiration of testicular exudate; histologic examination and culture of resected testis.

PROGNOSIS   Infection infrequently affects survival; testicular destruction is likely.

THERAPY   Specific antibiotics; orchiectomy.

OTHER INFORMATION   Mumps orchitis is usually unilateral; it results in some degree of testicular atrophy but sterility is uncommon.

Prostatitis

DESCRIPTION   Inflammatory disease of prostate, occurring as an acute or chronic bacterial infection, as a nonspecific component of prostatic hyperplasia, or as a specific or nonspecific granulomatous process.

DISEASE ENTITIES; SYNONYMS AND ACRONYMS   Acute bacterial prostatitis, chronic prostatitis, nonspecific nongranulomatous prostatitis, granulomatous prostatitis.

INCIDENCE   Common, especially complicating prostatic hyperplasia.

AGE   Older men.

ETIOLOGY, PATHOGENESIS, AND PREDISPOSING FACTORS   Spread of bacterial infection (*E. coli*, other gram-negative organisms) from urine; in chronic prostatitis, there may or may not be a history of previous episodes of acute prostatitis.

SITES INVOLVED   Prostate glands and stroma; coexisting posterior urethritis or cystitis is likely.

GROSS LESIONS   Acute prostatitis: edematous enlargement of gland with foci of suppuration, possibly abscesses; chronic prostatitis: enlargement of gland with nodularity and small calculi.

MICROSCOPIC LESIONS   Acute: suppuration mostly within glands and ducts, stromal edema; chronic: chronic inflammation and few PMNs around glands and ducts, dilated ducts containing inspissated secretions.

COMPLICATIONS   Urethral obstruction, which may compound the obstruction caused by coexisting prostatic hyperplasia; bacteremia and sepsis; bacteremia may be induced by prostatic massage or instrumentation.

SIGNS AND SYMPTOMS   Acute: dysuria, swollen and painful prostate, tenderness to palpation on rectal exam, fever; chronic: suprapubic or lower back pain, intermittent dysuria.

CLINICAL DIAGNOSIS AND OTHER CLINICAL FEATURES   Acute prostatitis is usually obvious in its presentation; prostatic massage should be avoided because of inducing bacteremia; chronic prostatitis may be subtle and give only intermittent problems.

LABORATORY DIAGNOSIS   Cultures of urine and prostatic secretions. In some cases of chronic prostatitis, cultures are negative; *Chlamydia trachomatis* or *Ureaplasma urealyticum* may be responsible in these cases.

PROGNOSIS   Acute prostatitis usually responds to antibiotics; in chronic prostatitis, recurrences are common.

THERAPY   Specific antibiotic therapy.

OTHER INFORMATION   Many cases of acute prostatitis follow instrumentation of the urethra or prostate, such as catheterization, cystoscopy, urethral dilatation, or transurethral resection.

Pathology Facts, by Richard C.
Harruff, J.B. Lippincott
Company, Philadelphia © 1994.

Chapter 18

Female Genital System and Breast

Carcinoma of Breast—In Situ

DESCRIPTION Primary malignant neoplasm of breast arising from the epithelium of the terminal duct lobular unit, contained within the basement membrane of the ducts without any invasion of the breast stroma.

DISEASE ENTITIES; SYNONYMS AND ACRONYMS Intraductal carcinoma, comedocarcinoma; lobular carcinoma-in-situ (CIS); intraductal papillary carcinoma.

INCIDENCE Pure in situ carcinoma is less common than invasive carcinoma; occurs along with invasive carcinoma.

AGE Same age range as for invasive carcinoma.

ETIOLOGY, PATHOGENESIS, AND PREDISPOSING FACTORS Same risk factors as for invasive carcinoma.

SITES INVOLVED Most commonly in the upper outer quadrant of breast, same as for invasive carcinoma.

GROSS LESIONS Intraductal: dilated ducts filled with expressible creamy substance, little surrounding fibrosis; lobular CIS: often grossly inapparent or indistinguishable from the associated fibrocystic disease.

MICROSCOPIC LESIONS Intraductal: ducts filled with large pleomorphic cells showing cribiform pattern and central necrosis; lobular CIS: lobules filled and expanded with smaller and more uniform cells.

COMPLICATIONS Invasive carcinoma develops in 30%; subsequent invasive carcinoma may occur in either breast; bilateral disease is common with lobular CIS; few cases that metastasize may have had undetected invasion.

SIGNS AND SYMPTOMS Lump or mass is not as obvious as with invasive carcinoma; its presence is often masked by coexistent fibrocystic disease.

CLINICAL DIAGNOSIS AND OTHER CLINICAL FEATURES Mammography can detect early cancers on the basis of microcalcification within neoplastic ducts or in surrounding fibrous tissue; mass may not be palpable or may feel like fibrocystic disease.

LABORATORY DIAGNOSIS Histologic examination of biopsy specimen; numerous sections must be examined to fully exclude invasion; fine needle aspiration cytology can not reliably distinguish in situ from invasive carcinoma.

PROGNOSIS Good; considered to be a nonmetastasizing carcinoma.

THERAPY Mastectomy with axillary dissection or a modified and more limited procedure; long-term follow-up.

OTHER INFORMATION Intraductal papillary carcinoma is an uncommon variant showing papillary formations of neoplastic cells within ducts.

Carcinoma of Breast—Invasive

DESCRIPTION Primary invasive malignant neoplasm of breast, nearly always adenocarcinoma; the most common type (70–80%) is the ductal type, followed by lobular carcinoma (5–10%); other variants are less frequent.

DISEASE ENTITIES; SYNONYMS AND ACRONYMS Ductal or lobular carcinoma, scirrhous carcinoma; medullary carcinoma, mucinous or colloid carcinoma.

INCIDENCE Affects 1 out of 11–13 women during their lifetime; causes 20% of female cancer deaths.

AGE Rare before age 25; increasingly common with age until menopause; slow increase thereafter.

ETIOLOGY, PATHOGENESIS, AND PREDISPOSING FACTORS Major risk factors: high socioeconomic status, family history, early menarche and late menopause, nulliparity or late age of first pregnancy, fibrocystic disease with epithelial hyperplasia, estrogen.

SITES INVOLVED Breast; upper outer quadrant in 50%, in the center of the breast in 20%, and in one of the other quadrants in 10% each; lobular type is likely to be bilateral or multicentric.

GROSS LESIONS Hard, irregular, whitish mass with consistency of cut unripe pear, extending projections of tumor into surrounding breast tissue; granules of calcification and focal yellow areas of necrosis.

MICROSCOPIC LESIONS Ductal: large pleomorphic cells arranged in glands, cords, nests, and sheets within dense fibrous stroma; lobular: single-file arrangement of small uniform cells in dense fibrous stroma.

COMPLICATIONS Widespread metastases, usually to lung, bone, and liver; also brain, adrenal, and ovary; commonly terminates with cachexia, malignant pleural effusions and carcinomatosis.

SIGNS AND SYMPTOMS Painless mass in the breast discovered by patient or examiner, fixed in position or movable; retraction of skin or nipple and peau d'orange are common findings; enlargement of axillary lymph nodes.

CLINICAL DIAGNOSIS AND OTHER CLINICAL FEATURES Hard irregular mass in the breast of a peri- or postmenopausal women is most likely cancer; any mass in any woman's breast may be cancer; mammography for screening; biopsy for definitive diagnosis.

LABORATORY DIAGNOSIS Histologic examination of biopsy, often frozen section prior to mastectomy; count of positive lymph nodes; estrogen receptor assay; aspiration cytology; flow cytometry.

PROGNOSIS 5-year survival by stage: I, 80%; II, 65%; III, 40%; IV, 10%. Late recurrences are common.

THERAPY Mastectomy with axillary dissection; antiestrogen therapy, radiation therapy, chemotherapy.

OTHER INFORMATION Stage I: tumor < 2 cm, no metastases; II: tumor 2–5 cm or axillary lymph node metastases; III: tumor > 5 cm, skin or chest wall invasion, axillary metastases with fixation; IV: distant metastases.

Carcinoma of Cervix

DESCRIPTION   Primary malignant neoplasm, most commonly squamous cell carcinoma, arising from cervical epithelium, invading surrounding structures and metastasizing to lymph nodes, distant organs, and bone.

DISEASE ENTITIES; SYNONYMS AND ACRONYMS   Squamous cell carcinoma of cervix, cervical carcinoma.

INCIDENCE   Most common gynecologic cancer; in US, 15/100,000/year; in undeveloped countries, up to 100/100,000.

AGE   Peak age is around 50 years, 10–20 years after the peak age of carcinoma-in-situ.

ETIOLOGY, PATHOGENESIS, AND PREDISPOSING FACTORS   Progression from carcinoma-in-situ (CIS); as with CIS, human papilloma virus (HPV), particularly types 16, 18, and 31, is currently the presumptive etiology; transmitted sexually.

SITES INVOLVED   Uterine cervix, initially in the transformation zone around the cervical os; in some cases, the carcinoma develops within the endocervical canal and is not visible until advanced.

GROSS LESIONS   Most commonly a fungating exophytic tumor; less frequently the lesion is ulcerative; invasion beyond the cervix occurs early.

MICROSCOPIC LESIONS   Squamous cell carcinoma of three subtypes: large cell nonkeratinizing carcinoma (most common), large cell keratinizing carcinoma, and small cell undifferentiated carcinoma.

COMPLICATIONS   Invasion of uterus and vagina; invasion of urinary bladder trigone with ureteral obstruction, hydronephrosis and renal failure; vesicovaginal and rectovaginal fistulas; local and distant metastases.

SIGNS AND SYMPTOMS   Vaginal discharge, postcoital bleeding, pain, dyspareunia; positive Pap smears.

CLINICAL DIAGNOSIS AND OTHER CLINICAL FEATURES   Cervical examination by direct visualization or by colposcopy; suspicious lesions require biopsy or at least scraping for cytologic examination.

LABORATORY DIAGNOSIS   Cytologic examination of cervical scrapings or histologic examination of biopsy, the latter being more accurate.

PROGNOSIS   Depends on stage, ranging from 90% 5-year survival for Stage I to 10% survival for Stage IV.

THERAPY   Surgery and radiation therapy.

OTHER INFORMATION   Stage 0: CIS; I: confined to cervix; II: invasion beyond cervix but not to pelvic wall or lower vagina; III: invasion to pelvic wall or lower vagina; IV: spread beyond pelvis or to bladder or rectum.

Carcinoma of Endometrium

DESCRIPTION Primary malignant neoplasm arising from endometrium, usually an adenocarcinoma; adenoacanthoma and adenosquamous carcinoma variants demonstrate squamous as well as glandular components.

DISEASE ENTITIES; SYNONYMS AND ACRONYMS Adenocarcinoma of endometrium, adenoacanthoma, adenosquamous carcinoma, secretory carcinoma, clear cell adenocarcinoma.

INCIDENCE Fairly common; second most common gynecologic cancer.

AGE Postmenopausal ages 55–65 years; rare under age 40.

ETIOLOGY, PATHOGENESIS, AND PREDISPOSING FACTORS Conditions with altered estrogen metabolism or hyperestrinism: obesity, diabetes mellitus, hypertension, infertility, menstrual irregularities, granulosa cell tumor, estrogen therapy.

SITES INVOLVED Initially endometrium with subsequent invasion of myometrium and cervix; spread through fallopian tubes to pelvic peritoneum; metastasis to regional lymph nodes and distant sites.

GROSS LESIONS Shaggy yellowish mass involving the endometrium with areas of necrosis and hemorrhage; invasion of myometrial wall progresses along a broad front.

MICROSCOPIC LESIONS Graded by FIGO (International Federation of Gynecology and Obstetrics) scheme: G1, well-differentiated glandular; G2, partly solid areas; G3, all solid or undifferentiated carcinoma.

COMPLICATIONS Invasion of surrounding structures (rectum, bladder, pelvis); metastasis to lung, peritoneum and omentum, ovary, liver, bowel, and vertebral bone.

SIGNS AND SYMPTOMS Vaginal bleeding and discharge (leukorrhea) usually forcing the woman to seek medical attention; thus, most endometrial carcinomas (80%) present at an early stage.

CLINICAL DIAGNOSIS AND OTHER CLINICAL FEATURES A likely diagnosis in a postmenopausal women with uterine bleeding; uterus may or may not be enlarged by palpation during pelvic exam; dilatation and curettage (D&C).

LABORATORY DIAGNOSIS Histologic examination of curettings from D&C; Pap smears have a fairly high false-negative rate in detecting endometrial carcinoma.

PROGNOSIS Depends on grade and stage ranging from 90% 5-year survival with Stage I to 20% with Stage III.

THERAPY Hysterectomy alone or in combination with radiation therapy.

OTHER INFORMATION Stage I: confined to uterus; II: extension to cervix; III: invasion outside uterus but confined to true pelvis; IV: extension beyond true pelvis, bladder, or rectum invasion, metastases.

Carcinoma of Ovary

DESCRIPTION Primary malignant tumors of ovary arising from surface epithelium; serous or mucinous and at least partly cystic, these tumors are the malignant counterparts of cystadenomas.

DISEASE ENTITIES; SYNONYMS AND ACRONYMS Serous or mucinous cystadenocarcinoma, endometrioid carcinoma, clear cell carcinoma (variant of endometrioid carcinoma).

INCIDENCE Third most common gynecologic cancer; serous type is the most common, followed by endometrioid type.

AGE Increasing incidence with age after 40 years.

ETIOLOGY, PATHOGENESIS, AND PREDISPOSING FACTORS Increased risk with family history of ovarian and other visceral cancers; ill-defined environmental factors may play a role; less common in multiparous women and in those taking oral contraceptives.

SITES INVOLVED Ovary; serous adenocarcinoma is bilateral in 65% of cases, mucinous adenocarcinoma in 20%, endometrioid carcinoma in 40%; simultaneous carcinoma of endometrium and endometrioid carcinoma may occur.

GROSS LESIONS Grossly all types are similar; partly solid and partly fluid-filled multicystic mass 10–15 cm or much larger; papillary and nodular structures protrude into the cyst cavity and from the surface.

MICROSCOPIC LESIONS Serous: papillary structures of neoplastic ciliated columnar cells, psammoma bodies; mucinous: papillary, mucinous cells; endometrioid: glandular structures similar to endometrial carcinoma.

COMPLICATIONS Direct serosal spread throughout the pelvic and abdominal peritoneum, encasing the intestines and viscera within the tumor mass; ascites; pseudomyxoma peritonei; distant metastases; cachexia.

SIGNS AND SYMPTOMS Lower abdominal pain, fullness, bloating; variable gastrointestinal and urinary symptoms; usually presents in advanced stages because there are no specific signs useful for early detection.

CLINICAL DIAGNOSIS AND OTHER CLINICAL FEATURES Suspicion regarding vague complaints of fullness in the lower abdomen; pelvic exam; ultrasonography, CT or MRI scans; paracentesis to collect fluid for cytologic study.

LABORATORY DIAGNOSIS Cytologic examination of ascites fluid; histologic examination of resected or biopsied mass; invasion of stroma is a major criterion to distinguish the malignant from borderline lesions.

PROGNOSIS Generally poor due to advanced stage when discovered; overall 5-year survival is less than 20%.

THERAPY Surgical resection if possible; chemotherapy.

OTHER INFORMATION Stage I: confined to one or both ovaries; II: extension beyond ovaries into pelvis; III: intraperitoneal spread beyond pelvis, retroperitoneal lymph node metastases; IV: distant metastases.

Carcinoma of Vagina and Vaginal Adenosis

DESCRIPTION   Adenosis refers to changes in the vaginal epithelium associated with in utero exposure to diethylstilbestrol (DES); in a small proportion of cases with adenosis, vaginal adenocarcinoma develops.

DISEASE ENTITIES; SYNONYMS AND ACRONYMS   Clear cell adenocarcinoma of vagina; vaginal adenosis and squamous metaplasia, DES-related changes.

INCIDENCE   Up to 2 million women were exposed to DES; one third developed adenosis, 0.1% developed carcinoma.

AGE   Adenosis is present throughout the lifetime; carcinoma develops between 14 and 22 years of age.

ETIOLOGY, PATHOGENESIS, AND PREDISPOSING FACTORS   DES interferes with the embryonic transition in the vagina occurring between 8 and 18 weeks gestation, resulting in persistence of glands that may undergo metaplasia or malignant transformation.

SITES INVOLVED   Vaginal epithelium; clear cell adenocarcinoma usually develops in the anterior wall of the upper third of the vagina.

GROSS LESIONS   Adenosis is best recognized with iodine stain; clear cell adenocarcinoma is an invasive and ulcerating tumor involving the vaginal wall and subjacent structures.

MICROSCOPIC LESIONS   Adenosis: mucinous glandular columnar cells replace normal squamous epithelium; surface undergoes squamous metaplasia; carcinoma: anaplastic cells with abundant clear cytoplasm containing glycogen.

COMPLICATIONS   Adenosis: recurrent infections, excessive secretion of mucus; carcinoma: local invasion (bladder, ureters, rectum), distant metastases, especially to lungs.

SIGNS AND SYMPTOMS   Adenosis presents with excess secretions or infection, or it may be asymptomatic, detected only by vaginal Pap smear; carcinoma presents with mass, pain, urinary symptoms, bloody discharge.

CLINICAL DIAGNOSIS AND OTHER CLINICAL FEATURES   Adenosis is visualized by the Schiller stain (iodine painted on the epithelium does not stain areas of adenosis); carcinoma appears as an indurated ulcerating mass that requires biopsy.

LABORATORY DIAGNOSIS   Histologic examination of biopsied lesion; the cytologic finding of columnar or metaplastic squamous cells in a vaginal scraping indicates adenosis.

PROGNOSIS   Poor for advanced carcinoma; screening programs detect early cancers that are curable.

THERAPY   Surgical resection and radiation therapy; pelvic exenteration for advanced carcinoma.

OTHER INFORMATION   DES is a synthetic estrogen prescribed during the years 1940–1971 for threatened abortion; the daughters of women so treated are at risk for vaginal adenosis and clear cell adenocarcinoma.

Carcinoma of Vulva

DESCRIPTION   Primary malignant neoplasm, nearly always squamous cell carcinoma, arising from epithelium of vulva; carcinoma-in-situ and squamous dysplasia are recognized as precursor lesions.

DISEASE ENTITIES; SYNONYMS AND ACRONYMS   Squamous carcinoma of vulva; vulvar intraepithelial neoplasia (VIN) is precursor lesion (dysplasia, carcinoma-in-situ).

INCIDENCE   Constitutes 3% of all gynecologic cancers.

AGE   Usually affects women over 60; recent increase in younger cases is associated with papilloma virus.

ETIOLOGY, PATHOGENESIS, AND PREDISPOSING FACTORS   Invasive carcinoma follows dysplasia and carcinoma-in-situ after several years; 80% of preinvasive lesions are positive for human papilloma virus (HPV-16).

SITES INVOLVED   Originates in vulvar epithelium and progresses to invasion of vagina, perivulvar skin, anus and rectum; metastasizes to inguinal, iliac, and pelvic lymph nodes.

GROSS LESIONS   VIN may show only redness or leukoplakia; invasive carcinoma is usually exophytic (70%) or less often ulcerative; verrucous carcinoma is a fungating mass resembling a giant condyloma.

MICROSCOPIC LESIONS   VIN shows cellular hyperplasia with nuclear atypia involving part or all of the epithelium but no invasion; invasive squamous cell carcinoma is usually well-differentiated with keratinization.

COMPLICATIONS   Constant bleeding and oozing; ulceration; secondary infections; stricture of urethra, vagina, and rectum; metastasis to lungs, liver, and other sites.

SIGNS AND SYMPTOMS   Itching, pain, ulceration, bleeding, dyspareunia; purulent discharge due to secondary infection.

CLINICAL DIAGNOSIS AND OTHER CLINICAL FEATURES   A raised or ulcerated vulvar lesion is suspicious for cancer; in-situ lesions are less obvious; diagnosis requires biopsy; inguinal nodes may be enlarged due to metastases or secondary infection.

LABORATORY DIAGNOSIS   Histologic examination of biopsied lesion; depth of invasion should be determined because of its importance for prognosis.

PROGNOSIS   Poor for advanced lesions; good for verrucous carcinoma; VIN may recur or progress to invasion.

THERAPY   Surgical excision of early lesions and for verrucous carcinoma; vulvectomy for advanced lesions.

OTHER INFORMATION   Stage 0: VIN; I: less than 2 cm diameter; II: greater than 2 cm; III: spread to urethra, vagina, anus, or limited lymph node metastasis; IV: rectal, bladder, bone involvement or distant metastasis.

Cervical Dysplasia

DESCRIPTION Abnormal proliferation and differentiation of cervical squamous epithelium, representing a stage in malignant transformation, characterized by nuclear atypia and loss of cytoplasmic maturation.

DISEASE ENTITIES; SYNONYMS AND ACRONYMS Cervical intraepithelial neoplasia (CIN); mild, moderate, or severe dysplasia; carcinoma-in-situ (CIS).

INCIDENCE Common; increased incidence with multiple sex partners and early age at first intercourse.

AGE Dysplastic lesions are first seen in young sexually active women; CIS is most common around age 30.

ETIOLOGY, PATHOGENESIS, AND PREDISPOSING FACTORS DNA of human papilloma virus (HPV) is found in nearly all CIN lesions, condylomas, and invasive carcinomas; HPV types 16, 18, 31, transmitted sexually, are highly associated with CIN and carcinoma.

SITES INVOLVED Confined to epithelium above the basement membrane; initially in the transformation zone around the cervical os where there is normally squamous metaplasia; at the squamocolumnar junction.

GROSS LESIONS Changes are not visible to the unaided eye but may be visualized by colposcopy or by the Schiller test (painting the cervix with iodine solution to reveal regions lacking glycogen).

MICROSCOPIC LESIONS Cytologic atypia (nuclear hyperchromatism, increased n/c ratio) in the lower third of the epithelium (mild dysplasia), lower two thirds (moderate), or entire epithelium (severe dysplasia and CIS).

COMPLICATIONS Invasive cervical carcinoma will develop in most women with CIS if it is left untreated; CIS progresses to invasion in 10–15 years and sometimes much sooner.

SIGNS AND SYMPTOMS CIN (the dysplasias and CIS) cause no symptoms, but there is likely coexistence of other sexually transmitted diseases (high-risk populations); usually detected by routine Pap smear.

CLINICAL DIAGNOSIS AND OTHER CLINICAL FEATURES Annual Pap smears for all women starting at age 18 or at the onset of sexual activity; frequency may be modified after several negative smears; colposcopic examination and biopsy for positive smears.

LABORATORY DIAGNOSIS Cytologic examination of cervical scrapings (Pap smears); histologic examination of cervical biopsy or conization; immunostaining or DNA hybridization for presence of HPV.

PROGNOSIS Good if treated; CIS is completely curable.

THERAPY Cryosurgery, electrocautery, laser ablation of dysplastic foci; cervical conization, hysterectomy.

OTHER INFORMATION Dysplasia and CIS are regarded as stages of CIN, as follows: mild dysplasia, CIN I; moderate, CIN II, severe dysplasia and CIS, CIN III. Overall, only a minority of CIN's progress to invasion.

Chorioamnionitis

DESCRIPTION   Infection of the placental membranes by bacteria ascending from the vagina, usually caused by premature and prolonged rupture of the membranes.

DISEASE ENTITIES; SYNONYMS AND ACRONYMS   Funisitis; villitis.

INCIDENCE   Common; an expected complication of premature rupture of the membranes.

AGE   Within the last few days of pregnancy.

ETIOLOGY, PATHOGENESIS, AND PREDISPOSING FACTORS   Prolonged rupture of membranes; *E. coli* and other gram-negative organisms, staphylococci, streptococci and *Gardnerella vaginalis* are organisms likely to be cultured from the infected amniotic fluid.

SITES INVOLVED   Fetal surface of the placenta, placental membranes, umbilical cord and umbilical cord blood vessels (funisitis).

GROSS LESIONS   Membranes appear cloudy or thickened with purulent exudate; exudate adherent to fetal surface of the placenta; cloudy amniotic fluid, often foul-smelling.

MICROSCOPIC LESIONS   Infiltration of PMNs on the surface of and within membranes and placental amnion; with funisitis there is PMN exudation in the walls of umbilical blood vessels and in Wharton's jelly.

COMPLICATIONS   Maternal sepsis, endometritis, pelvic inflammatory disease; neonatal pneumonia, gastroenteritis, peritonitis, skin and eye infections; forces premature delivery; may be associated with stillbirth.

SIGNS AND SYMPTOMS   Premature rupture of membranes, followed by rising fever; intrauterine fetal demise is indicated by absence of fetal movements and heartbeat.

CLINICAL DIAGNOSIS AND OTHER CLINICAL FEATURES   Fever developing in a pregnant woman with ruptured membranes; fetus may be immature, producing a predicament between premature delivery and risking sepsis due to chorioamnionitis.

LABORATORY DIAGNOSIS   Culture of amniotic fluid; blood culture; placental examination following delivery.

PROGNOSIS   Usually good but does increase morbidity for both mother and neonate.

THERAPY   Delivery or otherwise termination of pregnancy with evacuation of uterus; antibiotics.

OTHER INFORMATION   In the less common hematogenous infections, the villi are inflamed (villitis) but the membranes are clear.

Cystadenoma of Ovary and Tumors of Low Malignant Potential

DESCRIPTION Primary cystic tumors of ovary arising from surface epithelium; this group includes benign as well as borderline malignant tumors that, as a category, overlap with cystadenocarcinoma.

DISEASE ENTITIES; SYNONYMS AND ACRONYMS Serous cystadenoma, mucinous cystadenoma; tumors of low malignant potential or of borderline malignancy.

INCIDENCE Common; cystadenoma, particularly the serous type, is the most common benign tumor of ovary.

AGE Adult women under the age of 40–45 years; borderline tumors occur in a slightly higher age range.

ETIOLOGY, PATHOGENESIS, AND PREDISPOSING FACTORS Derived from surface epithelium, apparently due to its repeated disruption by ovulation; less frequent in multiparous women and users of birth control pills.

SITES INVOLVED Ovary; bilateral ovaries in 5–30% of cases, more frequently with the serous variety and with tumors of borderline malignancy.

GROSS LESIONS Thin-walled cystic mass from few to many centimeters in diameter; some are huge; multiloculation is more common with the mucinous type; papillary and solid areas are indicators of malignant potential.

MICROSCOPIC LESIONS Fibrous wall lined internally by ciliated columnar (serous type) or mucinous columnar cells; piling up of epithelial cells and nuclear atypia without wall invasion are features of borderline tumors.

COMPLICATIONS Compression of neighboring structures; ovarian torsion; tumors of borderline malignancy may spread throughout abdomen or metastasize; pseudomyxoma peritonei with mucinous borderline tumors.

SIGNS AND SYMPTOMS Lower abdominal pain; abdominal enlargement or bloating; gastrointestinal or urinary symptoms such as constipation or frequency; sudden intense pain may indicate torsion.

CLINICAL DIAGNOSIS AND OTHER CLINICAL FEATURES Usually palpable on pelvic examination; visualized be ultrasonography and CT scans; laparoscopy, laparotomy with biopsy or resection.

LABORATORY DIAGNOSIS Histologic examination of resected tumor; sampling of solid and papillary areas is important to assess the malignant potential.

PROGNOSIS Benign cystadenomas are cured with therapy; 10-year survival for borderline tumors is 70–75%.

THERAPY Surgical resection.

OTHER INFORMATION Cystadenofibroma and Brenner tumor are less common tumors of surface epithelium, both usually benign.

Dysfunctional Uterine Bleeding

DESCRIPTION   Abnormal uterine bleeding without an anatomic lesion of the uterus; most often caused by anovulatory cycles; defects in follicular or luteal phases of the menstrual cycle are less likely causes.

DISEASE ENTITIES; SYNONYMS AND ACRONYMS   DUB, anovulatory cycles, inadequate luteal phase.

INCIDENCE   The most common gynecological problem of women in their childbearing years.

AGE   From menarche to menopause; anovulatory cycles are common in adolescents and premenopausal women.

ETIOLOGY, PATHOGENESIS, AND PREDISPOSING FACTORS   With anovulatory cycles there is no corpus luteum to secrete progesterone and thus the endometrium fails to mature; other causes: prolonged or shortened follicular phase, inadequate luteal phase.

SITES INVOLVED   Endometrium, under the influence of hormonal secretions from the ovaries and pituitary; lesion of ovary (polycystic ovaries, granulosa-theca cell tumor) or pituitary (infarct, adenoma) may be present.

GROSS LESIONS   Irregular areas of hyperplastic endometrial thickening with foci of hemorrhage. With anovulatory cycles, corpus lutea are absent from the ovaries.

MICROSCOPIC LESIONS   Endometrium shows only proliferative changes; after the midcycle drop in estrogen, the stroma collapses and the endometrium becomes necrotic, hemorrhagic, and sloughs.

COMPLICATIONS   Estrogen secretion unopposed by progesterone leads to endometrial hyperplasia and predisposes to endometrial carcinoma; endometrial polyps; infertility.

SIGNS AND SYMPTOMS   Excessive bleeding during or between menstrual periods; virilism suggests polycystic ovaries or an ovarian tumor, which may be palpable; signs of other endocrine disease may be present.

CLINICAL DIAGNOSIS AND OTHER CLINICAL FEATURES   Absence of midcycle body temperature rise indicates anovulation; systemic, metabolic, or nutritional diseases, ovarian lesions, and thyroid, adrenal, or pituitary disease should be excluded.

LABORATORY DIAGNOSIS   Endometrial biopsy showing no secretory changes indicates anovulation; weak changes indicate inadequate corpus luteum function; prolactin may be elevated; vaginal hormonal cytology is seldom used.

PROGNOSIS   Often self-limited; anovulatory cycles naturally cease after ovarian maturation and after menopause.

THERAPY   Progesterone supplements, administered as oral contraceptives, allow proper endometrial cycling.

OTHER INFORMATION   Anatomic lesions that cause abnormal uterine bleeding include endometrial hyperplasia, polyps, carcinoma, endometritis, uterine leiomyomas, ectopic or intrauterine pregnancy.

Ectopic Pregnancy

DESCRIPTION   Any gestation that develops in a site other than the endometrium, usually within the fallopian tube, which eventually ruptures because of the expanding tubal pregnancy.

DISEASE ENTITIES; SYNONYMS AND ACRONYMS   Tubal pregnancy.

INCIDENCE   Common, at a rate of 1 case per 200 normal pregnancies.

AGE   Within the reproductive years; usually young women.

ETIOLOGY, PATHOGENESIS, AND PREDISPOSING FACTORS   Tubal scars caused by healed salpingitis (gonococcal and nongonococcal) impede conceptus passing through tube and promote tubal implantation; other causes: endometriosis, salpingitis isthmica nodosa.

SITES INVOLVED   Almost always within the fallopian tube, usually the distal or middle third; uncommon cases occur on the surface of ovary or pelvic peritoneum.

GROSS LESIONS   Fallopian tube is distended several centimeters by the placenta and fetus within amniotic sac; after rupture of the thin wall, the tube is filled with hemorrhage and the conceptus is expelled.

MICROSCOPIC LESIONS   Features of the fetus and placenta are normal for the gestational age; trophoblast of the placenta invades into the smooth muscle of the tube; tubal mucosa is decidualized.

COMPLICATIONS   Rupture of the fallopian tube, usually by the 12th week of gestation, causing intra-abdominal hemorrhage that can be life-threatening; infertility if the other tube is also damaged.

SIGNS AND SYMPTOMS   Abdominal pain that suddenly becomes severe; often presents as an intra-abdominal emergency (acute abdomen).

CLINICAL DIAGNOSIS AND OTHER CLINICAL FEATURES   Highly likely diagnosis in a young woman presenting with severe abdominal pain; pelvic examination and ultrasonography exclude intrauterine pregnancy and may detect the distended tube.

LABORATORY DIAGNOSIS   Human chorionic gonadotropin (HCG) is elevated, producing a positive pregnancy test; microscopically, endometrial curettings show hypersecretory changes (Arias-Stella reaction).

PROGNOSIS   Usually good, assuming diagnosis is made promptly and appropriate therapy is rendered.

THERAPY   Surgical resection of fallopian tube; fluid volume and/or blood replacement; treatment of shock.

OTHER INFORMATION   Ectopic pregnancy within the isthmus of the tube ruptures earlier (within 6 weeks) because this part is not as distensable as the ampulla.

Endometrial Hyperplasia

DESCRIPTION   Hyperplasia of glands and stroma of the endometrium in response to estrogen stimulation; the type of hyperplasia is described, or graded, by various terms that indicate its malignant potential.

DISEASE ENTITIES; SYNONYMS AND ACRONYMS   Simple, mild or cystic hyperplasia; complex, moderate, or adenomatous hyperplasia; atypical hyperplasia.

INCIDENCE   A common cause of abnormal menstrual bleeding.

AGE   Perimenopausal or postmenopausal ages.

ETIOLOGY, PATHOGENESIS, AND PREDISPOSING FACTORS   Excess estrogens due to anovulatory cycles, Stein-Leventhal syndrome (polycystic ovaries), granulosa-theca cell tumor, adrenocortical hyperfunction, obesity, estrogen therapy.

SITES INVOLVED   Endometrium; however, an ovarian disorder may be the primary lesion.

GROSS LESIONS   Thick, creamy tan endometrial mucosa; polypoid regions and focal hemorrhage are often present.

MICROSCOPIC LESIONS   The grade of hyperplasia depends on the glandular component; in simple hyperplasia, the glands are cystic, not crowded; in complex hyperplasia, there is glandular crowding with or without atypia.

COMPLICATIONS   Progression to adenocarcinoma; the risk of this depends on the type or grade of hyperplasia and the degree of glandular atypia; simple hyperplasia does not progress, complex hyperplasia does.

SIGNS AND SYMPTOMS   Abnormal or excessive uterine bleeding during or between menstrual periods; postmenopausal bleeding.

CLINICAL DIAGNOSIS AND OTHER CLINICAL FEATURES   Most likely diagnosis in a perimenopausal woman with abnormal uterine bleeding; an ovarian neoplasm should be considered; dilatation and curettage (D&C) is therapeutic and diagnostic.

LABORATORY DIAGNOSIS   Histologic examination of endometrial curettings from D&C; assessment should determine the type of hyperplasia (simple or complex) and the degree of atypia.

PROGNOSIS   Endometrial carcinoma develops in 5% of complex hyperplasia without atypia and in 30% with atypia.

THERAPY   D&C; if the hyperplasia recurs or if there is significant atypia, hysterectomy may be elected.

OTHER INFORMATION   The terminology of endometrial hyperplasia is confusing and varies with local tradition; the pathologic assessment must be translated into an estimate of the risk for developing cancer.

Endometriosis

DESCRIPTION   The presence of endometrial glands and/or stroma outside the uterus, usually implanted on the pelvic organs or pelvic peritoneum, producing infertility and pain.

DISEASE ENTITIES; SYNONYMS AND ACRONYMS   Endometrioma, chocolate cyst.

INCIDENCE   Common, particularly as a cause of infertility and excessive menstrual pain.

AGE   During the reproductive years, usually 20s and 30s.

ETIOLOGY, PATHOGENESIS, AND PREDISPOSING FACTORS   Favored theory is that endometrial tissue is regurgitated from the tubes to implant on sites in the pelvis; as this tissue undergoes cyclic menstrual changes, bleeding, pain, and adhesions develop.

SITES INVOLVED   Most commonly ovaries (80%) followed by uterine ligaments, pouch of Douglas, pelvic peritoneum, fallopian tube, uterine serosa; within surgical incision scars.

GROSS LESIONS   Small, reddish or rust-brown nodules on the surface of affected sites; fibrous adhesions often distort normal anatomy; tumorous masses (endometriomas) or blood-filled (chocolate) cysts may be present.

MICROSCOPIC LESIONS   Functionally active endometrial glands and stroma embedded in fibrous tissue; fresh hemorrhage reflects current menstruation; hemosiderin deposition is a result of previous bleeding.

COMPLICATIONS   Infertility, menstrual abnormalities, dyspareunia, intestinal adhesions; malignant transformation is rare.

SIGNS AND SYMPTOMS   Infertility is presenting complaint in 25% of cases; pelvic pain, especially before or during menstruation (dysmenorrhea); dyspareunia; painful defecation, and other gastrointestinal problems; dysuria.

CLINICAL DIAGNOSIS AND OTHER CLINICAL FEATURES   Severe pelvic pain worse during menstruation is highly suggestive; pelvic exam may encounter multiple painful foci; laparoscopy is successful in visualizing the lesions.

LABORATORY DIAGNOSIS   Histologic examination of biopsied lesion or resected organs, endometrioma, or chocolate cyst.

PROGNOSIS   Not a cause of mortality; often a chronic painful problem that persists until menopause.

THERAPY   Laparoscopic laser ablation, hysterectomy, salpingectomy, oophorectomy, hormone manipulation.

OTHER INFORMATION   Clear cell adenocarcinoma of ovary is associated with endometriosis.

Fibroadenoma of Breast

DESCRIPTION   A common benign primary tumor of breast, developing from the terminal duct lobular unit, composed of both fibrous stroma and glandular components.

DISEASE ENTITIES; SYNONYMS AND ACRONYMS   Giant fibroadenoma, juvenile fibroadenoma, tubular fibroadenoma, lactating fibroadenoma, fibroadenomatosis.

INCIDENCE   The most common benign neoplasm of breast.

AGE   During reproductive ages, usually 20–35 years; juvenile or giant fibroadenoma occurs in adolescents.

ETIOLOGY, PATHOGENESIS, AND PREDISPOSING FACTORS   Presumed to be increased sensitivity to estrogen within a localized region of the breast; fibroadenomas regress after menopause; lactating fibroadenomas develop postpartum.

SITES INVOLVED   Within breast tissue, usually in upper outer quadrant.

GROSS LESIONS   Well-circumscribed and demarcated from surrounding breast; rounded, firm and rubbery, not hard; usually 2–4 cm in diameter, ranging from 1 cm to 10–15 cm with the giant fibroadenoma.

MICROSCOPIC LESIONS   Glands lined by epithelial cells within a loose fibrous stroma; glands appear tubular in the pericanalicular pattern or elongated and slit-like in the intracanalicular pattern.

COMPLICATIONS   Rarely a carcinoma develops within a fibroadenoma; the vast majority are benign and are only of concern for aesthetic reasons or as a mass that needs to be differentiated from cancer.

SIGNS AND SYMPTOMS   Discovered by patient or examiner; palpable as a firm, well-rounded, and freely movable mass; may undergo size changes during menstrual period and enlarge during pregnancy.

CLINICAL DIAGNOSIS AND OTHER CLINICAL FEATURES   Patient age, characteristics on palpation, and mammography are usually accurate; biopsy is required to exclude cancer; a regressed, calcified fibroadenoma may present a hard mass in an elderly patient.

LABORATORY DIAGNOSIS   Histologic examination of biopsied lesion (usually the entire mass is removed as an excisional biopsy); fine-needle aspiration cytology is often diagnostic.

PROGNOSIS   In itself presents no significant risk; occasionally recurs.

THERAPY   Surgical excision.

OTHER INFORMATION   Regions microscopically similar to fibroadenoma, seen in fibrocystic disease, are called fibroadenomatosis.

Fibrocystic Disease of Breast

DESCRIPTION A common disorder of breast causing lumpiness, pain, and masses; characterized by a combination of fibrosis, cystic changes, and variable epithelial hyperplasia and metaplasia.

DISEASE ENTITIES; SYNONYMS AND ACRONYMS Fibrocystic changes, epitheliosis, ductal and florid papillomatosis, sclerosing adenosis.

INCIDENCE Very common; may be present to some degree in 50% of women, causing significant disease in 10%.

AGE Late 20s to mid-40s, peak incidence just before menopause; infrequently diagnosed after menopause.

ETIOLOGY, PATHOGENESIS, AND PREDISPOSING FACTORS Various hormonal imbalances; estrogen excess, absolute or relative; progesterone deficiency with anovulation; altered tissue responsiveness to estrogen; less common in women on oral contraceptives.

SITES INVOLVED Breast tissue, usually diffusely and bilaterally; fibrous stroma of breast, ductal and lobular epithelium.

GROSS LESIONS Cysts of various sizes ranging from microscopic up to a few millimeters, filled with clear or brown fluid (blue dome cyst), surrounded by dense fibrotic tissue, occasionally forming discrete masses.

MICROSCOPIC LESIONS Fibrosis, cysts, apocrine metaplasia of ductal epithelium; proliferation of glands (sclerosing adenosis); hyperplasia of ductal epithelium may be minimal or marked (papillomatosis) and atypical.

COMPLICATIONS Lumpiness and masses may be confused clinically with carcinoma; risk of carcinoma is increased in cases of fibrocystic disease that show epithelial hyperplasia, especially if atypia is present.

SIGNS AND SYMPTOMS Lumpiness throughout both breasts; pain, particularly prior to the menstrual period; a discrete mass is uncommon.

CLINICAL DIAGNOSIS AND OTHER CLINICAL FEATURES Breast palpation, feeling lumpiness throughout both breasts and history of pain prior to period help to differentiate from cancer; needle aspiration of cyst; mammography; some masses require biopsy.

LABORATORY DIAGNOSIS Fine needle aspiration cytology; histologic examination of breast biopsy, grading the epithelial hyperplasia; sclerosing adenosis is sometimes mistaken for carcinoma, particularly on frozen section.

PROGNOSIS Not a cause of mortality unless cancer develops but is often a chronic painful problem.

THERAPY Regular breast examination; biopsy of suspicious masses; occasionally mastectomy for florid cases.

OTHER INFORMATION Family history of breast carcinoma markedly increases the risk of developing carcinoma in the patient at all levels of epithelial hyperplasia.

Gestational Trophoblastic Disease

DESCRIPTION   A group of tumor-like conditions developing from aberrant pregnancy that may behave in a benign fashion (hydatidiform mole) or display malignant properties (invasive mole, choriocarcinoma).

DISEASE ENTITIES; SYNONYMS AND ACRONYMS   Hydatidiform mole, molar pregnancy; invasive mole, chorioadenoma destruens; choriocarcinoma.

INCIDENCE   In US, 1 mole in 1000 pregnancies; choriocarcinoma develops in 2% of moles; more common in Asia.

AGE   Greatest risk is for girls under 15 years; risk is also high and increases with ages over 40.

ETIOLOGY, PATHOGENESIS, AND PREDISPOSING FACTORS   Moles develop by androgenesis; its 46,XX karyotype is of paternal origin; the fetus dies and placental villi undergo hydropic degeneration; the trophoblastic tissue may acquire invasive properties.

SITES INVOLVED   Mole: chorionic villi of placenta, swollen like a bunch of grapes, fill uterine cavity; choriocarcinoma: trophoblastic tissue predominates, invading the wall of the uterus.

GROSS LESIONS   Mole: 1–2 liters or more of a stringy mass of swollen villi without fetus (complete mole) or with fetal parts (partial mole); choriocarcinoma: solid hemorrhagic necrotic tumor invading uterus.

MICROSCOPIC LESIONS   Mole: hydropic villi lacking blood vessels, trophoblast component is minor unless it is an invasive mole; choriocarcinoma: essentially all cytotrophoblast and syncytiotrophoblast without villi.

COMPLICATIONS   Development of choriocarcinoma, which metastasizes widely; uterine hemorrhage, infection, coagulopathy; embolism of trophoblast; perforation of uterus with invasive mole.

SIGNS AND SYMPTOMS   Presentation in 4th or 5th month with vaginal bleeding; sometimes molar fragments are passed; uterus is often enlarged more than expected for gestational age.

CLINICAL DIAGNOSIS AND OTHER CLINICAL FEATURES   Disparity between uterine size and gestational age is quite suspicious; ultrasound examination is diagnostic by showing the mole's vesicular image; evacuation of uterus yields typical mole.

LABORATORY DIAGNOSIS   Human chorionic gonadotropin (HCG) is important to measure at intervals following therapy; persistent HCG elevation or increasing HCG indicates recurrent invasive mole or choriocarcinoma.

PROGNOSIS   Usually good; even metastatic choriocarcinoma is curable with therapy.

THERAPY   Suction curettage for mole; hysterectomy for invasive mole; chemotherapy for choriocarcinoma.

OTHER INFORMATION   Placental site trophoblastic tumor is uncommon and differs from choriocarcinoma by a benign behavior and monomorphic trophoblastic population. Nongestational choriocarcinoma is resistant to therapy.

Granulosa-Theca Cell Tumors of Ovary

DESCRIPTION　Primary tumors of ovary arising from granulosa and/or theca cells that may contain one or both of these elements and are associated with sex steroid hormone secretion.

DISEASE ENTITIES; SYNONYMS AND ACRONYMS　Granulosa cell tumor, thecoma, granulosa-theca tumor, fibroma, fibrothecoma.

INCIDENCE　Fairly common; altogether this group accounts for 5–10% of all ovarian tumors.

AGE　Any age, usually postmenopausal.

ETIOLOGY, PATHOGENESIS, AND PREDISPOSING FACTORS　Neoplastic disease of unknown etiology; thecomas and fibromas are benign; granulosa cell tumors may be malignant; steroid hormones secreted by these tumors can cause clinical syndromes.

SITES INVOLVED　Ovary, usually unilateral.

GROSS LESIONS　Fairly large, solid, encapsulated mass with whorling pattern on cut surface; thecomas are yellow, fibromas are white; granulosa cell tumors lack the whorling and may be partly cystic.

MICROSCOPIC LESIONS　Thecomas and fibromas are composed of spindle-shaped cells; thecal cells are plumper and contain lipid; granulosa cell tumors have polygonal cells in cords and sheets and show Call-Exner bodies.

COMPLICATIONS　Precocious puberty in girls due to estrogen secretion; endometrial hyperplasia and carcinoma in adults; less often, virilization; cystic breast disease; granulosa cell tumor may be malignant.

SIGNS AND SYMPTOMS　Lower abdominal pain, fullness or palpable mass; abnormal uterine bleeding; 10–15% with functional tumors develop endometrial carcinoma; precocious sexual development in a girl.

CLINICAL DIAGNOSIS AND OTHER CLINICAL FEATURES　Investigation of pelvic mass; pelvic examination; ultrasonography; laparotomy; should be considered in a woman with endometrial hyperplasia or carcinoma.

LABORATORY DIAGNOSIS　Histologic examination of resected tumor; it is not possible to predict malignant behavior of granulosa cell tumors based on their appearance; differentiation of fibroma and thecoma may be difficult.

PROGNOSIS　From 5 to 25% of tumors with a large granulosa cell component are malignant; pure thecomas never are.

THERAPY　Surgical resection.

OTHER INFORMATION　These tumors constitute a spectrum in which granulosa cells, theca cells, and fibrocytes are present alone or in various combinations; with respect to estrogen production, fibromas are nonfunctional.

Leiomyoma of Uterus

DESCRIPTION Primary benign tumor of uterus arising from smooth muscle, well circumscribed and often multiple.

DISEASE ENTITIES; SYNONYMS AND ACRONYMS Myoma, fibroid.

INCIDENCE Most common tumor of uterus and most common tumor of women; present in 25% of women over 30 years.

AGE During the reproductive years; uncommon before age 20; common past 30; most regress after menopause.

ETIOLOGY, PATHOGENESIS, AND PREDISPOSING FACTORS Regarded as a hormone-dependent neoplasm; growth is dependent on estrogens.

SITES INVOLVED Myometrium; intramural (within uterine wall), subserosal (covered by a thin layer of serosa), or submucosal (covered by a layer of endometrium); may project into the endometrial cavity as a polyp.

GROSS LESIONS Round, firm, sharply circumscribed, and encapsulated mass ranging less than 1 cm to over 20 cm in diameter; whorling cut surface appearance; often multiple; frequently distorts the uterus.

MICROSCOPIC LESIONS Interlacing bundles of uniform, well-differentiated, elongated, spindle-shaped smooth muscle cells with very few mitoses and no anaplasia.

COMPLICATIONS Excessive bleeding during or between the normal menstrual periods (menorrhagia), infertility, abortion, postpartum hemorrhage; malignant transformation is rare (less than 0.01%).

SIGNS AND SYMPTOMS Pelvic pain, fullness or palpable mass; urinary frequency; abnormal uterine bleeding; may undergo rapid increase in size during pregnancy; many are asymptomatic.

CLINICAL DIAGNOSIS AND OTHER CLINICAL FEATURES Usually by palpation on pelvic examination; ultrasonography; during hysterectomy or surgical operation for other reasons.

LABORATORY DIAGNOSIS In nearly all cases, the diagnosis is grossly obvious; histologic examination is for documentation and to exclude leiomyosarcoma.

PROGNOSIS Good, except in cases when the tumor interferes with pregnancy and causes abortion or fetal death.

THERAPY Usually hysterectomy for symptomatic cases; occasionally myomectomy is done to preserve the uterus.

OTHER INFORMATION Leiomyosarcoma is usually larger and more fleshy, has irregular margins and expands into the uterine cavity; microscopically, there are anaplasia and at least 5 mitoses per 10 high power fields.

Mature Cystic Teratoma of Ovary

DESCRIPTION   Primary benign tumor of ovary originating from germ cells; the tumors are cystic and contain elements of all three embryonic germ cell layers, particularly skin, hair, and other skin appendages.

DISEASE ENTITIES; SYNONYMS AND ACRONYMS   Benign cystic teratoma, dermoid cyst.

INCIDENCE   Common; accounts for 25% of all ovarian tumors.

AGE   Young women of reproductive age, usually 20–30 years.

ETIOLOGY, PATHOGENESIS, AND PREDISPOSING FACTORS   Presumed parthenogenesis, a process whereby a pluripotent diploid cell develops from one haploid germ cell and then proliferates to produce a tumor with karyotype 46,XX.

SITES INVOLVED   Ovary; 10–15% are bilateral.

GROSS LESIONS   Cystic mass obliterating ovary; thin fibrous wall with a solid nodule at one aspect; contains sebaceous material and matted hair; tooth structures and a variety of other tissues may be found.

MICROSCOPIC LESIONS   Mature tissue elements representing all three germ cell layers may be present, including skin with adnexal structures, bone, cartilage, teeth, thyroid, bronchi, intestine, and neural tissues.

COMPLICATIONS   Rupture causing chemical peritonitis, torsion, infection; infertility; secretion of thyroid hormone causing hyperthyroidism (struma ovarii); carcinoid syndrome due to secretion of serotonin.

SIGNS AND SYMPTOMS   Lower abdominal pain, fullness or palpable mass; menstrual problems; gastrointestinal or urinary complaints.

CLINICAL DIAGNOSIS AND OTHER CLINICAL FEATURES   Palpation of adnexal mass on pelvic examination; x-rays, ultrasonography, CT scans; laparotomy.

LABORATORY DIAGNOSIS   Histologic examination of resected tumor.

PROGNOSIS   Good; cured with therapy; does not recur.

THERAPY   Surgical resection.

OTHER INFORMATION   Immature (malignant) teratoma is a similar but largely solid tumor containing embryonic components that occurs in adolescents; rare dermoid cysts develop malignancy, usually a squamous carcinoma.

Nonneoplastic Cysts of Ovary

DESCRIPTION Nonneoplastic cysts of the ovary derived from surface epithelium (nonfunctional cysts) or from specialized cells of the follicles (functional cysts).

DISEASE ENTITIES; SYNONYMS AND ACRONYMS Nonfunctional: serous (inclusion) cyst; functional: follicle cyst, corpus luteum cyst, theca lutein cyst.

INCIDENCE Very common.

AGE Any age; most likely during the reproductive ages.

ETIOLOGY, PATHOGENESIS, AND PREDISPOSING FACTORS Serous: inclusion of surface epithelium within stroma; follicle: derived from atretic follicle; corpus luteum: incomplete involution of corpus luteum; theca lutein: elevated gonadotropin levels.

SITES INVOLVED Ovary, sometimes bilateral.

GROSS LESIONS Single or multiple, thin-walled, diameter less than 1 cm up to several centimeters, containing clear fluid, smooth inner wall; golden border and bloody fluid likely with corpus luteum or theca lutein cysts.

MICROSCOPIC LESIONS Serous cyst: fibrous wall with cuboidal or columnar cell lining; follicle cyst: granulosa and theca cell linings; corpus luteum and theca lutein cyst: luteinization of lining granulosa or theca cells.

COMPLICATIONS With functional cysts: menstrual irregularities, precocious puberty in a child; any cyst: ovarian torsion, rupture, hemorrhage into cyst or into the abdominal cavity.

SIGNS AND SYMPTOMS Lower abdominal pain, menstrual abnormalities; sudden increase in pain to severe levels indicates rupture or torsion.

CLINICAL DIAGNOSIS AND OTHER CLINICAL FEATURES To be considered in a woman of child-bearing age presenting with lower abdominal pain; differentiate from ectopic pregnancy and pelvic inflammatory disease; pelvic exam; ultrasonography; laparotomy.

LABORATORY DIAGNOSIS No specific tests other than histologic examination of resected specimen to categorize the cyst and differentiate it from a cystic neoplasm, benign or malignant.

PROGNOSIS Good, but may result in loss of the ovary.

THERAPY Surgical resection.

OTHER INFORMATION Multiple bilateral ovarian cysts with amenorrhea, infertility, and hirsutism constitute the polycystic ovary syndrome.

Pelvic Inflammatory Disease

DESCRIPTION Infectious disease involving the female pelvic organs caused by *N. gonorrhoeae* and other organisms, resulting in purulent exudation and later scarring in and around the fallopian tubes and ovaries.

DISEASE ENTITIES; SYNONYMS AND ACRONYMS Salpingitis, pyosalpinx, gonorrhea, pelvic peritonitis, tubo-ovarian abscess.

INCIDENCE Common; a consequence of sexually transmitted disease.

AGE Most common in young women.

ETIOLOGY, PATHOGENESIS, AND PREDISPOSING FACTORS Sexually transmitted: *N. gonorrhoeae, Chlamydia trachomatis*; postpartum, postabortion, or postsurgical: polymicrobial (coliforms, staphylococci, streptococci, clostridia); IUD: actinomyces.

SITES INVOLVED Gonorrhea starts in the vulvar, periurethral, and endocervical glands and spreads through the endometrium to the fallopian tubes where the infectious process escapes into the pelvic cavity.

GROSS LESIONS Acute salpingitis: purulent exudate that may distend the tubes (pyosalpinx); tubo-ovarian adhesions with exudate within the complex (tubo-ovarian abscess); pelvic serosal exudate.

MICROSCOPIC LESIONS Acute inflammatory exudate within the lumen and wall of the fallopian tube with edema and focal abscesses; abscesses in the ovary; purulent exudate on serosa; later, scarring of involved structures.

COMPLICATIONS Infertility due to destruction and scarring of ovaries and tubes; peritonitis, more commonly with the nongonococcal organisms; bacteremia; intestinal adhesions with bowel obstruction.

SIGNS AND SYMPTOMS Pelvic or lower abdominal pain; occasionally generalized abdominal pain; dysmenorrhea; irregular menses; fever; cervical, uterine, and adnexal tenderness on pelvic examination.

CLINICAL DIAGNOSIS AND OTHER CLINICAL FEATURES Suspected in a young woman with pelvic pain; differential: ectopic pregnancy, ovarian cyst, endometritis, appendicitis, urinary tract infection; investigate by pelvic examination, pelvic ultrasound.

LABORATORY DIAGNOSIS Culture of swabs from endocervix and urethra; cytologic examination of cervical smears with immunofluorescent staining for Chlamydia.

PROGNOSIS Early infections usually respond to treatment; neglected infections cause permanent damage.

THERAPY Specific antibiotics; surgical resection is occasionally required for tubo-ovarian abscess.

OTHER INFORMATION Pelvic peritonitis can spread to the upper abdomen to cause atypical pain that may radiate to the shoulder and perihepatitis with liver function abnormalities (Fitz-Hugh-Curtis syndrome).

Polycystic Ovary Syndrome

DESCRIPTION A clinical syndrome of obesity, hirsutism, and secondary amenorrhea or oligomenorrhea with infertility due to anovulation, accompanied by multiple follicle cysts within both ovaries.

DISEASE ENTITIES; SYNONYMS AND ACRONYMS Stein-Leventhal syndrome.

INCIDENCE Fairly common as a cause of infertility.

AGE Young women after menarche.

ETIOLOGY, PATHOGENESIS, AND PREDISPOSING FACTORS Loss of hypothalamic control over pituitary LH and FSH; high LH causes excessive androgen synthesis by ovary; androgen is converted to estrone, which stimulates more LH secretion.

SITES INVOLVED Bilateral ovaries.

GROSS LESIONS Ovaries are enlarged and contain multiple cysts averaging 1 cm in diameter within the stroma.

MICROSCOPIC LESIONS Cysts are lined by granulosa and theca cells, the latter of which are often luteinized; stroma shows hyperthecosis and fibrosis.

COMPLICATIONS Infertility, hirsutism.

SIGNS AND SYMPTOMS Triad of obesity, hirsutism, and secondary amenorrhea. An identical syndrome can be produced by an androgen-secreting tumor of the ovary.

CLINICAL DIAGNOSIS AND OTHER CLINICAL FEATURES Recognition of presenting signs; patients often come to attention for infertility assessment; demonstration of loss of midcycle body temperature elevation points to anovulatory cycles.

LABORATORY DIAGNOSIS Elevated LH, decreased FSH, and loss of normal periodicity; histologic examination of wedge resection of ovaries.

PROGNOSIS Successful therapy reverses the process and restores fertility in many patients.

THERAPY Wedge (partial) resection of both ovaries; clomiphene, oral contraceptives.

OTHER INFORMATION The partial ovarian resection reduces the mass of tissue producing androgen in response to pituitary stimulation and apparently breaks the positive feedback cycle causing the syndrome.

Spontaneous Abortion

DESCRIPTION   Termination of pregnancy without external interference before the fetus is considered viable at 22 weeks gestation.

DISEASE ENTITIES; SYNONYMS AND ACRONYMS   Miscarriage.

INCIDENCE   Up to 15% of known pregnancies abort; an additional 20–30% abort before pregnancy is known.

AGE   Women of childbearing age; within the first two trimesters of pregnancy.

ETIOLOGY, PATHOGENESIS, AND PREDISPOSING FACTORS   Fetal factors: chromosomal abnormalities, abnormal development; maternal factors: infection, uterine abnormalities including leiomyomas and cervical incompetence, progesterone deficiency, trauma.

SITES INVOLVED   Uterus, endometrium, placenta, and fetus.

GROSS LESIONS   Bloody fluid or blood clots with fragments of placenta and fetus intermixed; grossly apparent fetal abnormalities may be seen; empty gestational sac indicates early fetal death (blighted ovum).

MICROSCOPIC LESIONS   Necrosis, hemorrhage, and inflammation in decidua; placental chorionic villi are normal or swollen (hydropic change); fetus may not be found grossly or microscopically, having been expelled and lost.

COMPLICATIONS   Persistent bleeding and acute endometritis due to retained placental fragments; pelvic inflammatory disease; secondary amenorrhea following severe endometritis (Asherman's syndrome).

SIGNS AND SYMPTOMS   Passage of blood clots and tissue fragments with little warning or following variable abdominal pain and spotting of blood; often preceded by urge to defecate with abortus passed into toilet.

CLINICAL DIAGNOSIS AND OTHER CLINICAL FEATURES   Diagnosis is obvious if pregnancy is known; if pregnancy status is unknown, passage of blood may be regarded as menstrual abnormality; dilatation and curettage (D&C) for diagnosis and therapy.

LABORATORY DIAGNOSIS   Histologic examination of expelled tissue and curettings from D&C; decidualized endometrium without gestational products may indicate ectopic pregnancy; karyotyping of fetal tissue.

PROGNOSIS   Good chance for successful subsequent pregnancy unless abortions are recurrent (habitual abortion).

THERAPY   No treatment may be required; D&C to control bleeding and to remove any retained placental parts.

OTHER INFORMATION   Maternal alcohol consumption during pregnancy increases the risk of spontaneous abortion.

Toxemia of Pregnancy

DESCRIPTION   A disorder of late pregnancy characterized by hypertension, proteinuria, and edema (pre-eclampsia) that may progress to eclampsia with coma, seizures, and disseminated intravascular coagulation (DIC).

DISEASE ENTITIES; SYNONYMS AND ACRONYMS   Eclampsia, pre-eclampsia.

INCIDENCE   Some degree of toxemia develops in 6% of pregnancies, more often in primiparas than in multiparas.

AGE   During the last trimester, usually after 32 weeks of gestation.

ETIOLOGY, PATHOGENESIS, AND PREDISPOSING FACTORS   Current hypotheses implicate placental ischemia that leads to decreased prostaglandin E synthesis, enhanced angiotensin sensitivity, endothelial damage, platelet activation, and DIC.

SITES INVOLVED   Placenta is the site that initiates toxemia; in eclampsia, small blood vessels throughout the body are involved, especially in liver, renal glomeruli, brain, and pituitary gland.

GROSS LESIONS   Placenta: infarcts, retroplacental hematomas; liver: focal hemorrhages; kidney: lesions ranging from microinfarcts to bilateral cortical necrosis; brain: focal hemorrhages.

MICROSCOPIC LESIONS   Fibrin thrombi occluding arterioles and capillaries in affected organs; secondary necrosis from infarction; uterine spiral arteries show fibrinoid necrosis and accumulation of foamy macrophages.

COMPLICATIONS   Convulsions and coma indicate the onset of eclampsia; DIC results in bleeding diathesis and organ failure, especially of kidney; hypertension can precipitate cerebral hemorrhage or heart failure.

SIGNS AND SYMPTOMS   Pre-eclampsia: headaches, visual disturbances; hypertension, ankle edema, proteinuria. Eclampsia: convulsions, coma.

CLINICAL DIAGNOSIS AND OTHER CLINICAL FEATURES   Recognition of clinical signs; regular prenatal examinations of blood pressure and urine are important to detect toxemia at an early stage.

LABORATORY DIAGNOSIS   Urinalysis, particularly for proteinuria; serum BUN and creatinine.

PROGNOSIS   Pre-eclampsia is usually managed successfully; eclampsia carries a significant mortality.

THERAPY   Pre-eclampsia: rest, antihypertensives; eclampsia: magnesium sulfate, anticonvulsants, delivery.

OTHER INFORMATION   Aspirin and other antiplatelet drugs are under investigation for their effectiveness in decreasing the incidence and severity of toxemia.

Vulvar Dystrophy

DESCRIPTION A classification of benign lesions of the vulvar epithelium usually seen after menopause; subtypes include lichen sclerosis and hyperplastic dystrophy (more recently called squamous hyperplasia).

DISEASE ENTITIES; SYNONYMS AND ACRONYMS Lichen sclerosis et atrophicus, kraurosis vulvae, atrophic vulvitis; squamous hyperplasia, leukoplakia.

INCIDENCE Common.

AGE Any age; most common in middle age to elderly, particularly after menopause.

ETIOLOGY, PATHOGENESIS, AND PREDISPOSING FACTORS Squamous hyperplasia may be a response to chronic inflammation; lichen sclerosis shows increased cell turnover, possible due to genetic, inflammatory, or hormonal factors.

SITES INVOLVED Squamous epithelium of vulva.

GROSS LESIONS Lichen sclerosis: thin, smooth, and dry vulvar skin with atrophy of labia and introitus; squamous hyperplasia: thickening of the skin with whitish discoloration, described as leukoplakia.

MICROSCOPIC LESIONS Lichen sclerosis: thinning of epidermis, hyperkeratosis, loss of rete pegs, dermal fibrosis and scant chronic inflammation; squamous hyperplasia: marked epithelial thickening with hyperkeratosis.

COMPLICATIONS Lichen sclerosis: dyspareunia, predisposition to infection; squamous hyperplasia: by itself of little significance except that it may be confused with a malignant or premalignant lesion.

SIGNS AND SYMPTOMS Itching, discomfort, dyspareunia; discovery of lesion on routine examination.

CLINICAL DIAGNOSIS AND OTHER CLINICAL FEATURES Visual appearance of lichen sclerosis is distinctive, biopsy is confirmatory; the leukoplakia of squamous hyperplasia is indistinguishable from other lesions and biopsy is required.

LABORATORY DIAGNOSIS Histologic examination of biopsied lesion. If the lesion shows squamous atypia plus hyperplasia, then it should be classified as squamous dysplasia or vulvar intraepithelial neoplasia (VIN).

PROGNOSIS Good; these lesions are not premalignant; lichen sclerosis causes considerable chronic discomfort.

THERAPY Removal of irritants; treatment of any infections; symptomatic treatment.

OTHER INFORMATION Leukoplakia is a descriptive term only; specific terms are preferable; chronic dermatitis, squamous dysplasia, carcinoma, Paget's disease, and vitiligo all cause lesions that appear as leukoplakia.

Pathology Facts, by Richard C.
Harruff, J.B. Lippincott
Company, Philadelphia © 1994.

Chapter 19

Blood Elements and Lymphoid Tissue

Acute Lymphoblastic Leukemia

DESCRIPTION   Neoplastic proliferation of bone marrow lympho-cyte precursor cells; classified morphologically (Types L1-L3) or immunologically (T-cell, B-cell, or null-cell).

DISEASE ENTITIES; SYNONYMS AND ACRONYMS   Acute lymphoid leukemia, acute lymphocytic leukemia, ALL; L1-L3 by the FAB classification.

INCIDENCE   Most common pediatric cancer; about 1800 cases per year in US; more common in whites and in males.

AGE   Peak age around 4 years; smaller peak in older adults; L1 most common in children, L2 in adults.

ETIOLOGY, PATHOGENESIS, AND PREDISPOSING FACTORS   Chro-mosomal abnormalities are common, especially translocations; Philadelphia chromosome is present in a few; high incidence in Down's syndrome and in twin sibling of a child with ALL.

SITES INVOLVED   Primarily bone marrow and blood; secondary infil-trates in spleen, liver, and lymph nodes; leptomeninges and testes are often involved; mediastinal mass is common with T-cell ALL.

GROSS LESIONS   Bone trabeculae and cortex may be rarefied; spleen is enlarged and diffusely infiltrated; lymph nodes are fleshy gray; leptomeninges are thickened and opaque pale gray; testes are diffusely enlarged.

MICROSCOPIC LESIONS   Leukemic cells infiltrate diffusely throughout affected tissues; classified as L1-L3 by morphologic criteria; most are B-cell by cell markers; all types show nuclear features of immature lymphoblasts.

COMPLICATIONS   Replacement of normal marrow cells by ALL cells results in anemia, infections due to granulocytopenia, and bleeding disorders due to thrombocytopenia; leukemic menin-gitis and hyperuricemia are common.

SIGNS AND SYMPTOMS   Pallor, fatigue, fever, infections, gingival bleeding, epistaxis, petechiae, and ecchymosis in a previously healthy child; meningeal infiltration may produce signs similar to bacterial meningitis.

CLINICAL DIAGNOSIS AND OTHER CLINICAL FEATURES   Signs of bleeding, pallor, susceptibility to infection rapidly appearing in a child is highly suspicious; workup needs to exclude viral in-fection (infectious mononucleosis) and confirm leukemia.

LABORATORY DIAGNOSIS   CBC; blood and marrow examination; white count may be high or low; cytochemical tests and im-munologic markers to type the leukemia; presence of TdT dif-ferentiates ALL from nonlymphoblastic leukemia.

PROGNOSIS   In childhood ALL, aggressive therapy achieves 5-year survival of 60%; adult ALL remains poor.

THERAPY   Multiple drug chemotherapy; antibiotics; transfusions.

OTHER INFORMATION   L1: small uniform cells, scant cytoplasm; L2: medium size cells, irregular nucleus, moderate cytoplasm; L3: large cells, round nucleus, abundant dark blue cytoplasm, same as Burkitt's lymphoma cells.

Acute Myeloblastic Leukemia

DESCRIPTION   Neoplastic proliferation of multipotent or committed hematopoietic precursor cells showing variable myeloblastic, monoblastic, or normoblastic differentiation but no cytoplasmic maturation.

DISEASE ENTITIES; SYNONYMS AND ACRONYMS   Acute myeloid leukemia, AML, acute nonlymphocytic leukemia, ANLL; M1–M7 by the FAB classification.

INCIDENCE   Constitute 20% of all leukemias, 85% of adult acute leukemias, and 20% of childhood leukemias.

AGE   Predominantly adults, aged 15–40 years.

ETIOLOGY, PATHOGENESIS, AND PREDISPOSING FACTORS   Exposure to myelotoxin (benzene, alkylating agents) or radiation explains a few cases; others develop from myeloproliferative disorders, aplastic anemia and paroxysmal nocturnal hemoglobinuria.

SITES INVOLVED   Primarily bone marrow and blood; secondary infiltration of liver, spleen, lymph nodes, skin, other organs; soft tissue masses (granulocytic sarcoma, chloroma); M4 and M5 tend to infiltrate gingiva.

GROSS LESIONS   Red marrow is expanded with areas of bone softening; hepatosplenomegaly is usually not prominent; chloroma appears greenish; other lesions are determined by the complications.

MICROSCOPIC LESIONS   Neoplastic cells are monomorphous with cytoplasmic differentiation as defined by the FAB categories; nuclei are primitive with delicate chromatin and 3-5 nucleoli; auer rods are often present.

COMPLICATIONS   Anemia, infections, and bleeding; leukostasis causes vascular occlusion; neurologic symptoms due to meningeal infiltration or hemorrhage; DIC with M3; hyperuricemia and renal stones.

SIGNS AND SYMPTOMS   Fatigue and pallor due to anemia; fever, infections or ulcers due to neutropenia; purpura, petechiae, epistaxis, or gingival bleeding due to thrombocytopenia; manifestations have a rapid onset.

CLINICAL DIAGNOSIS AND OTHER CLINICAL FEATURES   Bleeding disorders and nonhealing ulcers are highly suggestive, confirmation requires laboratory investigation; effort is directed toward accurate classification of the leukemia.

LABORATORY DIAGNOSIS   CBC, blood and bone marrow examination; white count may be high or low; thrombocytopenia and pancytopenia (aleukemic leukemia) are common; a variety of cytochemical tests are used for classification.

PROGNOSIS   Poor, despite initial remission; only 10–15% survive; infection is most common cause of death.

THERAPY   Chemotherapy; bone marrow transplantation.

OTHER INFORMATION   FAB classification: M1 and M2, myeloblastic; M3, promyelocytic (progranulocytic); M4, myelomonocytic; M5, monocytic; M6, erythroleukemia; M7, megakaryoblastic.

Anemia

DESCRIPTION   Reduction below normal limits of the blood's hemoglobin concentration, hematocrit, and circulating red cell mass, resulting in deficient oxygen delivery and consequent tissue hypoxia.

DISEASE ENTITIES; SYNONYMS AND ACRONYMS   Several types classified by etiology and morphology.

INCIDENCE   Very common; the most common hematologic abnormality; iron-deficiency anemia is most common.

AGE   Any age, more likely in older adults; growing children and pregnant women are at risk.

ETIOLOGY, PATHOGENESIS, AND PREDISPOSING FACTORS   Decreased rate of red cell production (bone marrow failure, lack of nutrients), increased rate of destruction (hemolytic anemia), blood loss (acute or chronic).

SITES INVOLVED   Defects in bone marrow normoblasts produce hypoproliferative anemias, including nutritional deficiency anemias; hemolytic anemias are caused by abnormalities intrinsic and extrinsic to the red cell.

GROSS LESIONS   Depends on etiology; in hemolytic anemia, red (hematopoietic) marrow is increased, splenomegaly may be present; in sickle cell anemia, spleen is fibrotic; in aplastic anemia, red marrow is absent.

MICROSCOPIC LESIONS   Red cell morphology may indicate etiology, e.g., hypochromic, microcytic = iron deficiency; megaloblastic = B_{12} or folate deficiency; spherocytosis, reticulocytosis = hemolytic anemia.

COMPLICATIONS   Severe anemia can cause heart failure and hypoxic damage of liver and kidney; other complications depend on the specific type of anemia.

SIGNS AND SYMPTOMS   Weakness, fatigue, dyspnea on exertion; headache, drowsiness, fainting, dim vision; pallor of skin, mucosa, and conjunctiva; tachycardia; ankle ulcers (sickle cell), koilonychia (iron deficiency).

CLINICAL DIAGNOSIS AND OTHER CLINICAL FEATURES   Signs and symptoms, especially pallor, may not be recognized unless the hemoglobin concentration is reduced to about half of normal; workup is directed at establishing the etiology of the anemia.

LABORATORY DIAGNOSIS   CBC, examination of blood smear and often bone marrow; determination of serum iron; reticulocyte count; sickle cell screen; hemoglobin electrophoresis; Coomb's test; G6PD assay; osmotic fragility.

PROGNOSIS   Depends on etiology; good for nutritional deficiency; more often poor for hemolytic anemia.

THERAPY   Depends on etiology; correction of nutritional deficiency; various attempts to reduce hemolysis.

OTHER INFORMATION   Acute blood loss does not affect the hematocrit for several hours. Red cell indices, MCV (mean cell volume), and MCHC (mean cell hemoglobin concentration) help classify the anemia morphologically.

Anemia of Chronic Disease

DESCRIPTION   Mild to moderate anemia associated with chronic inflammatory, infectious and neoplastic diseases, caused by several factors affecting iron metabolism, red cell production, and red cell survival.

DISEASE ENTITIES; SYNONYMS AND ACRONYMS   Anemia of chronic disease.

INCIDENCE   Common complication of various chronic diseases, e.g., rheumatoid arthritis, tuberculosis, cancer.

AGE   Any age but more likely in older adults because of higher frequency of chronic diseases.

ETIOLOGY, PATHOGENESIS, AND PREDISPOSING FACTORS   Multifactorial; macrophage defect in iron recycling and return to developing erythrocytes; decreased red cell survival; inadequate levels of erythropoietin; diminished response to erythropoietin.

SITES INVOLVED   Reticuloendothelial (monocyte-macrophage) system exhibits defective function as a response to the chronic disease state; bone marrow normoblasts are hypoproliferative; red cell survival is reduced.

GROSS LESIONS   No specific lesions other than the manifestations of the particular underlying chronic disease.

MICROSCOPIC LESIONS   Red cells are usually normocytic/normochromic, sometimes microcytic/hypochromic; marrow cellularity is normal or shows increased myeloid:erythroid ratio; stainable iron is normal or increased.

COMPLICATIONS   The anemia compounds the physical debilitation produced by the underlying chronic disease and places an additional burden on the cardiovascular system.

SIGNS AND SYMPTOMS   Pallor, fatigue, dyspnea, tachycardia; all may be overshadowed by the manifestations of the primary disease.

CLINICAL DIAGNOSIS AND OTHER CLINICAL FEATURES   Should be suspected in a patient with a chronic inflammatory, infectious or neoplastic disease; other causes must be excluded: iron deficiency, hemolytic anemia, bone marrow metastases, etc.

LABORATORY DIAGNOSIS   CBC, blood and bone marrow examination with iron stains showing adequate or increased iron stores; decreased serum iron, decreased iron binding capacity, and decreased iron saturation.

PROGNOSIS   Depends on control of the underlying condition.

THERAPY   Treatment of underlying disease; maintenance of adequate nutrition.

OTHER INFORMATION   Anemia with neoplasia may be due to several factors; myelophthistic anemia is a consequence of bone marrow metastasis; aplastic anemia is a common complication of cancer chemotherapy.

Aplastic Anemia

DESCRIPTION   Hematologic disorder characterized by anemia, neutropenia, and thrombocytopenia with hypocellular bone marrow; caused by failure of the myeloid precursor stem cells.

DISEASE ENTITIES; SYNONYMS AND ACRONYMS   Pancytopenia, bone marrow failure, bone marrow aplasia, aplastic marrow.

INCIDENCE   Fairly common; affects both sexes.

AGE   Any age.

ETIOLOGY, PATHOGENESIS, AND PREDISPOSING FACTORS   Drugs (chloramphenicol, alkylating agents), chemicals (benzene), radiation, viral infections (NANB hepatitis); half of cases are idiopathic and may be immunologically mediated; Fanconi's anemia.

SITES INVOLVED   Bone marrow primarily, reflected in peripheral blood cell counts; secondary changes occur throughout the body due to cytopenias.

GROSS LESIONS   Yellow marrow is increased, red marrow absent or markedly decreased; secondary changes are due to bleeding (ecchymosis, purpura) and infections (pneumonia, oral and skin ulcers).

MICROSCOPIC LESIONS   Bone marrow is nearly acellular and completely fatty with marked decrease in all cell lines; peripheral blood shows rare platelets and granulocytes; skin and oral ulcers show scant inflammation.

COMPLICATIONS   Bleeding due to thrombocytopenia, infections due to neutropenia; anemia occurs later causing heart failure; acute nonlymphocytic leukemia develops in 5% of cases.

SIGNS AND SYMPTOMS   Easy bruisability, bleeding after minor trauma and from gums; recurrent infections; oral or skin ulcers with little exudate and delayed healing; pallor, dyspnea, and tachycardia from anemia.

CLINICAL DIAGNOSIS AND OTHER CLINICAL FEATURES   Easy bruisability, bleeding, and indolent ulcers are prime indicators that should prompt blood studies, followed by bone marrow aspiration and biopsy.

LABORATORY DIAGNOSIS   CBC shows pancytopenia (anemia, neutropenia, thrombocytopenia); bone marrow biopsy shows fatty marrow with markedly decreased hematopoietic cells (aplastic marrow).

PROGNOSIS   Usually poor, especially with the idiopathic form.

THERAPY   Removal of myelotoxin; bone marrow transplant, immunosuppressive therapy, antithymocyte globulin.

OTHER INFORMATION   Pure red cell aplasia is associated with a thymoma or is secondary to neoplasms, infections, drugs, and autoimmune diseases; parvovirus infection causes aplastic crisis in hemolytic anemia.

Autommimune Hemolytic Anemia— Cold Antibody Type

DESCRIPTION Hemolytic anemia caused by autoantibodies of the IgM class that bind to red cell I/i antigens and fix complement at cool temperatures; associated with atypical pneumonia and malignant lymphomas.

DISEASE ENTITIES; SYNONYMS AND ACRONYMS Cold agglutinin disease.

INCIDENCE Common with lymphoid neoplasms; occurs with mycoplasma pneumonia and infectious mononucleosis.

AGE More common in older adults due to the increased incidence of lymphomas.

ETIOLOGY, PATHOGENESIS, AND PREDISPOSING FACTORS IgM antibodies bind to red cell I/i antigens and fix complement in the cool distal extremities; IgM dissociates in warmer blood, complement remains bound, opsonizing the red cell for phagocytosis.

SITES INVOLVED Red cell membrane, where I/i glycoproteins project from the surface; liver Kupffer cells (rather than spleen macrophages) attack the opsonized red cells and cause hemolysis.

GROSS LESIONS No specific lesion; liver may be somewhat enlarged; splenomegaly is not present, in contrast to warm antibody immune hemolytic anemia.

MICROSCOPIC LESIONS Peripheral blood film shows rouleaux formation and possibly spherocytosis; erythrophagocytosis by Kupffer cells lining the hepatic sinusoids may be present.

COMPLICATIONS Hemolytic anemia, usually of mild to moderate severity; vascular occlusion in parts exposed to cold; Raynaud's phenomenon.

SIGNS AND SYMPTOMS Depend on the severity of anemia and the nature of primary disease; Raynaud's phenomenon refers to blanching, pain, and cyanosis of the fingers on exposure to cold.

CLINICAL DIAGNOSIS AND OTHER CLINICAL FEATURES Except for the overt presentation of Raynaud's phenomenon, most cases are first recognized as laboratory abnormalities while doing blood tests for the primary disease.

LABORATORY DIAGNOSIS Red cells agglutinate in refrigerator but not at room temperature; rouleaux formation is noted on blood smear; Coomb's test is positive for complement; antibody associated with lymphoma is monoclonal.

PROGNOSIS Good if associated with mycoplasma; depends on prognosis of neoplasm if associated with lymphoma.

THERAPY Treatment of underlying condition; avoidance of cold exposure to extremities; plasmapheresis.

OTHER INFORMATION The rare paroxysmal cold hemoglobinuria, associated with syphilis and certain viral infections, is caused by a cold-reacting IgG antibody against red cell P antigen.

Autoimmune Hemolytic Anemia—
Warm Antibody Type

DESCRIPTION Hemolytic anemia mediated by autoantibodies directed against red cell Rh group membrane proteins, resulting in erythrophagocytosis by splenic macrophages and chronic hemolysis.

DISEASE ENTITIES; SYNONYMS AND ACRONYMS Immune hemolytic anemia, immunohemolytic anemia, AIHA.

INCIDENCE Fairly common, especially in association with lymphocytic neoplasms and autoimmune diseases.

AGE Usually in older adults due to their higher incidence of predisposing conditions.

ETIOLOGY, PATHOGENESIS, AND PREDISPOSING FACTORS Most cases are idiopathic; others are commonly associated with chronic lymphocytic leukemia, malignant lymphoma, autoimmune disease, viral infection, certain cancers, and inflammatory bowel disease.

SITES INVOLVED Red cell membrane, which is coated by anti-Rh autoantibodies and activated complement; opsonized red cells are attacked by macrophages; hemolysis occurs in the spleen.

GROSS LESIONS Spleen is usually markedly enlarged and congested.

MICROSCOPIC LESIONS Spherocytosis is present in the peripheral smear; erythrophagocytosis may be seen in the congested spleen.

COMPLICATIONS Severe intractable anemia with heart failure; infections; thromboembolism; other complications depend on any primary disorder or associated condition; hemolytic transfusion reactions.

SIGNS AND SYMPTOMS Jaundice and pallor of anemia; fatigue, dyspnea, tachycardia; course is unpredictable with remissions and relapses in the level of active hemolysis.

CLINICAL DIAGNOSIS AND OTHER CLINICAL FEATURES An anticipated complication of chronic lymphocytic leukemia or lupus erythematosus; anemia and jaundice indicate hemolysis; laboratory studies are required to establish immune etiology.

LABORATORY DIAGNOSIS Positive Coomb's (antiglobulin) test detects IgG and sometimes complement on the red cells; reticulocytosis, spherocytosis; unconjugated hyperbilirubinemia; cross-match may be impossible.

PROGNOSIS Often poor, progressing to intractable anemia or terminating in one of the other complications.

THERAPY Steroids, other immunosuppressive therapy, plasmapheresis; blood transfusions are difficult.

OTHER INFORMATION Certain drugs induce immune hemolytic anemia, notably penicillins, cephalosporins, alpha-methyldopa and quinidine; hapten formation and immune complexes mediate drug-induced immune hemolysis.

Chronic Lymphocytic Leukemia

DESCRIPTION Neoplastic disease of lymphocytes characterized by the accumulation of small mature lymphocytes in bone marrow and blood with secondary infiltration of lymph nodes, spleen, liver, and other tissues.

DISEASE ENTITIES; SYNONYMS AND ACRONYMS CLL; overlaps with small lymphocytic lymphoma and Waldenstrom's macroglobulinemia.

INCIDENCE Constitutes 25% of all leukemias in US and Europe; uncommon in Asia; male:female = 2:1.

AGE Older adults over 50 years; average age 60 years.

ETIOLOGY, PATHOGENESIS, AND PREDISPOSING FACTORS CLL lymphocytes proliferate slowly but are long-lived and thus accumulate in the marrow, replacing normal elements; via blood, they infiltrate other organs; chromosomal abnormalities are common.

SITES INVOLVED Primarily bone marrow and blood; secondarily lymph nodes, splenic white pulp, liver portal regions, and sinusoids; potentially any tissue or organ, usually with perivascular infiltration.

GROSS LESIONS Bone marrow changes are not appreciable; enlarged lymph nodes have a fleshy pale gray cut surface; splenic white pulp is prominent, sometimes forming tumor nodules; liver is diffusely enlarged.

MICROSCOPIC LESIONS CLL cells have small dark round nuclei and scant cytoplasm (mature lymphocytes); bone marrow shows nodular or diffuse infiltrates of lymphocytes; other tissues may be infiltrated by CLL lymphocytes.

COMPLICATIONS Anemia, infections, and bleeding due to replacement of normal marrow cells by CLL cells; hemolytic anemia; hypogammaglobulinemia; hypersplenism; development of large cell lymphoma (Richter's syndrome).

SIGNS AND SYMPTOMS Pallor, fatigue, weight loss; commonly lymphadenopathy and hepatosplenomegaly; infection, such as an episode of herpes zoster, may bring a patient to attention.

CLINICAL DIAGNOSIS AND OTHER CLINICAL FEATURES Many are asymptomatic and are discovered on physical examination to have enlarged lymph nodes and/or spleen; diagnostic evaluation is aimed at classification, staging, and monitoring for complications.

LABORATORY DIAGNOSIS CBC, blood and bone marrow examination; lymphocytosis (usually B-cells) may exceed 100,000/cmm; many smudge cells are seen on blood smear; monoclonal IgM or anti-Rh antibodies may be present.

PROGNOSIS From 2 to over 10 years survival, median 6 years; infections are the usual cause of death.

THERAPY Conservative chemotherapy; therapy does not affect survival and may compound risk of infections.

OTHER INFORMATION Rai stage 0: only lymphocytosis > 15,000/cmm; I: lymphocytosis with lymphadenopathy; II: with hepatosplenomegaly; III: with anemia; IV: with thrombocytopenia.

Chronic Myeloid Leukemia

DESCRIPTION Chronic myeloproliferative syndrome characterized by neoplastic proliferation of hematopoietic cells, predominantly the granulocytic series, associated with the Philadelphia chromosome.

DISEASE ENTITIES; SYNONYMS AND ACRONYMS Chronic myelogenous leukemia, CML, chronic granulocytic leukemia, CGL.

INCIDENCE Constitutes 15–20% of all leukemias; the most common myeloproliferative syndrome; male:female = 3:2.

AGE Ranges between 25 and 60 years; median age 45 years.

ETIOLOGY, PATHOGENESIS, AND PREDISPOSING FACTORS Philadelphia chromosome, a translocation of the long arm of chromosome 22 to chromosome 9, is present in all three hematopoietic cell lines; some cases are related to benzene or radiation exposure.

SITES INVOLVED Bone marrow, blood, and spleen; the chromosomal defect originates in multipotent stem cells; myeloblasts, normoblasts, megakaryocytes, and sometimes lymphocytes all carry the Philadelphia chromosome.

GROSS LESIONS Red marrow is expanded; spleen is markedly enlarged with a soft bloody cut surface lacking white pulp; spleen infarcts are common; hepatomegaly is likely.

MICROSCOPIC LESIONS Marked leukocytosis in blood smear with immature granulocytes, normoblasts, abnormally large platelets and many basophils; marrow is markedly hypercellular; spleen shows myeloid metaplasia.

COMPLICATIONS Replacement of normal marrow cells with leukemic cells leads to anemia, infections and bleeding disorders; most die after the leukemia enters a blast crisis; spleen can rupture with minimal trauma.

SIGNS AND SYMPTOMS Fatigue, weight loss, sweating, anorexia, feeling of fullness in the left abdomen, abnormal bleeding; as the disease progresses, infections and hemorrhage become particularly common.

CLINICAL DIAGNOSIS AND OTHER CLINICAL FEATURES Presenting signs and symptoms are often quite nonspecific; abnormal bleeding and marked splenomegaly are highly suspicious for CML.

LABORATORY DIAGNOSIS CBC, examination of blood and bone marrow; very high white count, often >100,000/cmm with predominance of immature forms; thrombocytosis, basophilia; low leukocyte alkaline phosphatase (LAP) score.

PROGNOSIS Poor; median survival of 3–4 years, ranging from 2 to 8 years.

THERAPY Chemotherapy alone or in conjunction with bone marrow transplantation.

OTHER INFORMATION Most cases terminate in acute leukemia (blast crisis), which shows features of either acute myeloid or lymphoblastic leukemia.

Disseminated Intravascular Coagulation

DESCRIPTION Hemostatic disorder characterized by uncontrolled activation of both coagulation and fibrinolytic systems, leading to fibrin deposition and consumption of platelets, fibrin, and coagulation factors.

DISEASE ENTITIES; SYNONYMS AND ACRONYMS DIC, consumption coagulopathy, defibrination syndrome.

INCIDENCE Common, particularly after shock, sepsis, obstetric complications, and massive trauma.

AGE Any age; often seen in young adults because of their high incidence of trauma.

ETIOLOGY, PATHOGENESIS, AND PREDISPOSING FACTORS Release of thromboplastic substances and diffuse endothelial damage; initially fibrin thrombi form in small blood vessels; later plasmin is activated and fibrin and fibrinogen are consumed.

SITES INVOLVED Microthrombi form within vessels of any organ, producing significant lesions in brain (infarcts, hemorrhage), lung (associated with ARDS), kidneys (renal cortical necrosis), adrenals (hemorrhage).

GROSS LESIONS Infarcts or small hemorrhages due to microthrombi may be seen in the first phase; petechiae, purpura, ecchymoses, hematomas, and mucosal surface bleeding occur after consumption of hemostatic elements.

MICROSCOPIC LESIONS Fibrin microthrombi within small blood vessels with secondary infarction or hemorrhage; infarcts range from small to extensive; diffuse bleeding may also be evident.

COMPLICATIONS DIC is itself a complication of a primary event; infarcts occasionally contribute to organ failure; more often, failure of hemostasis with uncontrolled bleeding occurs, which carries high mortality.

SIGNS AND SYMPTOMS Hemorrhagic diathesis developing in a patient with trauma, shock, heat stroke, obstetric complications, cancer, or infections, or gram-negative sepsis.

CLINICAL DIAGNOSIS AND OTHER CLINICAL FEATURES Hemostatic failure in a predisposed patient is usually obvious, as in acute DIC; chronic low-grade DIC complicating certain cancers (e.g., progranulocytic leukemia, adenocarcinomas) may be subtle.

LABORATORY DIAGNOSIS Decreased fibrinogen level and low platelet count; prolonged bleeding time, prothrombin time, partial thromboplastin time, and thrombin time; elevated levels of fibrin split products.

PROGNOSIS Often carries a high mortality; survival depends largely on control of the primary condition.

THERAPY Treatment of initiating condition; heparin anticoagulation; transfusion of fresh frozen plasma.

OTHER INFORMATION Microangiopathic hemolytic anemia can occur with DIC. Waterhouse-Friderichsen syndrome and Sheehan's syndrome are special manifestations of DIC; eclampsia is closely associated with DIC.

Folic Acid Deficiency Anemia

DESCRIPTION Macrocytic/megaloblastic anemia caused by deficiency of folic acid (folate, pteroylmonoglutamic acid); similar to vitamin B_{12} deficiency anemia but without the neurologic degeneration.

DISEASE ENTITIES; SYNONYMS AND ACRONYMS Megaloblastic anemia, macrocytic anemia.

INCIDENCE Common only in predisposed persons (malnutrition, alcoholism, chronic hemolytic anemia).

AGE Any age, depending on predisposing conditions; usually adults.

ETIOLOGY, PATHOGENESIS, AND PREDISPOSING FACTORS Primary malnutrition, overcooking of food, alcoholism, pregnancy, chronic hemolytic anemia (sickle cell disease), small bowel disease (sprue); dilantin, methotrexate therapy.

SITES INVOLVED Like B_{12} deficiency, folate deficiency affects all cells in the body by suppressing DNA synthesis; significant alterations are confined to the bone marrow and blood.

GROSS LESIONS Increased red marrow and decreased yellow marrow.

MICROSCOPIC LESIONS Hypercellular bone marrow with erythroid hyperplasia; megaloblastic normoblasts with immature nuclei (nuclear-cytoplasmic asynchrony); macrocytes and hypersegmented polys in the peripheral smear.

COMPLICATIONS Anemia with high output heart failure.

SIGNS AND SYMPTOMS Pallor, dyspnea, and tachycardia due to anemia.

CLINICAL DIAGNOSIS AND OTHER CLINICAL FEATURES Investigation of anemia would return results indicating megaloblastic anemia; vitamin B_{12} deficiency must be excluded before folate deficiency is diagnosed and treated.

LABORATORY DIAGNOSIS CBC, examination of peripheral blood and bone marrow; decreased serum levels of folate; increased urinary excretion of formiminoglutamic acid (FIGlu) after oral administration of histidine.

PROGNOSIS Depends on the effects of the predisposing condition; usually good without permanent damage.

THERAPY Oral supplementation of folic acid but only after vitamin B_{12} deficiency is excluded.

OTHER INFORMATION Folic acid therapy will reverse the megaloblastic anemia of vitamin B_{12} deficiency but will not arrest the neurologic degeneration of combined system disease.

Glucose-6-Phosphate Dehydrogenase (G6PD) Deficiency Anemia

DESCRIPTION   Hemolytic anemia due to deficiency of the enzyme G6PD, causing abnormal red cell sensitivity to oxidant injury; on exposure to ingested oxidants, hemoglobin is denatured and hemolysis occurs.

DISEASE ENTITIES; SYNONYMS AND ACRONYMS   G6PD-deficiency hemolytic anemia.

INCIDENCE   One genetic variant is present in 10–15% of US blacks; another is transmitted in Mediterraneans.

AGE   Defect is present from birth; ingestion of oxidant determines when the hemolysis occurs.

ETIOLOGY, PATHOGENESIS, AND PREDISPOSING FACTORS   X-linked recessive gene affecting males; inactive G6PD does not reduce glutathione and antioxidant protection is lost; exposure to an oxidant denatures red cell hemoglobin and leads to hemolysis.

SITES INVOLVED   Denatured hemoglobin precipitates in red cells as Heinz bodies; in spleen, Heinz bodies are pitted from the red cells, weakening their membranes and promoting hemolysis or phagocytosis.

GROSS LESIONS   Splenic enlargement may occur during a hemolytic crisis.

MICROSCOPIC LESIONS   Spherocytes in peripheral smear during hemolytic episodes; Heinz bodies appear as inclusions within red cells stained with crystal violet; erythroid hyperplasia in marrow during recovery from episode.

COMPLICATIONS   Ingestion of oxidant foods (fava beans) or drugs (chloroquine, atabrine, sulfonamides, and others) produces hemolysis; in severe cases, there may be shock and renal failure.

SIGNS AND SYMPTOMS   Jaundice developing within 2–3 days after ingestion of oxidant drug or food; fever and hypotension in severe cases; may be confused with hemolytic crisis of malaria when antimalarial drugs are given.

CLINICAL DIAGNOSIS AND OTHER CLINICAL FEATURES   Hemolytic crisis in a man of Mediterranean or African descent who has recently ingested certain foods, or antimalarial, sulfonamide, nitrofuran, or related drug; family history may be positive.

LABORATORY DIAGNOSIS   Hyperbilirubinemia, predominantly unconjugated; drop in hematocrit; hemoglobinemia, hemoglobinuria; Heinz bodies in red cells; decreased activity of red cell G6PD; reticulocytosis in recovery phase.

PROGNOSIS   Good with avoidance of offending agent; severe hemolytic crisis may be life-threatening.

THERAPY   Withdrawal of offending drug; transfusion if needed; supportive measures.

OTHER INFORMATION   In the G6PD A$^-$ variant (US blacks) the oldest red cells are most deficient in enzyme activity; in G6PD Mediterranean, all red cells are deficient and hemolytic episodes are more severe.

Hemophilia A

DESCRIPTION   Bleeding disorder characterized by spontaneous and excessive bleeding, due to deficiency of Factor VIII, inherited as a sex-linked recessive trait by which males are affected and females are carriers.

DISEASE ENTITIES; SYNONYMS AND ACRONYMS   Classic hemophilia, Factor VIII deficiency.

INCIDENCE   The most common inherited coagulation factor deficiency; affects males or homozygous females.

AGE   Present at birth; likely to cause death in childhood if untreated.

ETIOLOGY, PATHOGENESIS, AND PREDISPOSING FACTORS   Many different genetic lesions cause Factor VIII deficiency; 25% of cases are due to new mutations; Factor VIII is required to initiate the intrinsic coagulation pathway by activation of Factor X.

SITES INVOLVED   Factor VIII is synthesized in the liver and coded on chromosome 12; typical place for bleeding is into the large weight-bearing joints; also bleeding from wounds, soft tissue, and viscera.

GROSS LESIONS   Characteristic lesion is recurrent hemarthrosis which leads to progressive joint deformity; other lesions are hematomas that develop in soft tissue following minor trauma.

MICROSCOPIC LESIONS   Nonspecific evidence of old and recent hemorrhage; synovium in joint with hemarthrosis undergoes hyperplasia, and hemosiderin pigment accumulates within synovial macrophages.

COMPLICATIONS   Bleeding may be life-threatening even after minor trauma; recurrent hemarthrosis progresses to joint deformity; transmission of viral hepatitis and HIV infection by Factor VIII concentrates.

SIGNS AND SYMPTOMS   The severity of the bleeding disorder varies; severe cases are obvious at birth with spontaneous hemorrhage; mild cases show excessive bleeding only after traumatic injuries.

CLINICAL DIAGNOSIS AND OTHER CLINICAL FEATURES   Hemarthrosis rather than petechiae and purpura distinguish hemophilia from platelet disorders and von Willebrand's disease; the inheritance pattern is also distinctive.

LABORATORY DIAGNOSIS   Bleeding time is normal; partial thromboplastin time (PTT) is prolonged; immunoassay for Factor VIII finds reduced levels; antenatal detection of the gene is possible using DNA probes.

PROGNOSIS   Therapy prolongs life but longevity and quality of life are significantly reduced.

THERAPY   Factor VIII concentrates prepared from pooled plasma (now heat-treated to reduce HIV transmission).

OTHER INFORMATION   Heterozygous females may be affected in cases of "unfavorable lyonization." Hemophilia B (Christmas disease) due to Factor IX deficiency is clinically indistinguishable from hemophilia A.

Hereditary Spherocytosis

DESCRIPTION   Hereditary hemolytic anemia caused by a defect in the red cell cytoskeleton, making the cells spherical and less deformable, resulting in an accelerated rate of red cell destruction in the spleen.

DISEASE ENTITIES; SYNONYMS AND ACRONYMS   Hereditary spherocytosis.

INCIDENCE   Most common in North Europeans with a rate approaching 1 in 5000 in some groups.

AGE   Presents at birth or in early age with jaundice; mild cases may present later with anemia.

ETIOLOGY, PATHOGENESIS, AND PREDISPOSING FACTORS   Autosomal dominant genetic deficiency in the red cell membrane protein, spectrin; the deficient membrane produces spherocytes which are poorly deformable and are trapped and hemolyzed in the spleen.

SITES INVOLVED   Red cell membrane (structural abnormality), spleen (site of hemolysis), and bone marrow (compensatory hyperplasia for increased destruction of red cells).

GROSS LESIONS   Splenomegaly in the range of 500–1000 g due to increased sequestration of red cells. Red marrow is expanded.

MICROSCOPIC LESIONS   In the peripheral smear, red cells appear small, dark, and lack the normal central pallor; erythroid hyperplasia in the bone marrow; congestion in the splenic cords with erythrophagocytosis.

COMPLICATIONS   Anemia; hemolytic crises with massive hemolysis in spleen, producing shock in very severe cases; aplastic crisis with bone marrow failure due to parvovirus infection; cholelithiasis (pigment stones).

SIGNS AND SYMPTOMS   Triad of anemia, splenomegaly, and jaundice; neonatal hyperbilirubinemia is sometimes severe enough to require exchange transfusions.

CLINICAL DIAGNOSIS AND OTHER CLINICAL FEATURES   Family history, Scandinavian or Northern European ancestry; combination of jaundice and pallor of anemia indicates hemolytic anemia; splenomegaly is fairly distinctive.

LABORATORY DIAGNOSIS   CBC; blood and bone marrow examination; spherocytosis on peripheral smear; normocytic hyperchromic anemia indices; reticulocytosis as with any hemolytic anemia; increased red cell osmotic fragility.

PROGNOSIS   Good with treatment.

THERAPY   Splenectomy results in nearly complete reversal of the anemia and jaundice.

OTHER INFORMATION   Spherocytes can also be seen in immune hemolytic anemia; the direct antiglobulin test (Coomb's test) differentiates the two diseases.

Hodgkin's Disease

DESCRIPTION Neoplastic disease of lymphoid tissue characterized by the presence of Reed-Sternberg (RS) cells within a reactive cellular proliferation that determines the subclassification.

DISEASE ENTITIES; SYNONYMS AND ACRONYMS Hodgkin's lymphoma; nodular sclerosing (NS), lymphocyte predominance (LP) or depletion (LD), mixed cellularity (MC).

INCIDENCE Altogether not very common; NS is most common, especially in young women; second is MC in older men.

AGE One of the most common cancers in young people between ages 15 and 32 years; less frequent in elderly.

ETIOLOGY, PATHOGENESIS, AND PREDISPOSING FACTORS The RS cells and their variants, originating from lymphoid or dendritic-reticular cells, are the actual neoplastic cells; lymphocytes and other cells in the process are reactive nonneoplastic cells.

SITES INVOLVED Lymph nodes, usually cervical, supraclavicular, and mediastinal; spleen; progression involves adjacent lymph nodes, viscera (liver, lung, GI tract), and bone marrow.

GROSS LESIONS Lymph node enlargement and obliteration with "fish-flesh" tumor mass often extending into surrounding tissue; dense fibrous bands (esp. NS) and yellow areas of necrosis.

MICROSCOPIC LESIONS Identification of RS cells or their variants is essential for diagnosis; lacunar cells and fibrosis are characteristic of NS; LP, MC, and LD depend on the ratio of RS cells to reactive lymphocytes.

COMPLICATIONS Immune suppression caused by the disease or its therapy, compression or invasion of adjacent tissues, replacement of bone marrow; secondary cancers from chemotherapy (acute leukemia, lung cancer).

SIGNS AND SYMPTOMS Painless enlargement of lymph nodes, usually regional, especially in younger patients; constitutional symptoms of fever, night sweats, pruritis, and weight loss (Stage B symptoms).

CLINICAL DIAGNOSIS AND OTHER CLINICAL FEATURES Suspicion regarding persistent lymphadenopathy; lymph node biopsy; staging involves x-rays, CT scans, lymphangiography, liver and bone marrow biopsy, laparotomy, and splenectomy.

LABORATORY DIAGNOSIS Histologic examination of lymph node biopsy, resected spleen, liver, and bone marrow biopsies for diagnosis, classification, and staging. Modern therapy demands accurate classification and staging.

PROGNOSIS LP > NS > MC > LD depending on stage, therapy, age of patient (younger = better), and Stage B symptoms.

THERAPY Multiple-drug chemotherapy and radiation therapy; splenectomy may limit hematogenous dissemination.

OTHER INFORMATION Stage I: single lymph node group or extranodal region; II: >1 node groups on same side of diaphragm; III: involvement of nodes (or spleen) on both sides of diaphragm; IV: disseminated spread.

Iron-Deficiency Anemia

DESCRIPTION   Microcytic hypochromic anemia secondary to deficiency of iron required for hemoglobin synthesis; caused by inadequate dietary intake, increased demand or chronic blood loss.

DISEASE ENTITIES; SYNONYMS AND ACRONYMS   Microcytic hypochromic anemia, chronic blood loss anemia, hookworm anemia.

INCIDENCE   Very common; one of the most common medical disorders; more common in women and children.

AGE   Children, due to inadequate diet; young women, due to menstruation; elderly, due to GI bleeding.

ETIOLOGY, PATHOGENESIS, AND PREDISPOSING FACTORS   Dietary inadequacy plus increased demand (growth, pregnancy, menstruation), chronic blood loss (gynecologic and gastrointestinal disorders, hookworm), impaired absorption (gastrectomy, malabsorption).

SITES INVOLVED   Blood and bone marrow most importantly; tongue, esophagus, and stomach also show changes.

GROSS LESIONS   Bone marrow changes are not grossly apparent; tongue shows atrophic glossitis; esophageal webs are present in Plummer-Vinson syndrome; gastric mucosal atrophy, koilonychia, and alopecia may be present.

MICROSCOPIC LESIONS   Bone marrow: erythroid hyperplasia, decreased or absent iron in macrophages by the Prussian blue stain; peripheral blood: abnormally small and pale red cells with anisopoikilocytosis.

COMPLICATIONS   Heart failure due to anemia. Iron deficiency itself is a complication of diseases causing chronic blood loss, such as gastrointestinal cancer or peptic ulcer disease.

SIGNS AND SYMPTOMS   Pallor, fatigue, dyspnea, tachycardia due to anemia; atrophic glossitis, angular stomatitis, alopecia, koilonychia due to iron deficiency; other signs specific to the underlying process.

CLINICAL DIAGNOSIS AND OTHER CLINICAL FEATURES   Recognition of signs of anemia; diagnosis of iron-deficiency anemia should prompt an investigation to find the reason for the deficiency, particularly to exclude chronic blood loss.

LABORATORY DIAGNOSIS   CBC with peripheral smear; bone marrow examination with iron stain; decreased serum iron, increased total iron binding capacity (transferrin), decreased serum ferritin; stool exam for occult blood.

PROGNOSIS   Depends on the underlying condition; by itself the deficiency is easily corrected.

THERAPY   Iron supplementation; correction of the disorder causing chronic blood loss.

OTHER INFORMATION   Iron-deficiency anemia in an adult man or postmenopausal woman is usually caused by chronic blood loss; gastrointestinal or gynecologic cancer or other serious underlying disease may be present.

Lymphocytosis

DESCRIPTION   Elevated number of lymphocytes in the peripheral blood resulting in an increase in the absolute lymphocyte count beyond normal limits, often caused by a viral infection.

DISEASE ENTITIES; SYNONYMS AND ACRONYMS   Lymphocytic leukocytosis, atypical lymphocytosis.

INCIDENCE   Common with nearly any viral infection, particularly with infectious mononucleosis (IM).

AGE   Any age. Note: the normal absolute lymphocyte count is higher in children and infants than adults.

ETIOLOGY, PATHOGENESIS, AND PREDISPOSING FACTORS   Viral infections: Epstein-Barr infection (IM), cytomegalovirus etc.; other infections: Toxoplasmosis, pertussis, TB, brucellosis, rickettsiosis; chronic inflammatory conditions and immune reactions.

SITES INVOLVED   Blood lymphocytes, lymph nodes and spleen. In IM, the EBV-infected B-cells are immortalized and accumulate; T-cells react to the infection by proliferating as atypical lymphocytes.

GROSS LESIONS   Lymph nodes and spleen may be increased in size, especially in IM; splenic white pulp (lymphoid nodules) may be more prominent.

MICROSCOPIC LESIONS   Blood lymphocytes are increased in number; up to 20% may be atypical (large nucleus with nucleoli, abundant blue cytoplasm); lymph nodes and spleen show diffuse lymphoid hyperplasia of T-cell areas.

COMPLICATIONS   These are a function of the underlying infection or disease; splenic enlargement in IM predisposes to traumatic rupture; reactive atypical lymphocytosis may be confused with leukemia.

SIGNS AND SYMPTOMS   Fever, malaise, fatigue, sore throat, other manifestations specific to the particular infection; lymphadenopathy, generalized, or regional; splenomegaly.

CLINICAL DIAGNOSIS AND OTHER CLINICAL FEATURES   Recognition of signs of viral or other infection; lymphocytosis can help differentiate viral from bacterial infections; evaluation should exclude the possibility of leukemia.

LABORATORY DIAGNOSIS   CBC with differential count, blood smear examination; Mono-Spot and other serologic tests to evaluate the possibility of infection; bone marrow examination to exclude leukemia is rarely necessary.

PROGNOSIS   Good for reactive lymphocytosis; if leukemia, depends on the type.

THERAPY   Treatment and support as indicated for the specific infection.

OTHER INFORMATION   Atypical lymphocytosis seen with IM and other infections can usually be differentiated from leukemia by the appearance and heterogeneity of the atypical reactive lymphocytes.

Lymphoid Hyperplasia of Lymph Nodes

DESCRIPTION   Enlargement of lymph nodes caused by nonneoplastic proliferation of lymphocytes responding to an antigenic stimulus; may be follicular (B-cell), interfollicular (T-cell), or mixed.

DISEASE ENTITIES; SYNONYMS AND ACRONYMS   Reactive hyperplasia of lymph nodes, follicular or diffuse lymphoid hyperplasia, lymphadenopathy, chronic lymphadenitis.

INCIDENCE   Very common; represents normal function of lymph nodes responding to infection.

AGE   Any age, especially common in children as they are developing natural immunity.

ETIOLOGY, PATHOGENESIS, AND PREDISPOSING FACTORS   Follicular: viral or bacterial infections, rheumatoid arthritis, syphilis, toxoplasmosis, AIDS; interfollicular: infectious mononucleosis, varicella-zoster, measles, cytomegalovirus, lupus, dilantin.

SITES INVOLVED   Regional lymph node enlargement indicates localized infection, generalized enlargement indicates systemic disease; slightly enlarged cervical nodes in children and inguinal nodes in adults are normal.

GROSS LESIONS   Single lymph node or a group of several nodes are enlarged up to several cm in diameter; the lymph node capsule is completely intact; cut surface is fleshy, firm, and uniform.

MICROSCOPIC LESIONS   Follicular: hyperplasia of germinal centers with polarized mantles, pleomorphic reactive lymphocytes; interfollicular: diffuse hyperplasia in central nodal region with variety of reactive lymphocytes.

COMPLICATIONS   Depends on the disease to which the lymphoid tissue is reacting; may be confused with lymphoma or metastatic neoplasm; certain cases of atypical idiopathic hyperplasia progress to lymphoma.

SIGNS AND SYMPTOMS   Palpable enlargement of lymph nodes in a site except cervical in children and inguinal in adult indicates a pathologic process that may or may not be obviously connected to a local infection.

CLINICAL DIAGNOSIS AND OTHER CLINICAL FEATURES   History (recent infection, fever, vaccination) and physical examination, particularly of the region drained by the enlarged node(s); painful enlargement indicates acute lymphadenitis.

LABORATORY DIAGNOSIS   CBC with differential count, examination of peripheral smear; cultures and serologic tests for viral or bacterial infections; histologic examination of node biopsied because of persistent enlargement.

PROGNOSIS   Usually good; atypical hyperplasia and angioimmunoblastic lymphadenopathy may progress to lymphoma.

THERAPY   Treatment of underlying condition; excision for angiofollicular lymphoid hyperplasia.

OTHER INFORMATION   Acute or granulomatous lymphadenitis, sinus histiocytosis, metastatic neoplasm, primary malignant lymphoma, Hodgkin's and cat scratch diseases are other causes.

Malignant Lymphomas—Non-Hodgkin's

DESCRIPTION Primary neoplasms of lymphoid cells classified according to cell size, growth pattern, and T- and B-cell markers; also classified according to clinical grade.

DISEASE ENTITIES; SYNONYMS AND ACRONYMS Non-Hodgkin lymphoma, NHL; many varieties: small lymphocytic type, follicular lymphoma, diffuse large cell lymphoma, etc.

INCIDENCE Not common except in predisposed groups; certain subtypes are endemic in some areas of the world.

AGE Usually middle-aged adults; lymphoblastic lymphoma and African Burkitt's lymphoma occur in children.

ETIOLOGY, PATHOGENESIS, AND PREDISPOSING FACTORS Immunoblastic lymphoma: immunosuppression; autoimmune disease (Sjogren's); Burkitt's: Epstein-Barr virus; T-cell leukemia/lymphoma: HTLV-1; chromosome translocations are common.

SITES INVOLVED Usually lymph nodes first; also any extranodal lymphoid tissue, particularly spleen, thymus (especially lymphoblastic lymphoma), GI tract, and less often lung; secondary bone marrow invasion is common.

GROSS LESIONS Usually a solid white "fish-flesh" tumor mass obliterating lymph node and extending into soft tissue; yellow areas of necrosis and bands of fibrosis; splenic nodules.

MICROSCOPIC LESIONS Monomorphous population of lymphocytes growing in either a nodular (follicular) or diffuse pattern; cell size and growth pattern constitute basis of classification.

COMPLICATIONS Primary immune dysfunction; mass effect of tumor compressing other structures; invasion of mucosa with ulceration and bleeding; bone marrow infiltration and replacement of normal hematopoietic cells.

SIGNS AND SYMPTOMS Painless enlargement of lymph nodes, regional or generalized; splenomegaly; GI obstruction or bleeding with abdominal lymphoma; fever, pallor, fatigue, weight loss; skin lesions (mycosis fungoides).

CLINICAL DIAGNOSIS AND OTHER CLINICAL FEATURES Suspicion regarding persistent enlargement of lymph nodes without regional or systemic disease or infection; biopsy is required for diagnosis; extranodal lymphomas often present with abdominal mass.

LABORATORY DIAGNOSIS Examination of lymph node biopsy; spleen and bone marrow are examined for staging; the morphologic type is translated into an International Formulation clinical grade for prognosis and therapy.

PROGNOSIS Low-grade lymphomas are indolent and not affected by therapy; some high-grade lymphomas are curable.

THERAPY Aggressive chemotherapy for high-grade lymphomas; conservative therapy for low-grade lymphomas.

OTHER INFORMATION Low-grade: small cell lymphocytic, most follicular lymphomas; intermediate: diffuse and most large cell lymphomas: high-grade: large cell immunoblastic, lymphoblastic, and Burkitt's lymphomas.

Multiple Myeloma

DESCRIPTION Primary malignant neoplasm of plasma cells most often arising in bone marrow, characterized by secretion of abnormal immunoglobulins, destructive bone lesions, and replacement of normal marrow cells.

DISEASE ENTITIES; SYNONYMS AND ACRONYMS Plasma cell myeloma, plasmacytoma, plasma cell dyscrasia.

INCIDENCE Constitutes up to 15% of white cell neoplasms.

AGE Older age groups; peak age around 60 years.

ETIOLOGY, PATHOGENESIS, AND PREDISPOSING FACTORS Possibly prolonged antigenic stimulation with superimposed mutation; occasional chromosomal abnormalities are present; elderly persons often have monoclonal gammopathy but without obvious tumor.

SITES INVOLVED Initially bone and bone marrow: vertebra, ribs, skull, pelvis, femur are most common; later, spleen, liver, and many other organs; renal tubules are often damaged by light chains (myeloma nephropathy).

GROSS LESIONS Involved bone shows multiple areas of softening and replacement by reddish gelatinous tumor mass, giving a distinctive "punched out" x-ray appearance; other organs may show tumor masses.

MICROSCOPIC LESIONS Sheets of plasma cells replace normal marrow elements; individual plasma cells are either mature or immature with nucleoli and multinucleation; bone trabeculae that remain show osteoclastic activity.

COMPLICATIONS Infections due to abnormal immunoglobulin and neutropenia; renal failure; pathologic bone fractures; anemia, thrombocytopenia; amyloidosis, cryoglobulinemia, hyperviscosity syndrome; hypercalcemia.

SIGNS AND SYMPTOMS Bone pain most often in back, ribs, or legs; pathologic fractures; neurologic symptoms from spinal cord compression or direct invasion of nerve roots; weakness, pallor, fatigue; Raynaud's phenomenon.

CLINICAL DIAGNOSIS AND OTHER CLINICAL FEATURES Bone pain is the most common symptom; x-rays show distinctive lesions; investigation of anemia may lead to a diagnostic bone marrow biopsy or serum electrophoresis.

LABORATORY DIAGNOSIS M spike on serum electrophoresis, immunoelectrophoresis; red cell rouleaux formation on blood smear; Bence-Jones proteinuria; bone marrow biopsy; plasma cell leukemia may be seen in peripheral smear.

PROGNOSIS Poor; 30 months median survival; infections are most common cause of death.

THERAPY Chemotherapy with alkylating agent; solitary extramedullary plasmacytoma may be cured by excision.

OTHER INFORMATION Related plasma cell dyscrasias: Waldenstrom's macroglobulinemia, solitary plasmacytoma, heavy chain disease (intestinal lymphoma), AL amyloidosis, monoclonal gammopathy of undetermined significance.

Myeloproliferative Disorders

DESCRIPTION   Neoplastic disease of multipotent hematopoietic stem cells resulting in panhyperplasia of all three marrow cell lines; specific disorder is classified on the basis of the predominating cell line.

DISEASE ENTITIES; SYNONYMS AND ACRONYMS   Polycythemia vera (PV), chronic myelogenous leukemia (CML), myelofibrosis with myeloid metaplasia (MMM).

INCIDENCE   Uncommon, except for CML; essential thrombocythemia is a rare myeloproliferative disorder.

AGE   Ranges from 40 to 70 years; somewhat younger with chronic myelogenous leukemia than with the others.

ETIOLOGY, PATHOGENESIS, AND PREDISPOSING FACTORS   Largely unknown; bone marrow damage by myelotoxin (e.g., benzene) or radiation causes a few cases; the marrow fibrosis seen in these disorders may be mediated by platelet derived growth factor.

SITES INVOLVED   Primarily bone marrow; extramedullary hematopoiesis is usually present in spleen and liver; this is especially prominent in MMM and CML.

GROSS LESIONS   Red marrow is expanded; liver and spleen are enlarged; in MMM and CML, splenomegaly is massive and the parenchyma is soft and bloody; infarcts may be present.

MICROSCOPIC LESIONS   Hyperplasia of all marrow elements with excess of immature forms; granulocytic precursors predominate in CML; erythroid precursors and atypical normoblasts in PV; marrow fibrosis is prominent in MMM.

COMPLICATIONS   Neoplastic cells replace normal hematopoietic cells, leading to anemia, infections, and bleeding; thrombosis complicates PV; progression to acute leukemia is variable, most common with CML.

SIGNS AND SYMPTOMS   Fatigue, malaise, headache, dizziness; pruritis and gastric ulcers caused by histamine released from basophils; splenomegaly; patients are occasionally asymptomatic when discovered.

CLINICAL DIAGNOSIS AND OTHER CLINICAL FEATURES   Palpation of an enlarged spleen, manifestations of easy bruisability (e.g., purpura, ecchymosis), and bleeding are major indicators to be investigated further by examination of the blood.

LABORATORY DIAGNOSIS   CBC, examination of blood and bone marrow; peripheral smear may show elevated number of basophils, teardrop red cells, normoblasts, abnormally large platelets, and a spectrum of immature white cells.

PROGNOSIS   Generally poor; median survival is around 3–4 years with CML and MMM and over 10 years with PV.

THERAPY   Chemotherapy, bone marrow transplantation, transfusions; treatment of infections with antibiotics.

OTHER INFORMATION   CML and MMM can be differentiated by the leukocyte alkaline phosphatase test (positive in MMM) and Philadelphia chromosome (positive in CML; see pg. 313).

Neutropenia

DESCRIPTION Reduction in the number of PMNs in the blood, resulting in a decrease in the absolute neutrophil count, caused by inadequate production or increased destruction.

DISEASE ENTITIES; SYNONYMS AND ACRONYMS Polymorphonuclear leukopenia, granulocytopenia, agranulocytosis; occurs in aplastic anemia.

INCIDENCE Fairly common, especially in patients undergoing cancer chemotherapy.

AGE Any age depending on etiology.

ETIOLOGY, PATHOGENESIS, AND PREDISPOSING FACTORS Marrow toxicity (alkylating agent, chloramphenicol), irradiation, aplastic anemia, leukemia, lymphoma, metastatic tumor, alcoholism, sepsis, vitamin B_{12} deficiency, hypersplenism, cyclic neutropenia.

SITES INVOLVED Bone marrow myeloid stem cells are the usual site of abnormality; spleen, if enlarged, can sequester PMNs and cause their accelerated destruction.

GROSS LESIONS Bone marrow usually appears grossly normal; with bone marrow failure (aplastic anemia) red marrow is decreased and yellow marrow increased.

MICROSCOPIC LESIONS Depends on cause; with marrow suppression due to drugs, toxins, or radiation, the hematopoietic marrow is hypocellular or acellular; with increased peripheral destruction, marrow is hypercellular.

COMPLICATIONS Infections, becoming more likely with neutrophil counts less than 500/microliter, involving skin, oral mucosa, lungs, and respiratory tract, gastrointestinal tract and urinary system.

SIGNS AND SYMPTOMS Opportunistic infections, particularly within the oral cavity; oral ulcers are covered with a dark gray or greenish necrotic membrane; microscopically there is bacterial colonization and few PMNs.

CLINICAL DIAGNOSIS AND OTHER CLINICAL FEATURES Usually discovered during investigation of an infection or nonhealing ulcer; neutropenia is a predictable complication of cancer chemotherapy.

LABORATORY DIAGNOSIS CBC, examination of blood and bone marrow; microbiologic cultures and other studies directed at secondary infections.

PROGNOSIS Usually good if the neutropenia is only transient; poor if it persists.

THERAPY Antibiotics; granulocyte transfusions; granulocyte stimulating factor.

OTHER INFORMATION In many cases of neutropenia with marrow suppression, only the granulocyte precursors are decreased; in others, all elements are decreased, leading to pancytopenia as described for aplastic anemia (see pg. 309).

Neutrophilia

DESCRIPTION   Increased number of PMNs in the blood, producing an increased absolute neutrophil count, caused by proliferation of marrow precursors or mobilization from marrow and marginal storage pools.

DISEASE ENTITIES; SYNONYMS AND ACRONYMS   Neutrophilic or polymorphonuclear leukocytosis, granulocytosis, reactive leukocytosis.

INCIDENCE   Very common, especially with bacterial infections and tissue necrosis.

AGE   Any age.

ETIOLOGY, PATHOGENESIS, AND PREDISPOSING FACTORS   Any acute inflammatory condition: bacterial (pyogenic) infections, tissue necrosis (myocardial infarct, burns), endotoxin, hemorrhage, neoplasms, hereditary neutrophilia, myeloproliferative disorders.

SITES INVOLVED   Peripheral blood and bone marrow.

GROSS LESIONS   Depends on underlying condition.

MICROSCOPIC LESIONS   Blood smear shows increased PMNs often with immature forms (left shift); Dohle bodies and toxic granulations may be present; bone marrow is hyperplastic with increased myeloid:erythroid ratio.

COMPLICATIONS   Neutrophilia is a reaction to an underlying condition; any complications depend on that condition.

SIGNS AND SYMPTOMS   Fever, sometimes spiking fevers, tachycardia, shaking chills (rigors), and other acute phase reactions are systemic manifestations of inflammation; hyperemia, warmth, swelling, and pain are local signs.

CLINICAL DIAGNOSIS AND OTHER CLINICAL FEATURES   Along with the systemic and local manifestations, neutrophilia is a major indicator of inflammation; workup is directed at determining the cause of the inflammation.

LABORATORY DIAGNOSIS   CBC with differential count, examination of blood smear; bone marrow examination is usually not necessary unless there is a suspicion of leukemia.

PROGNOSIS   Usually good; indicates an appropriate response to infection or injury.

THERAPY   Treatment of the inflammatory condition, infarct, or infection.

OTHER INFORMATION   Leukemoid reaction is an intense neutrophilia that may be confused with leukemia; the leukocyte alkaline phosphatase test and bone marrow examination may be necessary to differentiate the two.

Polycythemia

DESCRIPTION   Increased red cell count, classified as relative (decreased plasma volume), absolute (increased red cell mass), primary (precursor cell abnormality), or secondary (excess erythropoietin).

DISEASE ENTITIES; SYNONYMS AND ACRONYMS   Erythrocytosis, Gaisbock's syndrome (stress polycythemia), polycythemia vera.

INCIDENCE   Relative polycythemia and secondary polycythemia are common; polycythemia vera is uncommon.

AGE   Any age, depending on cause: in infants, usually due to dehydration; in adults, many causes.

ETIOLOGY, PATHOGENESIS, AND PREDISPOSING FACTORS   Relative: dehydration, stress polycythemia; secondary: high altitude, congenital heart or chronic lung disease, excess androgens, renal cysts or hydronephrosis, erythropoietin-producing tumors.

SITES INVOLVED   Blood, bone marrow, red cell mass; erythropoietin-producing tumors in kidney (renal cell carcinoma), liver (hepatocellular carcinoma), or cerebellum (hemangioblastoma).

GROSS LESIONS   Depends on any primary lesion or tumor producing the secondary polycythemia; usually there is no gross lesion.

MICROSCOPIC LESIONS   With relative polycythemia the bone marrow is normal; with absolute polycythemia, the marrow is hyperplastic with a decreased myeloid/erythroid ratio.

COMPLICATIONS   Increased risk of thrombosis and thromboembolism. Polycythemia vera is a major predisposition for Budd-Chiari syndrome.

SIGNS AND SYMPTOMS   Ruddy complexion is typical of absolute polycythemia, e.g., inhabitants of high altitudes; cyanosis with congenital heart disease; vomiting and diarrhea may precede relative polycythemia.

CLINICAL DIAGNOSIS AND OTHER CLINICAL FEATURES   Often an incidental laboratory finding discovered in blood work requested for various purposes; workup is directed toward determining the cause for the polycythemia.

LABORATORY DIAGNOSIS   Elevated hemoglobin, hematocrit, and red cell count; red cell mass is determined by radioactive chromium (Cr-51) labeling; bone marrow exam is required for diagnosis of polycythemia vera.

PROGNOSIS   Depends on primary or underlying condition.

THERAPY   Treatment of underlying condition; repeated phlebotomy may be required for absolute polycythemia.

OTHER INFORMATION   Primary polycythemia (polycythemia vera) is a neoplastic condition described above in Myeloproliferative Disorders.

Sickle Cell Anemia

DESCRIPTION   Inherited hemoglobinopathy; abnormal hemoglobin (HbS) forms rigid tactoids when deoxygenated, producing hemolytic anemia and causing red cells to deform (sickle) and obstruct small blood vessels.

DISEASE ENTITIES; SYNONYMS AND ACRONYMS   Homozygous: sickle cell disease; heterozygous: sickle cell trait, sickle cell carrier state.

INCIDENCE   Common; up to 10% of US African-Americans carry the sickle cell trait.

AGE   Homozygous disease becomes obvious about 6–9 months when fetal hemoglobin is normally replaced.

ETIOLOGY, PATHOGENESIS, AND PREDISPOSING FACTORS   DNA mutation substitutes valine for glutamic acid in amino acid #6 of the beta hemoglobin chain; in the homozygote nearly all hemoglobin is HbS; in the heterozygote, HbS constitutes 30–40%.

SITES INVOLVED   Red cells, when sickled, occlude small blood vessels throughout body and cause infarcts in spleen, bone, lung, and other organs; bone marrow expands to compensate for increased red cell hemolysis.

GROSS LESIONS   Increased red marrow; small infarcts in several organs, especially bone and spleen; spleen becomes completely fibrotic (autosplenectomy); skin ulcers at the ankles are common.

MICROSCOPIC LESIONS   Erythroid hyperplasia of bone marrow; sickled and deformed red cells packed into small blood vessels; small infarcts; fibrotic spleen with dense hemosiderin.

COMPLICATIONS   Severe anemia; hemolytic crises, aplastic crises, vaso-occlusive (painful) crises; bacterial infections (pneumococcal pneumonia, salmonella osteomyelitis); iron overload; cholelithiasis; priapism.

SIGNS AND SYMPTOMS   Sickle cell disease is a devastating condition with recurrent crises leading to death usually before 30 years; sickle cell trait causes problems rarely (marked hypoxia, high altitudes).

CLINICAL DIAGNOSIS AND OTHER CLINICAL FEATURES   Family history is important; should be suspected in a black infant that becomes anemic after 6 months; early diagnosis of aplastic crises and bacterial infections is part of long-term care.

LABORATORY DIAGNOSIS   CBC; examination of blood and bone marrow; red cell sickling in vitro is used as a screening test; hemoglobin electrophoresis confirms the diagnosis; prenatal tests on fetal DNA are available.

PROGNOSIS   Poor for sickle cell disease; normal longevity for sickle cell trait.

THERAPY   Red cell transfusions, folic acid supplements, liberal use of antibiotics, maintenance of hydration.

OTHER INFORMATION   The heterozygous sickle cell gene provides protection against falciparum malaria, explaining the high frequency of the gene in certain African populations.

Splenomegaly

DESCRIPTION Enlargement of spleen due to infectious diseases, immunologic disorders, primary or secondary neoplasms, and storage diseases, as well as a consequence of passive congestion.

DISEASE ENTITIES; SYNONYMS AND ACRONYMS Splenitis, reactive hyperplasia, congestive splenomegaly.

INCIDENCE Very common due to the large number of predisposing conditions.

AGE Any age; more likely adults who have a greater possibility of predisposing conditions.

ETIOLOGY, PATHOGENESIS, AND PREDISPOSING FACTORS Infections involving blood (infectious mononucleosis, malaria, sepsis); lymphoma or leukemia; storage disease (Gaucher's); hematologic disorders (hemolytic anemia); portal hypertension (cirrhosis).

SITES INVOLVED Spleen; lymphoid tissue (white pulp) if splenomegaly is caused by infectious, inflammatory or immunologic disease; red pulp and sinusoids are expanded in splenomegaly due to passive congestion.

GROSS LESIONS Soft, enlarged spleen in most cases of acute infection and acute congestion; firmness indicates a chronic process; prominent white pulp with immune reactions; infarcts or tumor nodules may be present.

MICROSCOPIC LESIONS Congestive: sinusoids congested and/or fibrotic, Gamna-Gandy bodies (fibrotic nodules with hemosiderin); reactive: lymphoid hyperplasia and/or macrophages expand white pulp and infiltrate red pulp.

COMPLICATIONS Hypersplenism, in which the enlarged spleen traps and destroys normal blood cells, leading to anemia, neutropenia, and/or thrombocytopenia; splenic rupture may occur with minor blunt trauma.

SIGNS AND SYMPTOMS Palpable splenic mass in left upper quadrant under costal margin; pain indicates acute enlargement; other signs depend on etiology (e.g., ascites, jaundice, pallor of anemia, petechiae, fever, etc.)

CLINICAL DIAGNOSIS AND OTHER CLINICAL FEATURES History and physical examination may indicate etiology; x-rays, ultrasound, CT, or MRI scans to determine if the enlargement is diffuse or localized, solid or cystic; laparotomy with splenectomy.

LABORATORY DIAGNOSIS CBC with differential count and examination of blood smear may reveal a hematologic disorder; microbiologic and serologic studies may disclose an infection; histologic examination of resected spleen.

PROGNOSIS Depends on underlying condition; splenomegaly is often a sign of a serious disease.

THERAPY Depends on underlying condition; splenectomy may reverse anemia or other cytopenias.

OTHER INFORMATION Palpable splenomegaly occurs in 1–3% of the normal US population; in areas where malaria is endemic, splenomegaly may be present in half of the population.

Thalassemia

DESCRIPTION   Inherited anemia due to decreased synthesis of the beta chain of Hb (beta-thalassemia) or of the alpha chain (alpha-thalassemia) resulting in ineffective erythropoiesis and hemolysis.

DISEASE ENTITIES; SYNONYMS AND ACRONYMS   Beta-thalassemia, alpha-thalassemia; thalassemia major, Cooley's anemia; thalassemia minor.

INCIDENCE   Beta-thalassemia is most common; seen in Mediterranean populations, also some Africans and Asians.

AGE   Beta-thalassemia major presents at 6–9 months; alpha-thalassemia is present in utero with Hb Barts.

ETIOLOGY, PATHOGENESIS, AND PREDISPOSING FACTORS   Several defects in genes for globin synthesis causing deficiency of either beta or alpha chain; the unaffected chain, produced in relative excess, precipitates in the red cell and promotes hemolysis.

SITES INVOLVED   Chromosome 11 (beta) or 16 (alpha); Hb synthesis is impaired in bone marrow normoblasts; red cells are destroyed in spleen and liver; heart is affected by iron overload (hemosiderosis).

GROSS LESIONS   Red marrow is increased, yellow marrow decreased, and cortical bone thinned; enlargement of skull bones; marked splenomegaly and hepatomegaly; hemosiderosis, secondary hemochromatosis.

MICROSCOPIC LESIONS   Marked erythroid hyperplasia in the marrow; microcytic hypochromic red cells with anisopoikilocytosis and target cells; basophilic stippling of red cells; reticulocytosis.

COMPLICATIONS   Severe anemia with thalassemia major, requiring repeated blood transfusions; survival is not expected beyond the 20s; heart failure due to anemia and secondary hemosiderosis; cholelithiasis.

SIGNS AND SYMPTOMS   Beta-thalassemia presents at 6–9 months as Hb synthesis converts from the fetal form; alpha-thalass-emia is present at birth; the enlargement of the frontal skull produces a chipmunk-like face.

CLINICAL DIAGNOSIS AND OTHER CLINICAL FEATURES   Autosomal recessive inheritance of severe anemia; thalassemia minor produces only mild anemia sometimes confused with iron-deficiency anemia; skull x-ray shows "hair on end" with thalassemia major.

LABORATORY DIAGNOSIS   CBC, examination of blood and bone marrow; markedly increased fetal Hgb and increased HbA2 on hemoglobin electrophoresis; HbH and Hb Barts are seen with alpha-thalassemia.

PROGNOSIS   Poor with thalassemia major; thalassemia minor does not affect longevity or quality of life.

THERAPY   Blood transfusions; folic acid supplements; iron chelation therapy to reverse hemosiderosis.

OTHER INFORMATION   Alpha-thalassemia is much less common and often less severe unless there is complete suppression of the alpha chain; Hb Barts is tetramer of gamma chains, HbH is a tetramer of beta chains.

Thrombocytopenia

DESCRIPTION   Decrease in the platelet count below lower limits of normal caused by inadequate production from the bone marrow, increased destruction in the periphery, or splenic sequestration.

DISEASE ENTITIES; SYNONYMS AND ACRONYMS   Idiopathic thrombocytopenic purpura (ITP), thrombotic thrombocytopenic purpura (TTP), hemolytic uremic syndrome (HUS).

INCIDENCE   Common as a complication of leukemia, aplastic anemia, and aggressive cancer chemotherapy.

AGE   Depends on cause; acute ITP, children; TTP and chronic ITP, adults; HUS, children, pregnant women.

ETIOLOGY, PATHOGENESIS, AND PREDISPOSING FACTORS   Bone marrow failure (aplastic anemia); leukemia or metastatic cancer; AIDS; antiplatelet antibodies or immune complexes (ITP); endothelial damage (TTP, HUS, DIC); drugs; hypersplenism; transfusions.

SITES INVOLVED   Depends on etiology; either bone marrow or spleen are likely sites of primary disease; secondary bleeding occurs from small blood vessels in skin, mucosal surfaces, and brain.

GROSS LESIONS   Depends on cause; bone marrow may show decreased red marrow (aplastic anemia) or lytic areas (metastatic neoplasm); spleen may be diffusely enlarged (hypersplenism, ITP).

MICROSCOPIC LESIONS   Depends on cause: aplastic marrow, leukemic infiltrates, metastatic tumor; increased number of megakaryocytes with monolobulated immature forms indicates peripheral destruction, especially ITP.

COMPLICATIONS   Bleeding diathesis with major episode (e.g., intracranial hemorrhage) or chronic blood loss anemia and iron deficiency; microvascular thrombosis and microangiopathic hemolytic anemia with HUS and TTP.

SIGNS AND SYMPTOMS   Petechiae and/or purpura in skin and mucosa; easy bruisability; prolonged bleeding from gingiva or other sites following minor trauma; epistaxis, melena, hematuria, excessive menstrual bleeding.

CLINICAL DIAGNOSIS AND OTHER CLINICAL FEATURES   Recognition of bleeding disorder; differential includes diseases of blood vessels and coagulation factor deficiencies; petechiae are fairly specific for thrombocytopenia or platelet dysfunction.

LABORATORY DIAGNOSIS   CBC with platelet count, examination of blood and bone marrow; platelet-associated immunoglobulins are present in ITP; elevated LDH indicates microangiopathic hemolysis in TTP/HUS.

PROGNOSIS   Variable; often poor with leukemia and aplastic anemia; ITP, TTP, and HUS may respond to therapy.

THERAPY   Treatment of leukemia; steroids; exchange transfusion; platelet inhibitors; splenectomy for ITP.

OTHER INFORMATION   Drugs causing thrombocytopenia: quinidine, thiazides, methyldopa, meprobamate; TTP and HUS are mediated by as yet largely uncharacterized plasma factors that cause platelet activation.

Thrombosis

DESCRIPTION   Formation of a blood clot within the intact cardio-vascular system as a consequence of pathologic interactions of vascular endothelium, platelets, and coagulation enzymes.

DISEASE ENTITIES; SYNONYMS AND ACRONYMS   Thrombus; arterial thrombus, venous thrombus, mural thrombus; thrombotic vegetations of endocarditis.

INCIDENCE   Common, especially following trauma, surgery, or with atherosclerosis or heart failure.

AGE   Any age. More common in elderly because of increased risk factors.

ETIOLOGY, PATHOGENESIS, AND PREDISPOSING FACTORS   Athero-sclerosis, heart failure, trauma or surgery, tumors, pregnancy or birth control pills, defective fibrinolytic system. The classic triad is endothelial damage, stasis, and hypercoagulability.

SITES INVOLVED   Any artery, vein, or heart chamber. Important examples are coronary thrombus, leg vein thrombus, mural thrombus in aortic aneurysm, or mural thrombus in a left ventricular aneurysm.

GROSS LESIONS   Occlusive arterial thrombi show alternating gray and red lines of Zahn. Nonocclusive mural thrombi have prominent lines. Lines are absent or subtle in red occlusive venous thrombi.

MICROSCOPIC LESIONS   Fresh thrombus: clumps of platelets surrounded by leukocytes and red cells, all enmeshed within fibrin strands; organized and canalized thrombus: fibroblasts, connective tissue, and blood vessels.

COMPLICATIONS   Ischemia, infarction, and embolization; systemic embolus originates from mural thrombus or vegetations on heart valves; pulmonary embolus originates from venous thrombus.

SIGNS AND SYMPTOMS   Depend on organ involved; arterial thrombi cause ischemia, pain, infarcts, stroke, gangrene, sudden death; venous thrombi cause swelling, congestion, cyanosis, ischemia and hemorrhagic infarcts.

CLINICAL DIAGNOSIS AND OTHER CLINICAL FEATURES   Recognition of signs of ischemia: pain, dysfunction, swelling, pulselessness, discoloration of the organ supplied by the thrombosed vessel. Venography or arteriography may localize the lesion.

LABORATORY DIAGNOSIS   If infarction has occurred, studies are aimed at documenting necrosis. Less specific methods detect formation or degradation of fibrin.

PROGNOSIS   Depends on the size of the vessel involved and the presence of collateral circulation.

THERAPY   Anticoagulation; fibrinolytic (thrombolytic) agents; surgical thrombectomy or bypass.

OTHER INFORMATION   Thrombosis is a pathologic state similar to physiologic hemostasis. Prevention of thrombosis by eliminating predisposing conditions, e.g., early ambulation after surgery, is of major importance.

Vitamin B$_{12}$ Deficiency Anemia

DESCRIPTION   Macrocytic/megaloblastic anemia caused most often by malabsorption of vitamin B$_{12}$ because of lack of intrinsic factor (pernicious anemia) and less often because of dietary deficiency.

DISEASE ENTITIES; SYNONYMS AND ACRONYMS   Megaloblastic anemia, macrocytic anemia, pernicious anemia (PA); combined system disease.

INCIDENCE   Fairly common, especially in people with Northern European ancestry; slight male predominance.

AGE   In pernicious anemia, from 40 to 80 years.

ETIOLOGY, PATHOGENESIS, AND PREDISPOSING FACTORS   Intrinsic factor deficiency (PA), gastrectomy, small bowel disease (regional enteritis, lymphoma), fish tapeworm infestation, strict vegetarian diet, transcobalamin deficiency, carcinomatosis.

SITES INVOLVED   Vitamin B$_{12}$ deficiency affects all cells due to defective DNA synthesis; bone marrow, stomach, and central nervous system exhibit the major manifestations of PA.

GROSS LESIONS   Bone marrow: red marrow increased, yellow marrow decreased; stomach: flat atrophic mucosa, loss of rugal folds.

MICROSCOPIC LESIONS   Bone marrow: hypercellularity with erythroid hyperplasia, enlarged normoblasts (megaloblasts) with immature nuclei; macrocytes and hypersegmented polys in peripheral smear; chronic atrophic gastritis.

COMPLICATIONS   Anemia leading to high output heart failure; gastric ulcers and gastric carcinoma; myelin degeneration of posterior columns of spinal cord leading to ataxia and neuropathy (combined system disease).

SIGNS AND SYMPTOMS   Pallor, tachycardia, dyspnea; shiny, beefy-red tongue (atrophic glossitis); indigestion; ataxia, sensory loss, and spasticity in the distal extremities.

CLINICAL DIAGNOSIS AND OTHER CLINICAL FEATURES   Pallor and other signs of anemia should prompt blood studies; results indicating macrocytic anemia would be followed by investigations to determine the cause of B$_{12}$ or folate deficiency.

LABORATORY DIAGNOSIS   CBC, examination of peripheral blood and bone marrow; Schilling test; elevated serum LDH isozymes 1 and 2; gastric biopsy; stool exam; reticulocyte response to parenteral B$_{12}$ but not oral B$_{12}$.

PROGNOSIS   Usually good; better if corrected early before neurologic damage is advanced.

THERAPY   Parenteral injections of vitamin B$_{12}$.

OTHER INFORMATION   Major effects of B$_{12}$ deficiency are ineffective erythropoiesis and hemolysis. Chronic atrophic gastritis with achlorhydria and autoantibodies to parietal cells and intrinsic factor characterize PA.

Von Willebrand's Disease

DESCRIPTION   Inherited bleeding disorder caused by deficiency of von Willebrand's factor (vWF) which results in a prolonged bleeding time, excessive bleeding from wounds, and spontaneous bleeding from mucosa.

DISEASE ENTITIES; SYNONYMS AND ACRONYMS   Von Willebrand disease.

INCIDENCE   Second most common inherited bleeding disorder; autosomal dominant inheritance.

AGE   Present from birth; may become less severe with age.

ETIOLOGY, PATHOGENESIS, AND PREDISPOSING FACTORS   Most cases are due to reduced levels of vWF, synthesized by megakaryocytes and endothelial cells, coded on chromosome 12; normal function of vWF is to promote platelet adhesion and aggregation.

SITES INVOLVED   Platelets, blood vessel walls; vWF functions primarily to attach platelets onto subendothelial collagen at sites of endothelial damage. Bleeding from mucosa surfaces (especially GI) and from wounds.

GROSS LESIONS   Hemorrhage from GI mucosa and from other sites.

MICROSCOPIC LESIONS   Nonspecific evidence of hemorrhage in mucosal surfaces and at sites of trauma.

COMPLICATIONS   Excessive bleeding leads to shock, anemia, and iron deficiency; severe anemia can cause heart failure.

SIGNS AND SYMPTOMS   Bleeding from GI tract; epistaxis; prolonged and excessive bleeding from wounds; excessive menstrual bleeding; bleeding into joints is a feature of hemophilia but not von Willebrand's disease.

CLINICAL DIAGNOSIS AND OTHER CLINICAL FEATURES   Diagnosis is suspected because of the bleeding diathesis; differentiated from hemophilia by the pattern of bleeding and the mode of inheritance; laboratory confirmation is required.

LABORATORY DIAGNOSIS   Prolonged bleeding time with normal platelet count; low or absent ristocetin-induced aggregation of platelets; prolonged partial thromboplastin time.

PROGNOSIS   Usually good with therapy; condition may improve after adolescence.

THERAPY   Transfusion of fresh whole blood or platelet-rich plasma.

OTHER INFORMATION   Factor VIII complexes with vWF to activate Factor X which, in turn, activates the intrinsic coagulation pathway.

Pathology Facts, by Richard C.
Harruff, J.B. Lippincott
Company, Philadelphia © 1994.

Chapter 20

Endocrine System

Adrenocortical Insufficiency

DESCRIPTION   Acute or chronic hyposecretion of cortisol and usually aldosterone from the adrenal cortex, due to primary disease of the adrenal cortex or secondary to deficiency of ACTH.

DISEASE ENTITIES; SYNONYMS AND ACRONYMS   Primary chronic adrenocortical insufficiency: Addison's disease; primary acute: Waterhouse-Friderichsen syndrome.

INCIDENCE   Most common is iatrogenic suppression of ACTH by steroid therapy; the primary forms are uncommon.

AGE   Waterhouse-Friderichsen: children, young adults; Addison's and iatrogenic suppression: adults.

ETIOLOGY, PATHOGENESIS, AND PREDISPOSING FACTORS   Addison's: autoimmune destruction of adrenal cortex, tuberculosis; Waterhouse-Friderichsen: meningococcemia, other bacterial sepsis; secondary forms: pituitary lesion, withdrawal of steroid therapy.

SITES INVOLVED   Adrenal cortex and pituitary gland.

GROSS LESIONS   Autoimmune Addison's: marked adrenal atrophy; Addison's due to TB: caseous necrosis; Waterhouse-Friderichsen: bilateral diffuse hemorrhages or hematomas; secondary forms: cortical atrophy.

MICROSCOPIC LESIONS   Autoimmune Addison's: variable lymphocytic infiltrate, fibrous replacement; Waterhouse-Friderichsen: acute hemorrhage with variable necrosis; secondary forms: atrophic cortex, decreased thickness.

COMPLICATIONS   Acute insufficiency (Waterhouse-Friderichsen, Addisonian crisis): rapid development of shock, often fatal; chronic insufficiency: progressive weakness, salt wasting, hypotension, crisis, arrhythmias.

SIGNS AND SYMPTOMS   Waterhouse-Friderichsen: rapidly developing ecchymotic skin rash, cardiovascular collapse; Addison's: slowly developing weakness, nausea, vomiting, hypotension, hyperpigmentation of skin and mucosa.

CLINICAL DIAGNOSIS AND OTHER CLINICAL FEATURES   Acute insufficiency must be recognized quickly or the patient is lost; chronic insufficiency is difficult to recognize; should be anticipated in a patient recently withdrawn from steroid therapy.

LABORATORY DIAGNOSIS   Low serum sodium, chloride, bicarbonate, glucose, and urinary 17-ketosteroids; high serum potassium; ACTH high (primary) or low (secondary); positive blood cultures with Waterhouse-Friderichsen.

PROGNOSIS   Poor for Waterhouse-Friderichsen; in the chronic forms, therapy produces good recovery.

THERAPY   Replacement of steroid hormones; antibiotics for Waterhouse-Friderichsen; TB therapy if appropriate.

OTHER INFORMATION   Hyperpigmentation and salt wasting do not occur in secondary insufficiency; secondary adrenocortical insufficiency due to ACTH suppression is an important complication of steroid therapy.

Aldosteronoma

DESCRIPTION A functional adrenal cortical adenoma that secretes excessive aldosterone, resulting in hypertension, hypernatremia, hypokalemia, and edema.

DISEASE ENTITIES; SYNONYMS AND ACRONYMS Primary hyperaldosteronism, Conn's syndrome, low-renin hypertension, aldosterone-secreting adenoma.

INCIDENCE Uncommon; causes less than 1% of all cases of hypertension; more common in women.

AGE Adults, middle age.

ETIOLOGY, PATHOGENESIS, AND PREDISPOSING FACTORS Autonomous hypersecretion of aldosterone stimulates renal tubular resorption of sodium at the expense of potassium; the consequent elevations in blood pressure and fluid volume suppress renin.

SITES INVOLVED Adrenal cortex; secondary effects due to hypertension affect the blood vessels, heart, and kidneys.

GROSS LESIONS Yellow to orange circumscribed nodular nonencapsulated tumor arising from the adrenal cortex, usually less than 2 cm in diameter.

MICROSCOPIC LESIONS Neoplastic cells are similar to normal adrenal cortical cells; clear cells filled with foamy cytoplasm containing lipid vesicles are intermixed with compact cells without cytoplasmic lipid.

COMPLICATIONS Same as the complications of hypertension: arteriolosclerosis, cardiac hypertrophy, and hemorrhagic stroke. It is important to recognize this cause of hypertension because it can be cured.

SIGNS AND SYMPTOMS Moderate hypertension; edema; headaches, fatigue, weakness; neuromuscular abnormalities and electrocardiographic changes due to hypokalemia.

CLINICAL DIAGNOSIS AND OTHER CLINICAL FEATURES Differentiate from secondary hyperaldosteronism with high-renin hypertension (e.g., renal artery stenosis); CT scans and catheterization of each adrenal vein may localize the tumor.

LABORATORY DIAGNOSIS Elevated aldosterone, with marked difference in the levels from each adrenal vein; low plasma renin; electrolyte abnormalities (hypernatremia, hypokalemia, alkalosis).

PROGNOSIS Good if detected and treated before hypertensive damage occurs; a curable form of hypertension.

THERAPY Surgical resection of adrenal gland containing the adenoma.

OTHER INFORMATION Most adrenal adenomas are nonfunctional; only a minority cause hypercortisolism or hyperaldosteronism, even fewer cause virilization or feminization.

Carcinoma of Thyroid—Medullary

DESCRIPTION An uncommon primary malignant neoplasm of thyroid, considered a neuroendocrine tumor; some cases are familial as a part of a multiple endocrine neoplasia (MEN) syndrome.

DISEASE ENTITIES; SYNONYMS AND ACRONYMS Medullary carcinoma with amyloid stroma.

INCIDENCE Constitutes less than 10% of all thyroid cancers; most are sporadic, 10–15% are familial.

AGE Familial cases: young adults, even children; nonfamilial cases: middle-aged adults.

ETIOLOGY, PATHOGENESIS, AND PREDISPOSING FACTORS In familial cases, there is autosomal dominant transmission of genetic defect on chromosome 10; concurrent pheochromocytoma and parathyroid adenoma in MEN IIa; pheochromocytoma in MEN IIb.

SITES INVOLVED Thyroid gland; the neoplasm arises from the parafollicular C-cells that normally secrete calcitonin.

GROSS LESIONS Soft fleshy gray tumor with nodular growth pattern but irregular margins and no capsule; sporadic cases are usually single; familial cases are often multiple and bilateral.

MICROSCOPIC LESIONS Cuboidal or less often spindle-shaped cells arranged in nests, sheets, or ribbons; electron microscopy shows secretory granules; amyloid stroma is present in most cases.

COMPLICATIONS Local invasion and compression of neck structures; distant metastases to lung, liver, or bone; recurrence after resection.

SIGNS AND SYMPTOMS Palpation of neck mass or nodule over the thyroid; diarrhea due to calcitonin secretion; hypertension due to associated pheochromocytoma; other manifestations of associated hormone secretion.

CLINICAL DIAGNOSIS AND OTHER CLINICAL FEATURES Diarrhea and signs of multiple endocrinopathy serve to differentiate this one from other thyroid neoplasms; all members of a known affected family must be monitored closely for development of tumors.

LABORATORY DIAGNOSIS Histologic examination of resected tumor; immunohistochemical staining to demonstrate the presence of calcitonin and other hormones; calcitonin radioimmunoassay of serum to screen family members.

PROGNOSIS 5-year survival of 40%; much better in screened familial cases detected and treated early.

THERAPY Surgical resection; thyroidectomy may be performed prophylactically in familial cases.

OTHER INFORMATION Other hormones commonly secreted by medullary carcinoma are somatostatin, bombesin, and serotonin.

Carcinoma of Thyroid—Papillary and Follicular

DESCRIPTION   The two most common primary malignant neoplasms of thyroid arising from the follicular epithelium, both with the potential to invade surrounding neck structures and metastasize to distant sites.

DISEASE ENTITIES; SYNONYMS AND ACRONYMS   Papillary adenocarcinoma, follicular adenocarcinoma, mixed papillary and follicular carcinoma, angioinvasive adenoma.

INCIDENCE   Responsible for 0.4% of cancer deaths; female:male = 2–3:1; papillary is more common than follicular.

AGE   Papillary: adults 20–60 years, sometimes children; follicular: usually older ages, peak 40–60 years.

ETIOLOGY, PATHOGENESIS, AND PREDISPOSING FACTORS   Ionizing radiation; a high proportion of children receiving irradiation to the head and neck later developed thyroid cancers; high incidence in Japanese exposed to the Hiroshima/Nagasaki bombs.

SITES INVOLVED   Thyroid gland initially; papillary carcinoma usually spreads via lymphatics to cervical lymph nodes; the follicular type is more likely to spread hematogenously to lungs and bone.

GROSS LESIONS   Papillary: nodule of microscopic size up to several centimeters with invasive margins; may be sclerotic or partly cystic; follicular: either an apparently encapsulated mass or a hard diffusely invasive tumor.

MICROSCOPIC LESIONS   Papillary: cellular papillae, "orphan annie eye" nuclei, psammoma bodies; follicular: follicles of variable differentiation often with colloid, absence of papillary features.

COMPLICATIONS   Effects of local compression and invasion; distant metastases (lungs, bone, liver) more common and aggressive with follicular type; late recurrences with papillary type.

SIGNS AND SYMPTOMS   Palpable mass in neck over thyroid; may be nodular like an adenoma or nodular goiter, or hard and irregular; papillary carcinoma may present with cervical lymph node metastases and an occult primary.

CLINICAL DIAGNOSIS AND OTHER CLINICAL FEATURES   The mass may be obviously malignant (hard and irregular) but palpation is unreliable; most cancers are cold on scinitiscans but this method is not diagnostic; surgical biopsy is necessary.

LABORATORY DIAGNOSIS   Fine needle aspiration cytology may be diagnostic; histologic examination of biopsied lesion is most reliable; angioinvasive adenoma refers to follicular adenoma showing microscopic vascular invasion.

PROGNOSIS   Overall 5-year survival: papillary, 80–90%; follicular, 30–40%; depends also on stage.

THERAPY   Surgical excision; some follicular carcinomas concentrate sufficient radioiodine for treatment.

OTHER INFORMATION   Stage I: tumor within thyroid; II: cervical lymph node metastasis; III: invasion into soft tissue of neck; IV: distant metastasis. Any papillary features in mixed cancers indicate papillary behavior.

Cretinism

DESCRIPTION   Hypothyroidism in an infant or child; the hormone deficiency causes mental retardation, neuromuscular impairment and short stature; classified as endemic (iodine deficiency) or sporadic cretinism.

DISEASE ENTITIES; SYNONYMS AND ACRONYMS   Endemic cretinism, sporadic cretinism, neonatal or congenital goiter, neonatal hypothyroidism.

INCIDENCE   Common in iodine-deficient regions (endemic); uncommon in US where most cases are sporadic.

AGE   Present in the fetus and neonate with the endemic form; develops in infancy with sporadic forms.

ETIOLOGY, PATHOGENESIS, AND PREDISPOSING FACTORS   Endemic: maternal deficiency of dietary iodine; sporadic: thyroid agenesis or defect in one of the synthetic enzymes; neurologic impairment is usually more severe with endemic cretinism.

SITES INVOLVED   Thyroid gland primarily; secondary effects on all organs due to the hypometabolic state; nervous system and skeletal system are major targets for retarded development.

GROSS LESIONS   Thyroid gland is usually diffusely enlarged due to increased TSH stimulation; less often there is congenital defect of gland development (e.g., agenesis).

MICROSCOPIC LESIONS   Various patterns are seen: the follicles may be enlarged and distended with colloid, or small and excessively cellular with scant colloid. In agenesis, follicles are not present.

COMPLICATIONS   Irreversible neurologic damage with mental retardation, which is preventable if the condition is recognized and treated; dwarfism due to lack of skeletal growth at epiphyses.

SIGNS AND SYMPTOMS   May be subtle at birth and develop over weeks or months; failure to feed properly, slow weight gain, excessive sleeping, weak hoarse cry, enlarged tongue, protuberant abdomen, fontanelles remain open.

CLINICAL DIAGNOSIS AND OTHER CLINICAL FEATURES   It is crucial to recognize the condition as early as possible in the neonate to prevent neurologic damage; in the child, mental retardation is irreversible; in adolescents, epiphyses fail to close.

LABORATORY DIAGNOSIS   Elevation of TSH is the most sensitive finding; neonatal screening tests are based on detection of elevated TSH; depression of T3 and T4 may not be evident at birth.

PROGNOSIS   Good in many sporadic cases if detected and treated early; less is expected for endemic cases.

THERAPY   Synthetic thyroid hormone; iodine supplements (e.g., iodized salt) for prevention in endemic regions.

OTHER INFORMATION   In underdeveloped mountainous regions, cretinism is a significant public health problem; the word "cretin" originates from the mental retardation that renders them innocent or "Christian."

Cushing's Syndrome

DESCRIPTION   Syndrome related to excessive secretion of cortisol caused by: pituitary adenoma secreting ACTH; adrenal cortical neoplasm or hyperplasia; ectopic ACTH secretion; prolonged corticosteroid therapy.

DISEASE ENTITIES; SYNONYMS AND ACRONYMS   Hypercortisolism; pituitary Cushing's (Cushing's disease), adrenal Cushing's, ectopic Cushing's, iatrogenic Cushing's.

INCIDENCE   Iatrogenic Cushing's is by far the most common; then pituitary > adrenal > ectopic; female:male = 3:1.

AGE   Adults, middle aged and older.

ETIOLOGY, PATHOGENESIS, AND PREDISPOSING FACTORS   Pituitary adenoma or microadenoma secreting ACTH; hypothalamic dysfunction; adrenal cortical adenoma, nodular hyperplasia or carcinoma; lung cancer secreting ectopic ACTH; corticosteroid therapy.

SITES INVOLVED   Adrenal cortex is the source of excess cortisol except for iatrogenic cases; pituitary (basophilic adenoma) may be responsible for stimulating the adrenal cortex to hyperplasia and hyperfunction.

GROSS LESIONS   Adrenocortical adenoma: round yellow nodule, adjacent adrenal cortex atrophic; hyperplasia (either primary or secondary to ACTH): thickened cortex, often nodular; iatrogenic: thin cortex.

MICROSCOPIC LESIONS   Adenoma: disorganized mass of adrenocortical cells, poorly encapsulated, little pleomorphism; hyperplasia: diffuse increase in adrenocortical cells, often producing multiple cortical nodules.

COMPLICATIONS   Osteoporosis with pathologic fractures (femoral neck, vertebral compression); diabetes mellitus, obesity; poor wound healing, susceptibility to infections.

SIGNS AND SYMPTOMS   Moon face, buffalo hump, obesity, abdominal striae, easy bruisability, poor wound healing, hirsutism and menstrual abnormalities in women, impotence in men, psychological disturbances.

CLINICAL DIAGNOSIS AND OTHER CLINICAL FEATURES   Recognition of the classic signs of hypercortisolism, especially the peculiar distribution of obesity; Cushing's syndrome is an expected unfortunate complication of long-term steroid therapy.

LABORATORY DIAGNOSIS   Elevated plasma cortisol, loss of diurnal variation; high ACTH (pituitary or ectopic) or low (adrenal or iatrogenic); dexamethasone suppression and response to ACTH helps identify source of cortisol.

PROGNOSIS   Depends on the underlying disease and the ability to control the cortisol excess.

THERAPY   Resection of pituitary adenoma or adrenal adenoma; partial resection of hyperplastic adrenals.

OTHER INFORMATION   Cushing's may be less likely to complicate steroid therapy if doses are given on alternate days; withdrawal of steroids from a patient may produce Addison's disease.

Diabetes Mellitus

DESCRIPTION   A metabolic disease, involving mostly carbohydrate (glucose) and lipid, caused by absolute deficiency of insulin (Type I) or by resistance to insulin's action in the peripheral tissues (Type II).

DISEASE ENTITIES; SYNONYMS AND ACRONYMS   Type I: juvenile-onset, insulin dependent; Type II: adult or maturity-onset, non-insulin dependent.

INCIDENCE   Common, especially Type II; 7th leading cause of death in US; contributes to many others.

AGE   Type I: children and young adults; Type II: middle-aged and older adults.

ETIOLOGY, PATHOGENESIS, AND PREDISPOSING FACTORS   Type I: autoimmune destruction of beta cells triggered by viral infection, predisposition linked to HLA-DR on chromosome 6; Type II: deficiency of insulin receptors on target cells, obesity.

SITES INVOLVED   Type I: pancreatic islets, particularly beta cells; Type II: primary defect in target cell receptors although islets may show changes; secondary effects are common in blood vessels, eyes, and kidneys.

GROSS LESIONS   No gross lesion in the pancreas in primary diabetes mellitus; diabetes mellitus occurring with chronic pancreatitis is considered secondary diabetes and is not a part of this discussion.

MICROSCOPIC LESIONS   Variable and inconstant changes in islets: decreased numbers, lymphocytic infiltration or fibrosis (Type I); amyloidosis (Type II); hyaline arteriolosclerosis; Kimmelstiel-Wilson glomerular lesions.

COMPLICATIONS   Ketoacidosis with coma (Type I); nonketotic hyperosmolar coma (Type II); accelerated atherosclerosis with myocardial infarct, stroke, leg gangrene; retinopathy, neuropathy, renal failure, infections.

SIGNS AND SYMPTOMS   Classic triad includes polyuria, polyphagia, polydipsia; weight loss, fatigue, visual disturbances; dehydration, coma; most Type II diabetics are obese and hypertensive.

CLINICAL DIAGNOSIS AND OTHER CLINICAL FEATURES   Type I often presents suddenly; Type II is gradual; because symptoms can be confused with other conditions, diabetes should always be considered when evaluating middle-aged to elderly patients.

LABORATORY DIAGNOSIS   Fasting or random glucose; glucose tolerance test; urinalysis for sugar and acetone; therapy is best monitored by testing blood rather than urine; glycosylated hemoglobin reflects long-term control.

PROGNOSIS   Results in definite increased morbidity and mortality due to a variety of mechanisms.

THERAPY   Type I: definitely insulin, diet; Type II: diet, weight loss, hypoglycemic drugs, possibly insulin.

OTHER INFORMATION   Glycosylation of basement membrane collagen may cause the microvascular complications of diabetes; accumulation of polyols mediates cell damage; diabetic nephropathy includes several diseases.

Graves' Disease

DESCRIPTION Thyroid disease causing hyperthyroidism associated with diffuse goiter, caused by stimulation of growth and function of the gland by thyroid stimulating (TSI) and thyroid growth immunoglobulins (TGI).

DISEASE ENTITIES; SYNONYMS AND ACRONYMS Diffuse toxic goiter, primary hyperthyroidism, primary thyroid hyperplasia, thyrotoxicosis, thyroid storm.

INCIDENCE Fairly common, occurring in 0.4% of US population; female:male = 5–6:1.

AGE Commonly 30s–40s but may present at much older ages.

ETIOLOGY, PATHOGENESIS, AND PREDISPOSING FACTORS Autoantibodies (TGI and TSI) associated with HLA-DR3 immune response genes are directed at the TSH receptors causing enlargement and hyperfunction; other autoantibodies cause ophthalmopathy.

SITES INVOLVED Thyroid gland diffusely; eyes and periorbital tissues; skin of legs; lymphoid tissue throughout body is hyperplastic; lymph nodes, thymus, and white pulp of spleen are enlarged.

GROSS LESIONS Gland is diffusely moderately enlarged and meaty red-brown; normal waxy appearance is lost, reflecting loss of colloid; periorbital tissue is edematous; legs develop plaque-like areas of edema.

MICROSCOPIC LESIONS Hyperplasia of follicular epithelial cells; colloid is absent or greatly reduced; follicular cells are tall, crowded, and project folds into the lumen; treatment greatly modifies the appearance.

COMPLICATIONS Thyrotoxic crisis (thyroid storm) with hypermetabolism, fever, tachycardia and arrhythmias is fatal in 25% of cases; cardiomegaly and cardiomyopathy; ophthalmoplegia, ulceration of cornea.

SIGNS AND SYMPTOMS Hyperactivity, anxiety, muscle weakness, weight loss, heat intolerance, sweating, oligomenorrhea; tachycardia, palpitations, arrhythmias, tremor; lid lag, proptosis, exophthalmos; dermopathy; goiter.

CLINICAL DIAGNOSIS AND OTHER CLINICAL FEATURES Combination of diffuse goiter, ophthalmopathy, and typical symptoms of hypermetabolism is fairly diagnostic; dermopathy is often not present; palpation or auscultation of gland may reveal bruit.

LABORATORY DIAGNOSIS Elevations of T3 and T4; diffusely increased uptake of radioactive iodine; suppression of TSH; other autoantibodies and autoimmune diseases may be present; examination of resected gland.

PROGNOSIS Usually good; opthalmopathy persists despite control of hyperthyroidism.

THERAPY Suppression with iodine, thiouracil, or tapazole; radioactive iodine; subtotal thyroidectomy.

OTHER INFORMATION Elderly often present atypically with "apathetic hyperthyroidism" requiring laboratory diagnosis; other causes include toxic adenoma and toxic multinodular goiter.

Hashimoto's Thyroiditis

DESCRIPTION Autoimmune disease of thyroid that produces goiter and eventual hypothyroidism, which is mediated by thyroid growth and stimulating immunoglobulins (TGI, TGI) and by destruction of thyroid tissue.

DISEASE ENTITIES; SYNONYMS AND ACRONYMS Hashimoto's disease, struma lymphomatosa, lymphadenoid goiter, autoimmune thyroiditis.

INCIDENCE Fairly common, especially in women; female:male = 10:1.

AGE Usually in perimenopausal women; most cases between ages 30–50 years; some cases occur in children.

ETIOLOGY, PATHOGENESIS, AND PREDISPOSING FACTORS Genetic association with HLA-DR5; presumed deficiency of specific T-suppressor cells; autoantibodies (TSI, TGI, and TSH blocking) react with TSH receptor to produce glandular growth and dysfunction.

SITES INVOLVED Thyroid gland; TSH receptor is the major site for the autoimmune reaction; other autoantibodies are directed against follicular cell membranes and components of colloid.

GROSS LESIONS Diffuse symmetric moderate enlargement of gland, sometimes nodular; capsule is intact; cut surface is light gray and fleshy like lymph node; less commonly, gland is mildly enlarged and fibrotic.

MICROSCOPIC LESIONS Massive infiltration by all types of lymphocytes, including plasma cells; germinal centers present; normal follicles absent; remnants show scant colloid and Hurthle cell (oncocytic) degeneration.

COMPLICATIONS Eventually the lymphocytic infiltration and autoimmune reactions destroy enough functional gland to produce hypothyroidism; hyperthyroidism may occur earlier in the disease.

SIGNS AND SYMPTOMS Features of hypothyroidism, such as fatigue, lethargy, slowed speech, cold intolerance, dry skin, coarse hair, puffy face, myxedema; diffuse goiter.

CLINICAL DIAGNOSIS AND OTHER CLINICAL FEATURES Hypothyroidism in a middle-aged woman with diffuse goiter is likely to be Hashimoto's thyroiditis; an occasional patient presents with hyperthyroidism; other autoimmune diseases may coexist.

LABORATORY DIAGNOSIS Histologic examination of needle biopsy of thyroid; depending on the phase of the disease, T3 and T4 may be normal, low, or elevated; in later phases, T3 and T4 are depressed and TSH is elevated.

PROGNOSIS Good; despite progressive destruction of gland, euthyroid state can be maintained with therapy.

THERAPY Synthetic thyroid hormone supplementation; thyroidectomy is not usually indicated.

OTHER INFORMATION Grave's disease, Hashimoto's thyroiditis, and primary idiopathic myxedema are related by the presence of similar autoantibodies reacting with the TSH receptor but causing different effects.

Hyperparathyroidism

DESCRIPTION Hyperfunction of parathyroids; primary disease is caused by adenoma or by primary hyperplasia; secondary hyperparathyroidism is most often due to chronic renal failure.

DISEASE ENTITIES; SYNONYMS AND ACRONYMS Parathyroid adenoma; primary or secondary parathyroid hyperplasia.

INCIDENCE Secondary hyperparathyroidism is common in chronic renal failure; the primary form is uncommon.

AGE Usually adults; younger cases may occur with the multiple endocrine neoplasia (MEN) syndromes.

ETIOLOGY, PATHOGENESIS, AND PREDISPOSING FACTORS Adenomas and primary hyperplasia may be sporadic or familial, as in MEN syndromes Types I and IIa; chronic renal failure and other causes of hypocalcemia produce secondary hyperplasia.

SITES INVOLVED Parathyroids; adenoma usually involves only one gland, hyperplasia involves all four; secondary changes are important in bones and kidney; metastatic calcification may involve lungs and other sites.

GROSS LESIONS Adenoma: one gland is enlarged over normal, perhaps only a few millimeters up to a few centimeters; hyperplasia: all four glands are twice or several times larger than normal, although the enlargement may be asymmetric.

MICROSCOPIC LESIONS Adenoma: thinly encapsulated mass of usually chief cells compressing the surrounding gland; hyperplasia: glands are solidly cellular (either chief or clear cells) without the normal adipose tissue.

COMPLICATIONS Hypercalcemia with neuromuscular weakness, occasionally fatal; cystic bone lesions (osteitis fibrosa cystica); kidney stones; hypertension; peptic ulcers; pancreatitis; metastatic calcifications.

SIGNS AND SYMPTOMS Emotional changes, neuromuscular weakness, cardiovascular collapse indicate a crisis; kidney stones present with renal colic; bone lesions (also called brown tumors) with pathologic fracture.

CLINICAL DIAGNOSIS AND OTHER CLINICAL FEATURES Most cases are diagnosed early because of routine biochemical screening that includes calcium; x-rays may disclose multiple cystic bone lesions; an expected complication of chronic renal failure.

LABORATORY DIAGNOSIS Primary hyperparathyroidism: hypercalcemia, hypophosphatemia, hypercalciuria, elevated serum PTH; secondary: hypocalcemia, hyperphosphatemia, elevated PTH, other changes of underlying disease.

PROGNOSIS Usually good with therapy; often complicates management of chronic renal failure.

THERAPY Surgical exploration of all glands with biopsy; resection of adenoma if present.

OTHER INFORMATION Prolonged secondary hyperplasia, occurring in chronic renal failure can progress to autonomous primary hyperplasia, called "tertiary hyperparathyroidism."

Hypopituitarism

DESCRIPTION Hypofunction of adenohypophysis caused by intrinsic lesion or by a lesion in the hypothalamus; all hormones are usually deficient (panhypopituitarism); less often a single hormone (GH) is deficient.

DISEASE ENTITIES; SYNONYMS AND ACRONYMS Panhypopituitarism: Simmond's disease, pituitary cachexia, Sheehan's syndrome; GH deficiency only: pituitary dwarfism.

INCIDENCE Uncommon; Sheehan's syndrome, nonsecretory adenoma, and empty sella syndrome are most common.

AGE Any age, depending on cause; Sheehan's syndrome affects postpartum women.

ETIOLOGY, PATHOGENESIS, AND PREDISPOSING FACTORS Any destructive process in the hypothalamus or pituitary; postpartum infarction (Sheehan's); chromophobe adenoma; suprasellar tumors; infections; surgical excision; metastatic neoplasm.

SITES INVOLVED Pituitary, hypothalamus, or any space-occupying mass invading the sella turcica; 75% or more of the gland must be destroyed before panhypopituitarism develops.

GROSS LESIONS Infarcted gland is soft and pale or hemorrhagic; later there is contraction with scarring; adenoma is a rounded mass that obliterates the gland; glioma or craniopharyngioma can invade the sella.

MICROSCOPIC LESIONS Coagulative necrosis followed by fibrosis characterizes an infarct; chromophobe adenoma lacks cytoplasmic granules; craniopharyngioma resembles the embryonic tooth bud.

COMPLICATIONS Loss of tropic hormones leading to atrophy of target glands in the order: gonadotropins, GH, TSH, ACTH, PRL; thus hypogonadism, dwarfism in children, hypothyroidism, adrenocortical insufficiency.

SIGNS AND SYMPTOMS Amenorrhea in women; loss of pubic hair, gonadal atrophy, loss of libido and sterility in both sexes; weakness, fatigue, pallor, weight loss, hypotension; failure of lactation.

CLINICAL DIAGNOSIS AND OTHER CLINICAL FEATURES Infarction may go undiagnosed for years; tumors present signs due to mass effect; panhypopituitarism must be distinguished from failure of target glands; x-rays and CT scans may show abnormal sella.

LABORATORY DIAGNOSIS Radioimmunoassay of the tropic hormones (FSH, LH, TSH, ACTH) and of the target gland hormones (T3, T4, cortisol, estrogen, testosterone); specific deficiencies are variable.

PROGNOSIS Infarct: good, if recognized and treated early; tumor: generally poor.

THERAPY Specific hormone replacement; resection of any tumor invading sella.

OTHER INFORMATION GH deficiency causes pituitary dwarfism in children; there is normal mental development and proportion of features, in contrast to cretinism and achondroplasia.

Myxedema

DESCRIPTION   A condition of severe hypothyroidism in the adult caused by any lesion that destroys the thyroid gland or interferes with its function; primary myxedema refers to idiopathic atrophy of the thyroid.

DISEASE ENTITIES; SYNONYMS AND ACRONYMS   Primary idiopathic myxedema; hypothyroidism.

INCIDENCE   Severe hypothyroidism with myxedema is uncommon; mild hypothyroidism is fairly common.

AGE   Any age from late childhood on; may develop for years before it is clinically recognized.

ETIOLOGY, PATHOGENESIS, AND PREDISPOSING FACTORS   Resection or radioiodine ablation of thyroid for Grave's disease; TSH-blocking autoantibodies causing primary myxedema; Hashimoto's thyroiditis; iodine deficiency; pituitary disease.

SITES INVOLVED   Thyroid gland; secondary involvement of all organs and tissues due to the hypometabolic state; connective tissue and heart are noticeably affected.

GROSS LESIONS   Depends on primary lesion; usually the gland is markedly reduced in size; in some cases the gland is replaced by tumor; connective tissue shows myxoid degeneration; heart is dilated and flabby.

MICROSCOPIC LESIONS   In primary myxedema, there is extreme atrophy of follicles which appear small and sparsely distributed within connective tissue; other cases show features of the lesion that destroyed the gland.

COMPLICATIONS   Myxedema or hypothyroid cardiomyopathy with heart failure; myxedema coma; renal dysfunction, altered bowel motility; general slowing of muscular and mental activities.

SIGNS AND SYMPTOMS   Fatigue, apathy, lethargy, sluggishness, slowing of speech and mental functions; cold intolerance, enlarged tongue, coarse hair, dry skin, loss of lateral eyebrows, puffy pasty face, nonpitting edema.

CLINICAL DIAGNOSIS AND OTHER CLINICAL FEATURES   Recognition of the signs and symptoms of the hypometabolic state. In the elderly, hypothyroidism is sometimes mistaken for other conditions such as depression, dementia, and stroke.

LABORATORY DIAGNOSIS   Depression of T3 and T4; if due to thyroid disease, TSH is elevated; if due to pituitary or hypothalamic lesion, TSH is depressed.

PROGNOSIS   Good, but only if diagnosed and treated.

THERAPY   Synthetic thyroid hormone replacement (e.g., Synthroid).

OTHER INFORMATION   Deficient TSH due to hypothalamic or pituitary lesion causes trophoprivic hypothyroidism, in which adrenal cortical insufficiency is likely to coexist due to ACTH deficiency.

Neuroblastoma

DESCRIPTION   Primary malignant neoplasm that arises from immature cells of the adrenal medulla and secretes catecholamines; it occurs in children and presents with abdominal mass.

DISEASE ENTITIES; SYNONYMS AND ACRONYMS   Hutchinson-type neuroblastoma, ganglioneuroblastoma, ganglioneuroma.

INCIDENCE   One of the common tumors of childhood.

AGE   Usually under the age of 5 years; uncommon beyond 15 years.

ETIOLOGY, PATHOGENESIS, AND PREDISPOSING FACTORS   Most are sporadic tumors arising from primitive neural elements in adrenal medulla and other sites; some cases are familial; cytogenetic abnormalities are often present in the tumor cells.

SITES INVOLVED   Adrenal medulla or surrounding retroperitoneal region; few arise from posterior mediastinum, posterior cranial fossa or other sites; metastases are common in lymph nodes, liver, lung, and bone.

GROSS LESIONS   Solid, round, soft tumor mass, often large and obliterating adrenal gland; sometimes gray on cut surface but usually shows extensive hemorrhage and necrosis with cyst formation; focal calcification.

MICROSCOPIC LESIONS   Anaplastic, small, round-to-oval hyperchromatic cells with scant cytoplasm in sheets or forming Homer-Wright pseudorosettes; ganglion cells indicate maturation (ganglioneuroblastoma or ganglioneuroma).

COMPLICATIONS   Invasion of abdominal organs by direct spread; metastases to liver, lung, and bone; Hutchinson's neuroblastoma is one with extensive skull and orbital metastases that produce exophthalmos.

SIGNS AND SYMPTOMS   Abdominal mass, weight loss, decreased activity, poor feeding, fever; metastases may appear before the primary is apparent.

CLINICAL DIAGNOSIS AND OTHER CLINICAL FEATURES   The abdominal mass must be differentiated from Wilm's tumor and lymphoma; bone metastases can mimic Ewing's sarcoma or leukemia; biopsy is required for diagnosis.

LABORATORY DIAGNOSIS   Histologic examination of tissue; electron microscopy shows neurosecretory granules; detection in urine of elevated catecholamine metabolites, homovanillic or vanillylmandelic acid (HMA, VMA).

PROGNOSIS   Often poor; maturing tumors, age under 1 year, and absence of metastases indicate better survival.

THERAPY   Surgical resection; radiation therapy and chemotherapy.

OTHER INFORMATION   Stage I: confined to primary location; II: local invasion but not crossing midline; III: invasion across midline, local lymph node metastases; IV: distant metastases; IVs: age less than 1 year.

Nodular Goiter

DESCRIPTION   Enlargement of thyroid caused by excessive accumulation of colloid within enlarged follicles, caused by iodine deficiency, ingestion of goitrogens, or defects in synthesis or transport of hormone.

DISEASE ENTITIES; SYNONYMS AND ACRONYMS   Multinodular goiter, nontoxic goiter, colloid goiter, adenomatous goiter, simple goiter, struma, endemic goiter.

INCIDENCE   Common, particularly in mountainous regions far from the sea; more common in women.

AGE   May be present at birth; more often develops in adolescence and increases in size thereafter.

ETIOLOGY, PATHOGENESIS, AND PREDISPOSING FACTORS   Iodine deficiency (endemic goiter), goitrogenic drugs or foods (e.g., cassava), and defects in synthetic enzymes cause decreased T3 and T4; secondary elevation of TSH stimulates gland to enlarge.

SITES INVOLVED   Thyroid gland. Pituitary gland is involved as the source of TSH, stimulated by the decreased thyroid hormone.

GROSS LESIONS   Early cases show diffuse enlargement (simple, diffuse, or colloid goiter); in most clinically apparent cases, there are various sizes of nodules enlarging the gland up to several hundred grams.

MICROSCOPIC LESIONS   Follicles are distended with colloid; follicle lining cells are flattened; fibrosis, focal calcification, cystic changes, hemosiderin deposits and recent hemorrhage are present between nodules.

COMPLICATIONS   Compression of trachea and occasionally vena cava; mild to moderate hyperthyroidism with arrhythmias and possible heart failure; rarely hypothyroidism; confusion with neoplasia.

SIGNS AND SYMPTOMS   Visible enlargement of gland in neck, usually bilateral; a dominant nodule may present unilateral mass; episodic pain; choking sensation, dysphagia or stridor; venous engorgement.

CLINICAL DIAGNOSIS AND OTHER CLINICAL FEATURES   Inspection and palpation of gland is often sufficiently diagnostic; differentiation of dominant nodule from neoplasia may require radioiodine scintiscan, ultrasonography, CT scans, or surgery.

LABORATORY DIAGNOSIS   Examination of resected tissue; grossly, multiple nodules indicates nodular goiter rather than tumor; microscopically, distended follicles confirms diagnosis of goiter; T3 and T4 are usually normal.

PROGNOSIS   Usually good, except in infants who develop cretinism.

THERAPY   Surgical resection for cosmetic purposes or to relieve compressive effects; iodine replacement.

OTHER INFORMATION   Iodine should be replaced cautiously because hyperthyroidism may be produced. Infants of goitrous mothers are often cretins and suffer irreversible brain damage.

Pheochromocytoma

DESCRIPTION   Primary neoplasm of adrenal medulla in adults that secretes catecholamines and thereby causes hypertension; a similar tumor of autonomic ganglia is called extra-adrenal paraganglioma.

DISEASE ENTITIES; SYNONYMS AND ACRONYMS   Paraganglioma; carotid body tumor.

INCIDENCE   Uncommon; an infrequent cause of hypertension.

AGE   Adults, peaking in middle age.

ETIOLOGY, PATHOGENESIS, AND PREDISPOSING FACTORS   Most are sporadic; 10–20% are associated with at least four autosomal dominant familial syndromes, such as MEN IIa and b, also von Hippel-Lindau disease and neurofibromatosis.

SITES INVOLVED   Pheochromocytoma: adrenal medulla, often bilateral in familial cases; paraganglioma: retroperitoneum along the aorta, posterior mediastinum, dome of urinary bladder, carotid body.

GROSS LESIONS   Encapsulated round tumor mass with compressed adrenal at periphery; gray cut surface with variable hemorrhage; turns dark brown when exposed to oxidants (chromaffin reaction).

MICROSCOPIC LESIONS   Clusters of pleomorphic moderately large cells with basophilic cytoplasm in a vascular stroma; argentaffin stains are often positive; electron microscopy shows membrane-bound secretory granules.

COMPLICATIONS   Hypertension, episodic or sustained, often severe, leading to cardiac complications and stroke; catecholamine cardiomyopathy; metastasis is more common with paraganglioma than with pheochromocytoma.

SIGNS AND SYMPTOMS   Paroxysmal hypertension, accompanied by anxiety or other psychologic changes, precipitated by exercise, emotion, postural changes, urination, palpation of region of tumor, induction of anesthesia.

CLINICAL DIAGNOSIS AND OTHER CLINICAL FEATURES   Hypertensive attacks are highly suggestive; CT or MRI scans may localize the tumor; often laparotomy is required for diagnosis; surgical procedures may precipitate a hypertensive crisis.

LABORATORY DIAGNOSIS   Elevated catecholamines or metabolites (e.g., vanillylmandelic acid, VMA) in urine or plasma; histologic examination of tumor; immunohistochemistry may reveal several neuropeptides (bombesin, VIP etc.)

PROGNOSIS   Good if discovered and treated; many are discovered at autopsy after sudden death.

THERAPY   Resection of tumor; pharmacologic adrenergic blockade must be achieved before surgery.

OTHER INFORMATION   Pheochromocytoma and paraganglioma are essentially the same tumor arising in different sites; extra-adrenal tumors are more often malignant; histologic examination cannot predict malignant behavior.

Pituitary Adenoma

DESCRIPTION Primary neoplasm of anterior pituitary that produces systemic effects by secreting excess hormone and local effects (visual disturbances) by the tumor mass.

DISEASE ENTITIES; SYNONYMS AND ACRONYMS Acidophil, basophil, chromophobe adenoma; somatotropic, corticotropic adenoma, prolactinoma; microadenoma.

INCIDENCE Altogether uncommon; the most frequent cause of hyperpituitarism; male predominance.

AGE Usually between ages of 20 and 50 years.

ETIOLOGY, PATHOGENESIS, AND PREDISPOSING FACTORS Neoplastic disease of unknown etiology; syndromes are due to increased secretion of a single hormone, most commonly hyperprolactinemia, giantism or acromegaly (GH), or Cushing's syndrome (ACTH).

SITES INVOLVED Anterior pituitary initially; as the tumor enlarges, the entire pituitary may be destroyed; sella turcica is often enlarged; optic chiasm is frequently compressed; tumor may extend into base of brain.

GROSS LESIONS Pale or reddish rounded mass expanding within and beyond the sella turcica; capsule is poorly formed; extends into surrounding structures by pushing margins; hemorrhage and necrosis in large tumors.

MICROSCOPIC LESIONS Clusters of uniform cells similar to normal pituitary cells; basophil adenoma produces ACTH; acidophil, GH; chromophobe, PRL or nonsecretory; Crooke's hyaline is seen in basophil adenoma.

COMPLICATIONS Increased intracranial pressure; visual disturbances due to compression of optic chiasm; endocrinopathy; hypopituitarism with nonfunctional adenoma or after resection of tumor.

SIGNS AND SYMPTOMS Hyperprolactinemia: amenorrhea-galactorrhea and infertility in women; GH excess: acromegaly in adults (enlargement of hands, feet, mandible, and maxilla), giantism in children; ACTH: Cushing's disease.

CLINICAL DIAGNOSIS AND OTHER CLINICAL FEATURES Recognition of syndromes of hormone excess and local effect of tumor, particularly bilateral homonymous hemianopsia; local signs only with nonsecretory adenoma; enlarged sella on skull x-ray and scan.

LABORATORY DIAGNOSIS Elevated hormone by radioimmunoassay; failure of glucose to suppress GH secretion; histologic examination; electron microscopy; immunohistochemistry for specific peptide hormone.

PROGNOSIS Depends on size of tumor when discovered; often a prolonged downhill course.

THERAPY Transsphenoidal resection; radiation therapy; pharmacologic suppression of microprolactinoma.

OTHER INFORMATION In the familial multiple endocrine neoplasia syndrome (MEN I) there are adenomas of pituitary, thyroid, adrenal cortex, and pancreatic islets.

Thymoma

DESCRIPTION   Primary, usually benign neoplasm of thymus, arising from thymic epithelial cells and often associated with secondary autoimmune diseases, particularly myasthenia gravis and pure red cell aplasia.

DISEASE ENTITIES; SYNONYMS AND ACRONYMS   Benign thymoma, malignant thymoma, thymic carcinoma; myasthenia gravis, pure red cell aplasia.

INCIDENCE   Uncommon, but one of the most common tumors of the anterior mediastinum.

AGE   Adults; peak incidence in middle age; rare in children.

ETIOLOGY, PATHOGENESIS, AND PREDISPOSING FACTORS   Neoplastic disease of unknown etiology involving thymic epithelial cells; the accompanying lymphocytes are not neoplastic; secondary autoimmune diseases, myasthenia gravis, and pure red cell aplasia.

SITES INVOLVED   Thymus, epithelial cells; tumor mass is located in the superior anterior mediastinum; malignant thymoma may invade pleura, lung, trachea, heart, and great vessels.

GROSS LESIONS   Lobulated gray to tan mass with focal hemorrhagic and cystic areas; large tumors fill the anterior mediastinum and compress adjacent structures; invasion indicates a malignant thymoma.

MICROSCOPIC LESIONS   Round to oval cells with pale regular nuclei and moderate cytoplasm lacking distinct borders, surrounded by lymphocytes; recognized variants: round cell, spindle cell, and squamous cell types.

COMPLICATIONS   Local: compression or invasion (with malignant tumors) of mediastinal structures; systemic: myasthenia gravis, cytopenias (red cell aplasia), cancers, hypogammaglobulinemia, autoimmune diseases.

SIGNS AND SYMPTOMS   Cough, dyspnea, dysphagia, engorgement of veins of the face and neck (vena cava compression); muscle weakness; anemia or other hematologic disorder; infections; some are asymptomatic.

CLINICAL DIAGNOSIS AND OTHER CLINICAL FEATURES   Anterior mediastinal mass to be differentiated from Hodgkin's disease, malignant lymphoma, and germ cell tumor; x-rays, CT and MRI scans visualize mass; thoracotomy with biopsy confirms diagnosis.

LABORATORY DIAGNOSIS   Histologic examination of tissue; prominent lymphocyte component leads to confusion with Hodgkin's disease or lymphoma; electron microscopy and immunocytochemistry confirm epithelial origin.

PROGNOSIS   Poor for malignant thymoma or if there is associated systemic disease; benign thymoma is resectable.

THERAPY   Surgical resection of tumor.

OTHER INFORMATION   Malignant thymoma is differentiated from benign thymoma by gross evidence of invasion, not by microscopic criteria; thymic carcinoma is rare and displays obvious histologic anaplasia.

Thyroid Adenoma

DESCRIPTION   Benign neoplasm of thyroid arising from follicular cells or rarely from parafollicular cells, usually presenting as a solitary nodule.

DISEASE ENTITIES; SYNONYMS AND ACRONYMS   Follicular adenoma (micro- or macrofollicular, fetal, colloid, Hurthle cell, etc.), papillary adenoma, atypical adenoma.

INCIDENCE   Thyroid nodules are very common; however, only a minority of these are actually true adenomas.

AGE   Most common in middle age; nonneoplastic nodules also increase with age.

ETIOLOGY, PATHOGENESIS, AND PREDISPOSING FACTORS   Ionizing radiation involving the gland and exposure to radioactive fallout increase the incidence of nodules, adenomas and carcinomas several-fold; most cases, however, have no known exposure.

SITES INVOLVED   Thyroid gland, usually in a single site; multiple nodules in the gland probably represent multinodular goiter; a single nodule is more likely to be an adenoma.

GROSS LESIONS   Most often solitary, well-circumscribed and encapsulated rounded mass clearly demarcated from the surrounding gland; usually tan and sometimes focally hemorrhagic; papillary adenoma is partly cystic.

MICROSCOPIC LESIONS   Follicular adenoma is most common and shows different microscopic patterns; surrounding gland is compressed by the encapsulated tumor and shows no nodularity; Hurthle cell variant has a solid pattern.

COMPLICATIONS   Occasional adenomas may hyperfunction to cause thyrotoxicosis (toxic adenoma); otherwise, the main concern is to differentiate the lesion from cancer; risk of malignant transformation is probably low.

SIGNS AND SYMPTOMS   Palpable single nodule in the neck over the thyroid less than 3–4 cm in diameter; pain and sudden enlargement indicate bleeding into the adenoma; pressure effects on neck structures may occur.

CLINICAL DIAGNOSIS AND OTHER CLINICAL FEATURES   Most palpable nodules prove to be a dominant nodule of a nodular thyroid or nodular goiter; adenomas are usually "cold" on scintiscan but nonneoplastic nodules may also be cold.

LABORATORY DIAGNOSIS   Tissue examination; if surrounding gland is not nodular, the lesion is probably a neoplasm to be further categorized histologically; preoperative aspiration cytology may help to exclude malignancy.

PROGNOSIS   Good; does not recur after complete excision.

THERAPY   Surgical excision with surrounding margin of normal gland for diagnosis and definitive treatment.

OTHER INFORMATION   Papillary adenoma is uncommon, poorly encapsulated, and may represent low-grade carcinoma. Atypical adenoma, composed of spindle cells and possibly of parafollicular cell origin, is not precancerous.

Pathology Facts, by Richard C. Harruff, J.B. Lippincott Company, Philadelphia © 1994.

Chapter 21

Musculoskeletal System

Denervation Muscle Atrophy

DESCRIPTION Atrophy of skeletal muscle following loss of motor innervation; indicates a lesion of the lower motor neuron or its axon.

DISEASE ENTITIES; SYNONYMS AND ACRONYMS Neurogenic atrophy; peripheral neuropathy, amyotrophic lateral sclerosis (ALS), poliomyelitis, Werdnig-Hoffmann disease.

INCIDENCE An invariable complication of diseases damaging the lower motor neurons or motor nerves.

AGE Depends on underlying disease; Werdnig-Hoffmann affects infants, ALS affects middle age.

ETIOLOGY, PATHOGENESIS, AND PREDISPOSING FACTORS Loss of axon or its synaptic connection at the motor endplate causes degeneration and atrophy of the muscle fiber due to loss of tropic effects provided by the axonal connection.

SITES INVOLVED The primary disease is within the cranial or spinal motor neurons or within the motor nerves; reinnervation may be established with surviving nerve axons.

GROSS LESIONS Affected muscles are reduced in mass and show an increase in adipose tissue.

MICROSCOPIC LESIONS Pathognomonic pattern is type grouping, where the normal mosaic distribution of Type I and II fibers is replaced by groups of same type fibers; angulated atrophic fibers and target fibers may be seen.

COMPLICATIONS Progressive muscle weakness that leads to disability and incapacitation; generalized and progressive weakening of the chest muscles and diaphragm leads to respiratory failure.

SIGNS AND SYMPTOMS Depends on disease process: ALS, generalized muscle weakness and fasciculations; Werdnig-Hoffmann, "floppy infant"; alcoholic and diabetic neuropathies affect extremities.

CLINICAL DIAGNOSIS AND OTHER CLINICAL FEATURES Needs to be differentiated from primary muscle diseases and from diseases affecting the upper motor neuron; most cases develop gradually; Guillain-Barré neuropathy (polyneuritis) presents suddenly.

LABORATORY DIAGNOSIS Muscle biopsy with enzyme histochemistry shows characteristic type grouping; atrophic fibers are both Types I and II and stain darkly with esterase stain; serum creatine kinase is moderately elevated.

PROGNOSIS Depends on disease; ALS is fatal; muscle may recover after localized and minor nerve damage.

THERAPY Primarily supportive therapy; corticosteroids are occasionally used to slow neuronal destruction.

OTHER INFORMATION Muscle atrophy due to upper motor neuron disease (e.g., following stroke) shows selective atrophy of Type II fibers; this pattern is also seen with disuse, wasting, and long-term steroid therapy.

Duchenne Muscular Dystrophy

DESCRIPTION   Primary muscle disease, inherited as a recessive sex-linked defect or occurring as a new mutation, which affects a cytoskeletal protein of muscle and results in severe progressive muscle weakness.

DISEASE ENTITIES; SYNONYMS AND ACRONYMS   Progressive muscular dystrophy, Duchenne type; Becker variant.

INCIDENCE   The most common muscular dystrophy; affects 1 in 3500 male births; two thirds inherited; one third new mutations.

AGE   Present at birth but not evident until 3–4 years; total disability by age 10–15; death by age 20.

ETIOLOGY, PATHOGENESIS, AND PREDISPOSING FACTORS   Defective gene on short arm of X chromosome, normally coding for the protein dystrophin, a component of the cell membrane skeleton that may be involved with control of muscle contraction/relaxation.

SITES INVOLVED   Proximal muscles initially, particularly the pelvic and shoulder girdles; legs, trunk, and arm muscles; cardiac muscle is also involved.

GROSS LESIONS   Progressive replacement of the skeletal muscle mass by fibrofatty tissue which occupies more volume than the original muscle, thus resulting in the pseudohypertrophy seen clinically.

MICROSCOPIC LESIONS   Early: combination of enlarged, degenerating fibers with contraction bands, necrotic fibers infiltrated by macrophages, and regenerating fibers with central nuclei; late: replacement of muscle by fat.

COMPLICATIONS   Progressive muscle weakness that produces complete disability in adolescence; certain death before adulthood, caused by failure of respiratory muscles or by cardiac arrhythmia.

SIGNS AND SYMPTOMS   Weakness becomes apparent at age 3–4; child has difficulty standing and does so by pulling himself up with his hands on the legs; soon he cannot walk and is confined to wheelchair, then to bed.

CLINICAL DIAGNOSIS AND OTHER CLINICAL FEATURES   Maternal family history is often negative because one third of cases are due to mutations, not inherited; the pattern and progression of muscle weakness is distinctive; muscle biopsy for confirmation.

LABORATORY DIAGNOSIS   Elevated serum creatine kinase; muscle biopsy preferably taken from the quadriceps during an early phase of the disease shows characteristic microscopic features.

PROGNOSIS   Poor; progresses to complete incapacitation and certain death.

THERAPY   Supportive only; trials of genetic therapy and transplantation of myoblasts are in progress.

OTHER INFORMATION   The genetic defect in Duchenne muscular dystrophy results in complete deficiency of dystrophin; in the milder Becker variant, functional fragments of dystrophin are produced.

Fibrous Dysplasia

DESCRIPTION   Benign disorder of bone characterized by lesions where soft fibrous tissue containing small spicules of abnormally formed bone replace medullary structure of one or several bones.

DISEASE ENTITIES; SYNONYMS AND ACRONYMS   Monostotic fibrous dysplasia, polyostotic fibrous dysplasia, osteitis fibrosa disseminata, Albright's syndrome.

INCIDENCE   Uncommon; monostotic variant is more common; Albright's syndrome affects predominantly females.

AGE   Occurs in adults or children; cases in childhood may arrest at puberty or progress into adulthood.

ETIOLOGY, PATHOGENESIS, AND PREDISPOSING FACTORS   Presumed developmental abnormality; neither neoplastic nor hereditary; morphology of lesions suggests aberrant maturation and organization of bone formation.

SITES INVOLVED   Medullary cavity of femur, ribs, skull (including maxilla and mandible), humerus, tibia, pelvis, and others, with the frequency of involvement varying between the monostotic and polyostotic types.

GROSS LESIONS   Soft brown gritty tissue replaces the medullary trabeculae; cortex is thin and often expanded outward; affected bones are deformed by expansion, bowing and fractures.

MICROSCOPIC LESIONS   Cellular mass of regular fibroblasts arranged in whorling patterns with small spicules of woven bone interspersed; osteoblasts are not present; the bone appears to arise directly from fibroblasts.

COMPLICATIONS   Disfigurement of skull or crippling deformities due to distortion of bone structure; pathologic fractures; sarcoma development, especially if radiated; premature closure of epiphysis; endocrinopathy.

SIGNS AND SYMPTOMS   Visible expansion of bone (e.g., mandible, maxilla); pain over affected bone; fracture with minimal trauma; sexual precocity or other endocrine manifestation; pigmented skin lesions.

CLINICAL DIAGNOSIS AND OTHER CLINICAL FEATURES   X-rays show characteristic radiolucent lesions with a ground glass pattern, thin overlying cortex, and expansion of bone cavity; skin lesions appear as cafe-au-lait spots, often over affected bones.

LABORATORY DIAGNOSIS   Histologic examination of resected or biopsied tissue; microscopic features must be correlated with x-ray appearance to avoid confusing the lesion with tumor or callus.

PROGNOSIS   Unpredictable; extensive disease results in severe disability.

THERAPY   Curettage of lesions and packing them with bone chips to encourage proper bone growth.

OTHER INFORMATION   In Albright's syndrome, which occurs in less than 5% of polyostotic disease, there are pigmented skin macules and endocrine disorders (precocious puberty, Cushing's syndrome, hyperthyroidism).

Gout

DESCRIPTION Diseases associated with hyperuricemia; deposition of urate crystals in joints produces attacks of painful arthritis that may progress to chronic arthritis with tophus formation.

DISEASE ENTITIES; SYNONYMS AND ACRONYMS Urate gout, gouty arthritis, tophaceous gout; primary or secondary gout; metabolic or renal gout; urate nephropathy.

INCIDENCE Hyperuricemia may be present in 10% of adults but gout in less than 0.5%; predominantly in males.

AGE In men over 30 years; in women after menopause; children with leukemia may develop hyperuricemia.

ETIOLOGY, PATHOGENESIS, AND PREDISPOSING FACTORS Abnormal urate production from xanthine via purine nucleic acid metabolism; in some cases genetic enzyme defects are known; decreased renal excretion of urate; increased urate production from tumors.

SITES INVOLVED Joints: urate crystals elicit inflammatory response of PMNs and macrophages; initially one joint (often the great toe), later several joints; kidney: urate crystals in interstitium; uric acid calculi.

GROSS LESIONS Acute attacks are characterized by prominent signs of acute inflammation; chronic arthritis shows fibrosis of periarticular tissues and powdery, chalky-white deposits of sodium urate crystals (tophi).

MICROSCOPIC LESIONS In established lesions, needle-shaped crystals of urate salts are surrounded by foreign-body giant cell granulomas and fibrosis; in acute gouty arthritis, there are PMNs and synovial proliferation.

COMPLICATIONS Loss of joint mobility and disability due to chronic arthritis; renal failure due to urate nephropathy in chronic gout and in secondary hyperuricemia without arthritis; urate nephrolithiasis.

SIGNS AND SYMPTOMS Extreme pain, redness, and swelling of one great toe (podagra) typifies early acute attacks; precipitated by ethanol, overeating or stress; tophi around joints and ear helix are seen in chronic gout.

CLINICAL DIAGNOSIS AND OTHER CLINICAL FEATURES Early acute attacks remit (intercritical gout) and recur with involvement of additional joints; tophi develop only after several years; x-rays show lytic juxta-articular lesions.

LABORATORY DIAGNOSIS Elevated serum uric acid; synovial fluid examination shows birefringent uric acid crystals and excludes septic arthritis; albuminuria and azotemia indicate renal involvement.

PROGNOSIS Good with therapy; otherwise progressive joint destruction and renal failure are likely.

THERAPY Allopurinal to inhibit xanthine oxidase production of uric acid; colchicine for acute attacks.

OTHER INFORMATION Two types of gout involving specific enzyme defects are x-linked; saturnine gout is due to reduced renal clearance of urate in chronic lead poisoning.

Osteitis Fibrosa Cystica

DESCRIPTION   The end-stage of osteopenic bone disease caused by primary or secondary hyperparathyroidism; if secondary to chronic renal failure, renal osteodystrophy is a better term.

DISEASE ENTITIES; SYNONYMS AND ACRONYMS   Skeletal disease of hyperparathyroidism, von Recklinghausen's disease of bone; brown tumors; renal osteodystrophy.

INCIDENCE   Early forms are fairly common; the end-stage is uncommon due to early recognition and treatment.

AGE   Any age depending on cause; more common in adults.

ETIOLOGY, PATHOGENESIS, PREDISPOSING FACTORS   Hyperparathyroidism causes mobilization of calcium from bone with resorption of trabeculae and cortex; progresses to complete resorption of trabeculae, marrow fibrosis, hemorrhage, and cyst formation.

SITES INVOLVED   All bones are affected; frequently best appreciated in skull, phalanges, metacarpals, and tooth sockets; osteoclastic activity occurs at the endosteum and periosteum and around trabeculae.

GROSS LESIONS   Extreme rarefaction of marrow trabeculae with multiple soft brown cystic cavities throughout medulla; fractures, old and recent hemorrhage.

MICROSCOPIC LESIONS   Early: demineralization; later: osteoclastic hyperplasia, thin trabeculae, marrow fibrosis; end-stage: loss of trabeculae, irregular fibrosis with giant cells, hemosiderin-containing macrophages.

COMPLICATIONS   Fractures with minor trauma, skeletal deformity, disability; metastatic calcification in soft tissues and organs, gastrointestinal disorders and kidney stones complicate the hypercalcemia.

SIGNS AND SYMPTOMS   Presents with complications related to hypercalcemia and bone resorption; bone disease is rarely advanced because routine chemical screening is likely to disclose early changes in calcium metabolism.

CLINICAL DIAGNOSIS AND OTHER CLINICAL FEATURES   Recognition of the "bones, stones, moans and groans" of primary hyperparathyroidism; skeletal x-ray changes may be diagnostic; renal osteodystrophy is a common complication of chronic renal failure.

LABORATORY DIAGNOSIS   Hypercalcemia with primary hyperparathyroidism; hypocalcemia and hyperphosphatemia if secondary to renal failure; elevated PTH; brown tumor must be differentiated from giant cell tumor.

PROGNOSIS   Lesions are potentially reversible over a long period following treatment.

THERAPY   Resection of parathyroid adenoma; subtotal resection of all glands for parathyroid hyperplasia.

OTHER INFORMATION   In renal osteodystrophy, there are additional skeletal changes (especially osteomalacia) due to concomitant vitamin D deficiency and hypocalcemia. Brown tumors are not truly neoplastic.

Osteoarthritis

DESCRIPTION A condition affecting the large weight-bearing joints, characterized by degeneration of the articular cartilage and progressive destruction and remodeling of the joint structures.

DISEASE ENTITIES; SYNONYMS AND ACRONYMS Degenerative joint disease; primary osteoarthritis; secondary osteoarthritis.

INCIDENCE Very common; eventually affects most of the population; more common in women.

AGE Increasing incidence with age, particularly after 55 years; a common disease of the elderly.

ETIOLOGY, PATHOGENESIS, AND PREDISPOSING FACTORS Primary: adverse biomechanical and biochemical influences affecting the joint cartilage, increased stiffness of subchondral bone, obesity; secondary: previous injury to or abnormality of the joint.

SITES INVOLVED Vertebra, hips, and knees are most often involved; Heberden's nodes commonly form about the distal interphalangeal joints, but disabling involvement of hands is uncommon.

GROSS LESIONS Late stages of the disease show eburnation of the joint surface, remodeling of the joint surface, osteophytes around the lateral margins of the joint, subchondral bone cysts, and bone sclerosis.

MICROSCOPIC LESIONS Early: loss of metachromatic staining and fibrillation of cartilage; late: loss of articular cartilage, bone resorption, irregular and variable new bone and cartilage formation.

COMPLICATIONS Pain and loss of joint mobility in hips, knees, and sometimes hands; potential disability; vertebral osteophytes may compress nerve roots to cause neuromuscular problems.

SIGNS AND SYMPTOMS Joint pain and stiffness, worse in morning, easing after activity, and becoming worse again after long exertion; Heberden's nodes at distal interphalangeal joints.

CLINICAL DIAGNOSIS AND OTHER CLINICAL FEATURES Pain affects the back, hips, and knees most commonly; there are minimal local or systemic signs of inflammation; x-rays show joint narrowing, osteophytes (spurs, lips), and subchondral bone cysts.

LABORATORY DIAGNOSIS No specific tests except negative results indicating absence of inflammatory activity and thus excluding rheumatoid arthritis; resected femoral head for hip replacement usually shows advanced disease.

PROGNOSIS Slowly progressive joint degeneration that contributes to disability in old age.

THERAPY Balance of rest and exercise; weight loss, analgesics, NSAIDs; prosthetic joint replacement.

OTHER INFORMATION The etiology of primary osteoarthritis is not understood; abnormal chondrocyte growth and function, alterations in cartilage and proteoglycans, and collagenase activation may all play a role.

Osteomalacia and Rickets

DESCRIPTION   Reduced mineralization of the osteoid organic bone matrix, caused by vitamin D deficiency and resulting in osteopenia, weak bones and, in the growing child, skeletal deformities.

DISEASE ENTITIES; SYNONYMS AND ACRONYMS   Rickets (childhood); osteomalacia (adults).

INCIDENCE   Osteomalacia complicates senile osteoporosis and renal failure; primary rickets is uncommon in US.

AGE   Rickets refers to the disease in children, osteomalacia in adults; in US, most common in elderly.

ETIOLOGY, PATHOGENESIS, AND PREDISPOSING FACTORS   Poor bone mineralization due to hypocalcemia, caused by dietary or endogenous vitamin D deficiency; malabsorption (Crohn's, sprue, cystic fibrosis); renal disease; vitamin D-resistance.

SITES INVOLVED   All bones are affected, notably their epiphyseal growth plate and osteoid seams; vitamin D acts on intestine, bone, and renal tubules in conjunction with parathyroid hormone to maintain calcium levels.

GROSS LESIONS   Rickets causes frontal bossing of skull, pigeon breast deformity, rachitic rosary, bowing of legs, lumbar lordosis, poor dentition; osteomalacia causes osteopenia similar to osteoporosis.

MICROSCOPIC LESIONS   Rickets: thickened growth plate with irregular masses of cartilage intermixed with poorly formed osteoid; hemorrhage and callus due to fractures; osteomalacia: increased thickness of osteoid seams.

COMPLICATIONS   In the child, rickets causes skeletal deformities that are lifelong; in adults, osteomalacia predisposes to hip fractures and vertebral collapse and contributes to disability and mortality.

SIGNS AND SYMPTOMS   In rickets the typical skeletal deformities are evident; other signs of malnutrition or malabsorption are likely; osteomalacia may be asymptomatic until fracture occurs.

CLINICAL DIAGNOSIS AND OTHER CLINICAL FEATURES   Rickets should be obvious; the cause needs to be identified (often malabsorption or renal failure in US); osteomalacia is difficult to differentiate from osteoporosis; they often coexist.

LABORATORY DIAGNOSIS   Serum calcium is low in severe cases; in borderline cases of osteomalacia, calcium may be normal; bone biopsy morphometry differentiates between osteoporosis and osteomalacia.

PROGNOSIS   Good if diagnosed and treated early before deformity, fractures, and disability have occurred.

THERAPY   Vitamin D supplements; combined with calcium, this supplement provides a diagnostic test.

OTHER INFORMATION   Osteomalacia and osteoporosis frequently coexist and are difficult to separate in the elderly patient; thus calcium and vitamin D supplements are reasonable to prescribe in treating osteoporosis.

Osteomyelitis

DESCRIPTION Infection of bone, produced by hematogenous spread of bacteria or by direct inoculation of bone medulla, resulting in suppuration and bone necrosis and often progressing to chronic osteomyelitis.

DISEASE ENTITIES; SYNONYMS AND ACRONYMS Acute: suppurative osteomyelitis, pyogenic or Brodie's abscess; chronic osteomyelitis, Garre's sclerosing osteomyelitis.

INCIDENCE Common complication of trauma, particularly compound fractures; hematogenous infection is uncommon.

AGE Any age when due to trauma; children are more likely to develop hematogenous infection.

ETIOLOGY, PATHOGENESIS, AND PREDISPOSING FACTORS Bacterial contamination of devitalized bone; bacteremic spread to metaphyseal vessels establishes infection that spreads in the marrow, tracks through the cortex and dissects under the periosteum.

SITES INVOLVED Ends of long bones are typical for hematogenous infection in children; vertebral bodies are more likely in adults; posttraumatic osteomyelitis affects the region of fracture or surgery (e.g., hip).

GROSS LESIONS Suppuration within marrow and along cortex under periosteum; necrotic bone (sequestrum) becomes trapped in the midst of new bone formation (involucrum); Brodie's abscess shows localized suppuration.

MICROSCOPIC LESIONS PMN exudate in marrow; bone necrosis and bone resorption; new bone formation with osteoblastic proliferation; in Garre's osteomyelitis, chronic new bone formation produces dense bone sclerosis.

COMPLICATIONS Chronic osteomyelitis; delayed fracture healing; pathologic fracture; infective arthritis; draining skin sinuses that develop squamous carcinoma; septicemia, endocarditis; amyloidosis.

SIGNS AND SYMPTOMS Pain, redness, and swelling in affected region; tenderness on palpation; fever, malaise; osteomyelitis may be occult in an infant.

CLINICAL DIAGNOSIS AND OTHER CLINICAL FEATURES Recognition of signs that may be subtle; often found during investigation of unexplained fever; x-rays show changes of bone resorption and formation; nuclear bone scans show increased uptake at site.

LABORATORY DIAGNOSIS Blood cultures are often positive for the causative organism; histologic examination may be needed in cases where tumor cannot be excluded clinically.

PROGNOSIS Good if treated early; chronic osteomyelitis may be incurable and produce lifetime disability.

THERAPY High-dose intravenous antibiotics; surgical drainage, debridement, and removal of sequestrum.

OTHER INFORMATION Microorganisms include *S. aureus, E. coli, N. gonorrhea, H. influenzae,* salmonella (sickle cell disease); anaerobes (trauma); TB osteomyelitis is granulomatous and causes Pott's disease in the spine.

Osteonecrosis

DESCRIPTION Necrosis of bone and bone marrow without infection, often involving the femoral head, due to a variety of factors causing vascular insufficiency and in many cases due to unknown mechanisms.

DISEASE ENTITIES; SYNONYMS AND ACRONYMS Avascular necrosis, aseptic necrosis; Legg-Calvé-Perthes disease, Kohler's disease.

INCIDENCE Fairly common.

AGE Depends on cause; Legg-Calvé-Perthes disease causes osteonecrosis of the femoral head in children.

ETIOLOGY, PATHOGENESIS, AND PREDISPOSING FACTORS Often idiopathic; trauma (hip fracture, surgery); embolism, thrombosis of local vessels; sickle cell disease; Gaucher's disease, gout, polycythemia; steroid therapy, radiation; decompression sickness.

SITES INVOLVED Bone; cortex, trabeculae, and marrow; may occur at any site; often involves femoral head in both adults and children; Kohler's disease is necrosis of the navicular bone.

GROSS LESIONS Pale yellow discoloration of cortex and underlying trabecular bone, often with a vague wedge shape, outlined by a hemorrhagic border; necrotic region collapses below the adjacent cortex.

MICROSCOPIC LESIONS Necrosis of bone and marrow; the latter may show saponification; repair reaction with intertrabecular fibrovascular proliferation; osteoclastic bone resorption and osteoblastic new bone formation.

COMPLICATIONS Osteoarthritis of the femoral head after collapse and healing of the necrotic subchondral bone; pathologic fracture; bone growth disturbance if epiphysis is affected in children.

SIGNS AND SYMPTOMS Pain, disability, inability to walk; bone infarcts produce some of the painful crises that are frequent in sickle cell disease.

CLINICAL DIAGNOSIS AND OTHER CLINICAL FEATURES Suspected in cases with disabling pain in the hips or other sites; may complicate hip fractures, even after repair; x-rays show radiodense region conforming to the necrotic bone.

LABORATORY DIAGNOSIS Histologic examination of resected femoral head; cause of necrosis may be evident from microscopic study; primary or metastatic tumor must be excluded.

PROGNOSIS Contributes to mortality by complicating hip fractures in elderly; causes disability.

THERAPY Immobilization, fixation; hip replacement; hydration and transfusion in sickle cell crisis.

OTHER INFORMATION Avascular necrosis is a complication of steroid therapy; however, it may occur in systemic lupus erythematosus independent of steroid therapy.

Osteoporosis

DESCRIPTION   Reduction of total skeletal mass due to increased bone resorption, results in predisposition to pathologic fracture; mpst often idiopathic (primary), associated with advancing age.

DISEASE ENTITIES; SYNONYMS AND ACRONYMS   Primary osteoporosis, senile osteoporosis, postmenopausal osteoporosis; secondary osteoporosis.

INCIDENCE   Very common, especially in thin elderly white women; contributes to 40–50,000 deaths annually.

AGE   Begins after 40–50 years, apparent 10 years after menopause; affects 15% of white women over 65.

ETIOLOGY, PATHOGENESIS, AND PREDISPOSING FACTORS   Factors contributing to primary osteoporosis: low peak skeletal mass, estrogen or androgen deficiency, physical inactivity, vitamin D and calcium deficiency, age-dependent reduction in growth hormone.

SITES INVOLVED   All bones, cortex and trabeculae, are involved; worse in vertebral bodies, femoral neck, metacarpals, proximal radius, humerus, tibia, pelvis; hip, wrist, and vertebral crush fractures are common.

GROSS LESIONS   Thin cortex; thin trabeculae and reduction in their number, resulting in increased medullary space; obvious fractures with healing and deformity; collapse of vertebral bodies with kyphoscoliosis.

MICROSCOPIC LESIONS   Thin but normally formed cortex and trabeculae; normal calcification; trabeculae very slender; microfractures and fracture healing may be evident.

COMPLICATIONS   Femoral neck (hip) fractures lead to disability and directly contribute to mortality; wrist fractures; vertebral compression fractures (crush fractures), producing spinal deformity and disability.

SIGNS AND SYMPTOMS   Back pain, loss of height, kyphoscoliosis; skeletal fracture after minor fall or other insignificant trauma; usually asymptomatic until fracture occurs.

CLINICAL DIAGNOSIS AND OTHER CLINICAL FEATURES   Predisposed patient is thin, elderly, sedentary, white woman; x-rays show osteopenia which cannot be distinguished from osteomalacia without special scans or by biopsy; fracture may be evident.

LABORATORY DIAGNOSIS   Morphometry of bone biopsy; serum calcium, phosphate, and alkaline phosphatase are normal; hyperparathyroidism, hyperthyroidism, Cushing's disease, and neoplasia (e.g., myeloma) must be excluded.

PROGNOSIS   Cannot be reversed; therapy is aimed at retarding further skeletal loss.

THERAPY   Exercise, estrogen replacement, vitamin D, and calcium; control of any underlying conditions.

OTHER INFORMATION   Causes of secondary osteoporosis include a variety of nutritional and endocrine disorders, chronic and metabolic diseases, neoplasia involving bone marrow, steroid therapy, and anticonvulsants.

Osteosarcoma

DESCRIPTION   Primary malignant neoplasm of bone that originates in the medullary cavity and invades outward; most occur during active bone growth; others develop in later years at the site of other bone disease.

DISEASE ENTITIES; SYNONYMS AND ACRONYMS   Osteogenic sarcoma; primary osteosarcoma, secondary osteosarcoma; juxtacortical (parosteal) osteosarcoma.

INCIDENCE   The most common primary bone cancer; more common in males.

AGE   Most common between 10 and 20 years; older ages develop osteosarcoma secondary to other bone diseases.

ETIOLOGY, PATHOGENESIS, AND PREDISPOSING FACTORS   Retinoblastoma gene, radiation, active bone growth; secondary osteosarcomas develop in association with Paget's disease, fibrous dysplasia, chronic osteomyelitis, multiple enchondromas, etc.

SITES INVOLVED   Usually at the metaphyseal end of long bones; most occur around the knee (lower femur, upper tibia); in older ages, osteosarcoma may develop in flat bones (skull, pelvis).

GROSS LESIONS   Firm whitish mass enlarging within the medullary cavity of the metaphysis adjacent to the epiphyseal growth plate; invades through the cortex and lifts up the periosteum to invade soft tissue.

MICROSCOPIC LESIONS   Anaplastic cells of various sizes, round or polygonal and sometimes elongated, with hyperchromatic nuclei embedded in amorphous eosinophilic osteoid; abnormal cartilage may also be present.

COMPLICATIONS   Local mass effect; pathologic fracture; metastases often occur early, usually to the lung.

SIGNS AND SYMPTOMS   Swelling, pain, and tenderness over the affected site; pathologic fracture; previous sites of chronic bone disease (e.g., Paget's disease) may develop osteosarcoma.

CLINICAL DIAGNOSIS AND OTHER CLINICAL FEATURES   X-rays are often nearly diagnostic although biopsy is required for confirmation; starburst pattern and Codman's triangle are classic x-ray signs; CT and MRI scans visualize extent of tumor invasion.

LABORATORY DIAGNOSIS   Histologic examination of biopsy tissue; identification of osteoid produced by malignant neoplastic cells is critical; alkaline phosphatase is often elevated and provides a marker for recurrences.

PROGNOSIS   Generally poor although early discovery and aggressive therapy can produce a 60% 5-year survival.

THERAPY   Surgical amputation, radiation therapy, and chemotherapy.

OTHER INFORMATION   Secondary osteosarcomas (e.g., developing in Paget's disease) are more malignant than the regular type; juxtacortical osteosarcoma develops on the periosteal surface and has a better prognosis.

Paget's Disease of Bone

DESCRIPTION   Bone disease affecting one or many bones; initial phase of bone resorption, a second phase of active bone formation plus resorption, and a final inactive phase of bone sclerosis.

DISEASE ENTITIES; SYNONYMS AND ACRONYMS   Osteitis deformans; osteolytic stage, osteolytic-osteoblastic stage, osteosclerotic stage.

INCIDENCE   Common in white populations of Northern European and English origin; rare in Africans and Asians.

AGE   Increasing incidence with age, starting after 40 years.

ETIOLOGY, PATHOGENESIS, AND PREDISPOSING FACTORS   Speculated paramyxovirus infection of osteoclasts, stimulating them to hyperplasia and bone resorption; reactive osteoblastic activity attempts bone repair, resulting in dense, abnormally formed bone.

SITES INVOLVED   In polyostotic disease, simultaneous involvement of several bones (most frequently spine, pelvis, femur, skull, tibia, and humerus); in the less common monostotic form, only a single bone is involved.

GROSS LESIONS   Affected bones show thickened cortex and trabeculae, causing reduction in medullary cavity; porosity and softening of bones are features of the early phases, increased density in the late phase.

MICROSCOPIC LESIONS   Abnormal mosaic pattern of bone trabeculae, enhanced with polarized light; large osteoclasts with numerous hyperchromatic nuclei; prominent osteoblasts, depending on phase; intertrabecular fibrosis.

COMPLICATIONS   Fractures due to abnormal bone; vertebral collapse with spinal or nerve compression; enlargement of skull with narrowing of foramen magnum; secondary osteoarthritis; osteosarcoma; heart failure.

SIGNS AND SYMPTOMS   Pain in region of affected bone; increase in head size due to enlarged skull; bowing of legs; hearing loss, visual disturbances, and other manifestations of complications; most remain asymptomatic.

CLINICAL DIAGNOSIS AND OTHER CLINICAL FEATURES   Usually diagnosed radiologically during investigation of skeletal pain; x-rays show bone thickening and focal lucency early, then irregular sclerosis in later phases; osteosarcoma develops in 1%.

LABORATORY DIAGNOSIS   Histologic examination of bone biopsy, particularly to diagnose a secondary osteosarcoma; elevated serum alkaline phosphatase; elevated urinary hydroxyproline; elevated serum calcium in early phase.

PROGNOSIS   Causes disability; mortality is infrequent unless an osteosarcoma develops.

THERAPY   Incurable; trials involve calcitonin, diphosphonates, mithramycin to suppress osteoclastic activity.

OTHER INFORMATION   Bone turnover is accelerated at least 20 times over normal; high output heart failure results from excessive vascularization of the affected bone; other sarcomas besides osteosarcoma may develop.

Polymyositis-Dermatomyositis

DESCRIPTION A group of chronic inflammatory diseases of unknown etiology involving skeletal muscle and often skin, frequently associated with autoimmune diseases or with visceral cancers.

DISEASE ENTITIES; SYNONYMS AND ACRONYMS Polymyositis, myositis, dermatomyositis.

INCIDENCE Uncommon; increased in SLE, systemic sclerosis, and Sjogren's syndrome; most common in females.

AGE Different clinical presentations occur in different ages: young women, older adults, children.

ETIOLOGY, PATHOGENESIS, AND PREDISPOSING FACTORS Presumed autoimmune etiology; many patients form antinuclear antibodies (ANAs) particularly against transfer RNA; possibly a virus (Coxsackie B) triggers the process mediated by sensitized T-cells.

SITES INVOLVED Skeletal muscle and skin; multiple other organs may be involved with vasculitis; initially involves proximal muscles of extremities (pelvic and shoulder girdles).

GROSS LESIONS Early, muscle shows edema from inflammation; with advanced disease, there is muscle atrophy and yellow discoloration; the skin rash, seen in about half of cases, shows erythema, edema, and scaling.

MICROSCOPIC LESIONS Focal or diffuse infiltrates of lymphocytes and macrophages between muscle fibers and around blood vessels; degenerating, necrotic, and regenerating fibers; in late disease there is fat replacement.

COMPLICATIONS Progressive muscle weakness with disability; dysphagia; Raynaud's phenomenon; finger stiffness due to dermal fibrosis; pulmonary fibrosis; underlying cancer in adults.

SIGNS AND SYMPTOMS Muscle pain and proximal muscle weakness that may start slowly or suddenly; typical skin rash appears as a lilac discoloration of the upper eyelids with periorbital edema and scaling of skin.

CLINICAL DIAGNOSIS AND OTHER CLINICAL FEATURES Age, sex, skin rash, pattern of involvement, and biopsy differentiate myositis from muscular dystrophies; an autoimmune disease may coexist; visceral cancer may be occult, often primary lung cancer.

LABORATORY DIAGNOSIS Muscle biopsy usually reveals the inflammatory etiology; with focal muscle involvement, changes may be nonspecific; elevated serum creatine kinase; elevated ESR; ANAs frequently present.

PROGNOSIS Progresses to disability and death without therapy; responds well to therapy.

THERAPY Corticosteroids; relapses are common and continuous long-term therapy may be required.

OTHER INFORMATION Eosinophils in the inflammatory infiltrate indicate trichinosis; eosinophilic myositis is otherwise rare; granulomas indicate sarcoidosis involving muscle if infection is excluded.

Rhabdomyosarcoma

DESCRIPTION   Primary malignant neoplasm arising within soft tissue; exhibits a variable degree of skeletal muscle differentiation.

DISEASE ENTITIES; SYNONYMS AND ACRONYMS   Classified as embryonal, botryoid, alveolar, and pleomorphic rhabdomyosarcomas.

INCIDENCE   The most common soft tissue sarcoma in children, especially the embryonal type; uncommon in adults.

AGE   Children and young adults; the pleomorphic variant occurs in older adults.

ETIOLOGY, PATHOGENESIS, AND PREDISPOSING FACTORS   Neoplastic disease of unknown etiology; since most do not arise within skeletal muscle, undifferentiated mesenchymal cells or embryonal rests of rhabdomyoblasts are likely cells of origin.

SITES INVOLVED   Head and neck, including nasopharynx and orbit; genitourinary tract, especially bladder and vagina (sites of the botryoid type); skeletal muscle of extremities (usually alveolar or pleomorphic type).

GROSS LESIONS   Fleshy red, gray, or yellow mass that is either obviously invasive or shows pseudoencapsulation; the botryoid variant exhibits soft multilobulated polypoid masses projecting from the bladder or vagina.

MICROSCOPIC LESIONS   Embryonal and botryoid: elongated strap cells with cross striations; alveolar: honeycomb fibrous septa filled with anaplastic cells; pleomorphic: large anaplastic cells with rhabdomyoblasts.

COMPLICATIONS   Invasion and compression of local structures, particularly orbit, sinuses, cervical vertebra, and pelvic organs (bladder, rectum, ureters); metastasis to viscera (lung, heart, brain, bone marrow).

SIGNS AND SYMPTOMS   Enlarging mass within the head, neck or extremities; mass of grape-like projections from vagina; urinary symptoms from urinary bladder tumor; at least a quarter have metastases at presentation.

CLINICAL DIAGNOSIS AND OTHER CLINICAL FEATURES   A likely diagnosis of a head/neck mass in a child; morphology of botryoid variant is distinctive; CT and MRI scans visualize extent of invasion; cystoscopy to diagnose bladder tumors.

LABORATORY DIAGNOSIS   Histologic examination of tumor; diagnostic cross-striations may not be evident in poorly differentiated tumors; electron microscopy and immunohistochemical stains for desmin and myoglobin are useful.

PROGNOSIS   Generally poor (median survival 3–5 years); localized tumors treated aggressively may be cured.

THERAPY   Surgical wide excision or amputation; chemotherapy; radiation therapy.

OTHER INFORMATION   The benign counterpart, rhabdomyoma, is rare and usually occurs in the heart; most cardiac rhabdomyomas occur with tuberous sclerosis and are considered hamartomas rather than neoplasms.

Rheumatoid Arthritis

DESCRIPTION An inflammatory condition, often associated with rheumatoid factor (RF); affects mainly the small joints of hands and feet; results in pain and progressive deformity and disability.

DISEASE ENTITIES; SYNONYMS AND ACRONYMS RA; rheumatoid synovitis.

INCIDENCE Common, affecting at least 1% of the population; female: male = 3:1.

AGE Usually adults in the young to middle age range; juvenile RA affects children under age 16.

ETIOLOGY, PATHOGENESIS, AND PREDISPOSING FACTORS Possibly an autoimmune disease triggered by a viral infection; linked to HLA-DW4/DRW4; RF is IgM or IgG antibody against the Fc portion of IgG; reactive synovium (pannus) causes joint destruction.

SITES INVOLVED Most often small joints of hands and feet, usually symmetric; synovium becomes inflamed and hyperplastic, forming pannus, which spreads over joint surfaces and erodes articular cartilage.

GROSS LESIONS Early: villous and hyperemic pannus covers joint surfaces, eroding cartilage; late: fibrous scarring of joint structures and periarticular tissues; fibrous or bony ankylosis may occur.

MICROSCOPIC LESIONS Early: hyperplastic highly vascular synovium containing lymphocytes, plasma cells, and lymphoid nodules constitutes pannus that invades cartilage and bone; late: fibrosis replaces normal structures.

COMPLICATIONS Early: joint immobility due to swelling and pain of acute inflammation; late: progressive joint deformity and disability due to scarring, muscle atrophy, and ankylosis; secondary osteoarthritis.

SIGNS AND SYMPTOMS Early: episodes of joint swelling and pain often with fever and malaise; late: knobby deformity of joints, ulnar deviation of fingers due to fibrosis and contraction of periarticular tissues.

CLINICAL DIAGNOSIS AND OTHER CLINICAL FEATURES Typically, recurrent acute episodes alternate with remissions, progressing over 4–5 years to a chronic "burnt-out" phase of permanent joint deformity; x-ray changes include juxta-articular osteopenia.

LABORATORY DIAGNOSIS RF is present in 80% of cases; may be present in other diseases besides RA; synovial fluid forms poor mucin clot and may contain PMNs and other inflammatory cells but is sterile on culture.

PROGNOSIS Difficult to predict; quite variable in presentation, severity, progression, and ultimate outcome.

THERAPY Aspirin, nonsteroid anti-inflammatory drugs; corticosteroids; immunosuppressive agents; gold salts.

OTHER INFORMATION Rheumatoid nodules and vasculitis complicate some cases. Variants of RA include ankylosing spondylitis, psoriatic arthritis, Reiter's syndrome, arthritis with Sjogren's syndrome, and others.

Pathology Facts, by Richard C.
Harruff, J.B. Lippincott
Company, Philadelphia © 1994.

Chapter 22

Skin

Acne

DESCRIPTION   A disorder of the pilosebaceous unit, characterized by excessive sebum production, plugging of follicles, and an inflammatory response to the contents of ruptured follicles.

DISEASE ENTITIES; SYNONYMS AND ACRONYMS   Acne vulgaris, pimples, comedones; cystic acne.

INCIDENCE   Very common; affects both sexes but usually more common in males.

AGE   Adolescence; late teenage to early adult years.

ETIOLOGY, PATHOGENESIS, AND PREDISPOSING FACTORS   Androgen stimulates excess sebum production which becomes trapped in follicle plugged with keratin; Propionibacterium acnes proliferates and causes lipolysis; follicle ruptures, causing PMN exudation.

SITES INVOLVED   Skin, sebaceous hair follicle; face, chest and back; inflammatory reaction occurs in dermis.

GROSS LESIONS   Dilated follicles with dark keratin plugs (open comedones, blackheads); follicular papules without inflammatory changes (closed comedones, whiteheads); inflammatory nodules, papules, and pustules.

MICROSCOPIC LESIONS   Noninflammatory comedones show dilated follicle distended with sebum and keratin debris; with rupture, there are intense PMN exudation and infiltrates of lymphocytes and macrophages; later, fibrosis.

COMPLICATIONS   Cosmetic disfigurement with psychological injury; dermal and subcutaneous abscesses; extensive scar formation, keloids.

SIGNS AND SYMPTOMS   Variety of lesions ranging from blackheads, papules, pustules, red nodules, dermal cysts, and scars; all types of lesions or only one type may be present; skin is oily and glistening.

CLINICAL DIAGNOSIS AND OTHER CLINICAL FEATURES   Usually obvious in a teenager presenting with typical lesions; other acneiform eruptions include reactions to steroids and other drugs, perioral dermatitis, chloracne, and acne rosacea.

LABORATORY DIAGNOSIS   Rarely requires laboratory confirmation of diagnosis.

PROGNOSIS   Usually good with therapy; condition resolves with maturity.

THERAPY   Topical benzoyl peroxide, retinoic acid; systemic tetracycline, isotretinoin.

OTHER INFORMATION   Genetic factors may be involved, autosomal dominant with variable expression or polygenic. Pathogenesis involves increased sensitivity of sebaceous glands to androgens.

Basal Cell Carcinoma

DESCRIPTION   Malignant tumor of skin arising from basal cells of epidermis; tumor is invasive, ulcerative, and locally destructive but does not metastasize.

DISEASE ENTITIES; SYNONYMS AND ACRONYMS   BCC, basal cell epithelioma, rodent ulcer.

INCIDENCE   Common; one of the most common malignant tumors of humans.

AGE   Middle age to elderly.

ETIOLOGY, PATHOGENESIS, AND PREDISPOSING FACTORS   Excessive sun exposure (but one third occur on sun-unexposed sites); light-skinned people; increased incidence with immunosuppression and in defective DNA repair syndromes (xeroderma pigmentosa).

SITES INVOLVED   Skin, sun-exposed regions; face, upper chest, upper extremities; arises from basal cell layer and invades dermis.

GROSS LESIONS   Dome-shaped papule or nodule, pearly white or pink, telangiectasia on surface; advanced lesions are centrally ulcerated with raised, rolled margins; variants are plaque-like, multifocal, or pigmented.

MICROSCOPIC LESIONS   Nests of small, uniform, basophilic cells with scant cytoplasm, surrounded by mucinous connective tissue; invasion of dermis; tumor cell nests show characteristic palisading at their periphery.

COMPLICATIONS   Ulceration and enlargement can continue indefinitely, leading to invasion of bone, facial sinuses, eye; metastasis is extremely rare.

SIGNS AND SYMPTOMS   Pearly nodule on face or other exposed site in an older person with sun-damaged skin; ulcerative lesions are painless.

CLINICAL DIAGNOSIS AND OTHER CLINICAL FEATURES   The pearly nodular lesions are usually distinctive; multifocal superficial variants may resemble eczema or keratosis; pigmented variant resembles nevus or melanoma; excision for diagnosis and cure.

LABORATORY DIAGNOSIS   Histologic examination of excised lesion; margin of clear normal tissue needs to be confirmed microscopically; Moh's procedure involves microscopic examination of tumor excised by layers.

PROGNOSIS   Good; usually cured by excision; invasion of orbit or bone can lead to poor outcome.

THERAPY   Excision; Moh's microscopic controlled surgery for recurrent tumors and those invading around eye.

OTHER INFORMATION   In the autosomal dominant basal cell nevus syndrome, numerous basal cell carcinomas develop at an early age in association with skeletal and other abnormalities.

Contact Dermatitis

DESCRIPTION   An acute or chronic skin inflammation caused by exposure to a chemical, physical, or biologic agent; inflammation may be caused by an irritant action or by allergic mechanisms.

DISEASE ENTITIES; SYNONYMS AND ACRONYMS   Allergic contact dermatitis; irritant contact dermatitis; eczematous contact dermatitis; poison ivy.

INCIDENCE   Common; one of the most common skin diseases; 20% are allergic contact dermatitis.

AGE   Any age; in elderly, pattern of reaction is different and more likely of the irritant type.

ETIOLOGY, PATHOGENESIS, AND PREDISPOSING FACTORS   Delayed hypersensitivity; hapten of allergen binds to Langerhans cells that sensitize T-cells; these proliferate and mediate inflammation; irritant dermatitis predisposes to allergic dermatitis.

SITES INVOLVED   Skin; depends on area of exposure and thickness of skin; thin skin is more sensitive; cornified skin is resistant; face, eyelids; forearms, hands; feet, ankles; trunk; intertriginous regions.

GROSS LESIONS   Acute stage: eczematous dermatitis with papules, oozing vesicles, crusted erythematous lesions, occasionally bullae; chronic: thickened skin, scales, fissure, pigmentation changes.

MICROSCOPIC LESIONS   Edema of dermis and epidermis; intraepidermal edema separates squamous cells (spongiosis); infiltrate of lymphocytes, macrophages and eosinophils; chronic: epidermal hyperplasia and hyperkeratosis.

COMPLICATIONS   Widespread involvement; exfoliative dermatitis; secondary infection.

SIGNS AND SYMPTOMS   Acute: intense pruritis with red vesicles appearing 1–2 days after exposure in previously sensitized person, often identified as poison ivy; chronic: scaly thickened skin in sites of exposure.

CLINICAL DIAGNOSIS AND OTHER CLINICAL FEATURES   History, physical examination for clues of exposure; inquiries about occupation, hobbies, clothing, jewelry, cosmetics, fingernails, drug therapy; patch tests to attempt identification of allergen.

LABORATORY DIAGNOSIS   Histologic examination of biopsied skin, which is rarely needed for the acute form but may be necessary for chronic contact dermatitis.

PROGNOSIS   Good; acute lesions resolve in 3 weeks; chronic lesions persist until removal of agent.

THERAPY   Cool compresses; zinc oxide mixtures; topical anesthetics; steroids, topical or sometimes systemic.

OTHER INFORMATION   Common causes of allergic contact dermatitis are toxicodendron (poison ivy), paraphenylenediamine, nickel, rubber, acrylic nails, formalin, cosmetics and perfumes, epoxy, shoe leather constituents.

Dermatitis Herpetiformis

DESCRIPTION A vesicular and urticarial skin disease associated with gluten-sensitivity enteropathy and IgA immune complexes deposited in dermal papillae; blisters form at the dermal-epidermal interface.

DISEASE ENTITIES; SYNONYMS AND ACRONYMS Celiac disease, sprue, gluten-sensitivity enteropathy.

INCIDENCE Rare; most common in white males.

AGE Any age after weaning; most common in middle ages; onset usually from 20–40 years.

ETIOLOGY, PATHOGENESIS, AND PREDISPOSING FACTORS Gluten-sensitivity enteropathy; HLA-B8/DRW3; gluten/gliadin pass from intestine into blood and complex with IgA antibodies at tips of dermal papillae; lytic PMN enzymes cleave epidermis from dermis.

SITES INVOLVED Skin, preferentially extensor surfaces; elbows, knees, scapular, and sacral regions of back; lesions tend to be symmetric; disruption occurs in the dermis, under the basement membrane zone.

GROSS LESIONS Polymorphous erythematous lesions: papules, urticarial plaques, small vesicles, larger bullae; lesions cluster in groups (like herpes); excoriation produces crusted ulcers.

MICROSCOPIC LESIONS Dense aggregates of PMNs at tips of dermal papillae; detachment of the epidermis from the dermal papillae; rete ridges remain attached in the dermis; eosinophils are present in late lesions.

COMPLICATIONS Secondary infection; scarring; hyperpigmentation; celiac disease causes malabsorption and may develop intestinal lymphoma.

SIGNS AND SYMPTOMS Groups of lesions that appear similar to herpes vesicles; intensely pruritic and patients may scratch the lesions so that they present as crusted ulcers; malabsorption may be apparent or subclinical.

CLINICAL DIAGNOSIS AND OTHER CLINICAL FEATURES Recognition of pruritic vesicular dermatitis that is often associated with gastrointestinal disease; response to gluten-free diet; prompt response to therapeutic agents; skin biopsy.

LABORATORY DIAGNOSIS Histologic examination of skin biopsy; microabscesses at the tips of dermal papillae are distinctive; immunofluorescence shows granular IgA at tips of papillae; HLA typing; small bowel biopsy.

PROGNOSIS Responds rapidly to therapy.

THERAPY Avoidance of gluten; dapsone, sulfapyridine.

OTHER INFORMATION T-cells that normally function to remove circulating immune complexes may be deficient in the HLA-B8/DWR3 haplotype, predisposing individuals to develop immune complex tissue damage.

Erythema Nodosum

DESCRIPTION   An inflammatory reaction occurring in the subcutaneous fibroadipose tissue, resulting in raised tender nodules; associated with certain infections and reactions to drugs.

DISEASE ENTITIES; SYNONYMS AND ACRONYMS   Panniculitis, septal panniculitis; drug eruption.

INCIDENCE   Fairly common; more common in women.

AGE   Most common between 20 and 30 years.

ETIOLOGY, PATHOGENESIS, AND PREDISPOSING FACTORS   Infectious causes: streptococcal upper respiratory infections, TB, fungal infections; noninfectious: drugs (sulfonamides, oral contraceptives), sarcoidosis, inflammatory bowel disease.

SITES INVOLVED   Skin, subcutaneous tissue; inflammation involves the septa of subcutaneous fat; most common on anterior part of lower legs.

GROSS LESIONS   Erythematous nodules within the skin; multiple lesions appear in crops; nodules resolve to leave a bruised region that eventually fades.

MICROSCOPIC LESIONS   Early: PMNs, fibrin, and edema involving septa of fat lobules; later: lymphocytes, granulomas with giant cells, degeneration of collagen, fibrosis of septa, occasional eosinophils.

COMPLICATIONS   Systemic symptoms are usually not clinically significant; erythema nodosum is often associated with a serious infection.

SIGNS AND SYMPTOMS   Tender, raised skin nodules over the anterior lower legs, erupting in successive groups; fever, malaise, and arthralgia often accompany the eruption.

CLINICAL DIAGNOSIS AND OTHER CLINICAL FEATURES   Recognition of painful skin nodules; evaluation is directed toward exclusion of infectious disease and identification of drug causing the reaction; deep skin biopsy.

LABORATORY DIAGNOSIS   Histologic examination of skin biopsy; biopsy must be deep enough to include subcutaneous fat; cultures and special stains to exclude infectious granuloma.

PROGNOSIS   Good; usually resolves in 3–6 weeks.

THERAPY   Avoidance of offending drug; treatment of infection; potassium iodide.

OTHER INFORMATION   Other forms of panniculitis include erythema induratum, which originates as a vasculitis, and Weber-Christian disease (relapsing febrile nodular panniculitis).

Kaposi's Sarcoma

DESCRIPTION Malignant neoplasm originating in the skin, characterized by abnormal vascular proliferation and associated most commonly with AIDS.

DISEASE ENTITIES; SYNONYMS AND ACRONYMS Kaposi's sarcoma associated with AIDS; classical Kaposi's sarcoma, non-AIDS type.

INCIDENCE AIDS type: common; about 20% of AIDS patients develop Kaposi's sarcoma; non-AIDS type: rare.

AGE AIDS type: young adult male homosexual; non-AIDS type: elderly male.

ETIOLOGY, PATHOGENESIS, AND PREDISPOSING FACTORS Undetermined agent, possibly virus, stimulates neoplastic proliferation of vascular tissue throughout thickness of skin.

SITES INVOLVED Skin, predominantly dermis; non-AIDS type: mostly on the lower extremities; AIDS type: multiple lesions on several sites of skin and oral mucosa; dissemination to internal organs.

GROSS LESIONS Red to blue or brown macules, papules, plaques, and nodules; ranging in size from few mm to several cm.

MICROSCOPIC LESIONS Cellular mass of spindle cells with slit-like spaces containing red cells; in subtle forms, spindle cells interdigitate among dermal collagen bands; hemosiderin and inflammatory cells are present.

COMPLICATIONS AIDS type is aggressive and spreads widely to all organs; GI bleeding; organ dysfunction; cachexia; opportunistic infections develop due to AIDS.

SIGNS AND SYMPTOMS Multicentric discolored lesions in a patient with proven HIV infection or within a high-risk group.

CLINICAL DIAGNOSIS AND OTHER CLINICAL FEATURES Recognition of lesions in a predisposed individual; lesions may first appear like bruises; skin biopsy to confirm diagnosis.

LABORATORY DIAGNOSIS Histologic examination of skin biopsy; early lesions are difficult to diagnose.

PROGNOSIS With the AIDS type, poor.

THERAPY Treatment of AIDS; chemotherapy.

OTHER INFORMATION The non-AIDS type affects elderly men, Ashkenazi Jews and Africans; the disease is not as aggressive as with the AIDS type.

Lichen Planus

DESCRIPTION   A self-limited inflammatory skin disease characterized by violaceous, flat-topped, polygonal papules, often on the flexor aspect of wrist and forearms, and a distinctive lymphocytic dermal infiltrate.

DISEASE ENTITIES; SYNONYMS AND ACRONYMS   Lichen planopilaris.

INCIDENCE   Fairly common.

AGE   Mostly middle age; 30–70 years.

ETIOLOGY, PATHOGENESIS, AND PREDISPOSING FACTORS   Undefined alteration of the basal cell layer leading to humoral and cell-mediated immune reaction; associated with other immune diseases and with certain drugs.

SITES INVOLVED   Skin; flexor aspects of wrists and forearms are characteristic; sacrum, medial thighs, genitalia, lower extremities; oral mucosa; lichen planopilaris affects hair follicles to cause alopecia.

GROSS LESIONS   Flat-topped, violaceous papules, without scale, that may coalesce to form plaques and nodules; tiny white dots or lines on papules (Wickham's striae); white net-like pattern of lesions on oral mucosa.

MICROSCOPIC LESIONS   Dense band-like (lichenoid) lymphocytic infiltrate within upper dermis, obscuring the dermal-epidermal interface; saw-tooth pattern of rete ridges; degeneration of basal cells with fibrillary bodies.

COMPLICATIONS   Scarring, postinflammatory hyperpigmentation; cicatricial alopecia; development of carcinoma at sites of chronic mucosal lichen planus.

SIGNS AND SYMPTOMS   Polygonal, purple, flat-topped papules and plaques that are usually pruritic, located most characteristically on ventral wrists; lesions may develop at sites of trauma (Kobner's phenomenon).

CLINICAL DIAGNOSIS AND OTHER CLINICAL FEATURES   Recognition of characteristic pruritic lesions at typical sites; may be associated with certain drugs and diseases mediated by immune mechanisms (e.g., ulcerative colitis, primary biliary cirrhosis).

LABORATORY DIAGNOSIS   Histologic examination of skin biopsy; band of lymphocytes and degeneration of basal cell layer are most characteristic; epidermal thickening and hyperkeratosis occur in chronic lesions.

PROGNOSIS   Good; most acute lesions resolve within 1–2 years; chronic lesions persist up to 10 years.

THERAPY   Steroids, topical or systemic; isotretinoin; photochemotherapy; antipruritics.

OTHER INFORMATION   The band-like infiltrate of lymphocytes is so distinctive that the term "lichenoid" is used to describe this pattern in other diseases.

Lupus Erythematosus

DESCRIPTION   A chronic autoimmune disease with a variety of autoantibodies; in systemic lupus, there is multisystem organ involvement; in cutaneous (discoid) lupus, only the skin is involved.

DISEASE ENTITIES; SYNONYMS AND ACRONYMS   Discoid lupus erythematosus, DLE; cutaneous lupus erythematosus; systemic lupus erythematosus, SLE.

INCIDENCE   Fairly common; most commonly affects white women.

AGE   Young adult to middle age.

ETIOLOGY, PATHOGENESIS, AND PREDISPOSING FACTORS   Autoimmune disease associated with antinuclear autoantibodies; immune complexes are formed and deposited along the basement membrane, producing injury to the basal cell layer.

SITES INVOLVED   Skin; face and scalp with DLE; malar "butterfly rash" on the face with SLE; upper chest, back, and arms in a few cases; immune complexes are deposited in a band along the basement membrane zone.

GROSS LESIONS   DLE: raised, erythematous, well-demarcated, scaly discoid plaques with hyperkeratotic margins and depigmented center; SLE: diffuse erythematous rash, typically over cheeks of face.

MICROSCOPIC LESIONS   Vacuolization of basal cell layer; thickened basement membrane; thinned epidermis, loss of rete ridges; keratin plugs in follicles; lymphocyte infiltrates at dermal-epidermal border and deep dermis.

COMPLICATIONS   Disfiguring scar formation with the discoid lesions; cicatricial alopecia; follicular plugging, telangiectasia, atrophy of skin, depigmentation; a small proportion of DLE will develop SLE.

SIGNS AND SYMPTOMS   DLE: raised, papular, erythematous, scaly, disc-like plaques on face and sun-exposed upper body that progress to atrophic hypopigmented scars; alopecia. SLE: erythematous rash rather than discoid.

CLINICAL DIAGNOSIS AND OTHER CLINICAL FEATURES   DLE is recognized by the skin lesions without systemic involvement; SLE skin lesions are often less apparent than in DLE but may be identical; photosensitivity is common.

LABORATORY DIAGNOSIS   Histology of skin biopsy; basal layer vacuolization and dermal lymphocyte infiltrates are characteristic; immunofluorescence shows granular immune deposits along basement membrane (lupus band test).

PROGNOSIS   DLE: chronic, disfiguring but not life-threatening; SLE: chronic, progressive, high mortality.

THERAPY   DLE: steroids, topical or intralesional; SLE: systemic steroids, immunosuppressive therapy.

OTHER INFORMATION   Important lesions of SLE involve kidney; anti–double-stranded DNA favors systemic involvement; anti-ribonucleoprotein favors skin photosensitivity; most DLE patients have no autoantibodies in serum.

Malignant Melanoma

DESCRIPTION   Malignant tumor of melanocytes, which show radial and vertical growth patterns within the skin; radial growth is characteristic of spreading types and vertical growth characterizes nodular melanoma.

DISEASE ENTITIES; SYNONYMS AND ACRONYMS   Superficial spreading melanoma, nodular melanoma, lentigo maligna melanoma, acral lentiginous melanoma.

INCIDENCE   Fairly common in whites; uncommon in blacks; superficial spreading type is the most common.

AGE   Most common between 30 and 60 years; median 50 years.

ETIOLOGY, PATHOGENESIS, AND PREDISPOSING FACTORS   Excessive sun exposure on sensitive white skin; hereditary factors; dysplastic nevus or changing nevus; congenital giant nevus.

SITES INVOLVED   Sun-exposed skin; upper back in men, back and legs in women; acral lentiginous melanoma, the most common type in blacks, involves palmar, plantar, subungal, and mucosal sites.

GROSS LESIONS   Superficial spreading: larger than 10 mm, irregular border, and pigmentation; nodular type: elevated lesion from skin surface with irregular pigmentation, often arising from superficial spreading type.

MICROSCOPIC LESIONS   Superficial: large atypical variably pigmented cells in epidermis and papillary dermis, lymphocytic reaction; nodular: masses of tumor cells forming nodule in dermis and invading deeper dermis.

COMPLICATIONS   Metastatic melanoma; spreads first to regional lymph nodes, then hematogenous metastasis to all organs.

SIGNS AND SYMPTOMS   Change in a pre-existing skin lesion; itching or tenderness; rapidly growing irregular pigmented lesion; surface crusting or ulceration; pigmented lesion on sole of foot, palm, or under nail.

CLINICAL DIAGNOSIS AND OTHER CLINICAL FEATURES   Suspicious features are asymmetry; irregular border; uneven color with pink or light blue areas; flat ones indicate radial growth phase; nodular ones are in vertical growth phase; excisional biopsy.

LABORATORY DIAGNOSIS   Histologic examination of excised lesion; Clark's level of invasion and total thickness of lesion are important for prognosis.

PROGNOSIS   Good if excised in radial growth phase; poor for nodular growth; 75% mortality if thicker than 4 mm.

THERAPY   Excision with wide margin; regional lymph node dissection; chemotherapy, immunotherapy.

OTHER INFORMATION   Clark level I: epidermis above basement membrane; II: within normal papillary dermis; III: expansion of papillary dermis; III: reticular dermis invasion; V: invasion into fat.

Melanocytic Nevus

DESCRIPTION   Benign neoplasm of melanocytic cells in the skin, classified as junctional nevus, compound nevus, and dermal nevus.

DISEASE ENTITIES; SYNONYMS AND ACRONYMS   Nevus; mole; nevocellular nevus; acquired nevus.

INCIDENCE   Very common; the average person has several nevi.

AGE   Nevi arise during childhood, enlarge until adulthood, mature, and disappear with age.

ETIOLOGY, PATHOGENESIS, AND PREDISPOSING FACTORS   Sunlight stimulates melanocyte hyperplasia (lentigo) that progresses to neoplasm at the base of the epithelium; with further progression the neoplastic cells migrate and proliferate within the dermis.

SITES INVOLVED   Skin; particularly on sun-exposed surfaces of the body.

GROSS LESIONS   Brownish macule or slightly raised nodule; circular or oval, with regular smooth margins and even pigmentation; usually less than 6 mm in diameter.

MICROSCOPIC LESIONS   Nevus cells are small regular, finely pigmented cells forming nests at tips of rete ridges in junctional nevus; dermal masses of nevus cells in dermal nevus; nests and dermal masses in compound nevus.

COMPLICATIONS   Uncommon; a nevus may occasionally be cosmetically undesirable or becomes subject to trauma or irritation; dysplastic nevi are likely to progress to malignant melanoma.

SIGNS AND SYMPTOMS   Skin lesion of variable appearance; flat, dome-shaped, pedunculated; skin-colored, brown or black; hairy or hairless.

CLINICAL DIAGNOSIS AND OTHER CLINICAL FEATURES   Usually obvious from gross inspection; to be differentiated from ephelis (freckle), wart, seborrheic keratosis, lentigo, skin tag, and malignant melanoma; excisional biopsy for suspicious lesions.

LABORATORY DIAGNOSIS   Histologic examination of lesion; benign nevi show orderly junctional nests (if there is a junctional component), maturation of intradermal nevus cell growth pattern, and no cytologic atypia.

PROGNOSIS   Good for ordinary melanocytic nevi.

THERAPY   Usually not required; excision for cosmetic purposes or to evaluate suspicious lesions.

OTHER INFORMATION   Dysplastic nevus shows cytologic atypia and abnormal growth pattern; other types of nevi: congenital giant pigmented nevus, blue nevus, halo nevus, and Spitz nevus.

Mycosis Fungoides

DESCRIPTION   Malignant lymphoma primarily involving the skin that later spreads to lymph nodes, blood, and internal organs; the disseminated form is called Sézary syndrome.

DISEASE ENTITIES; SYNONYMS AND ACRONYMS   Cutaneous T-cell lymphoma; Sézary syndrome.

INCIDENCE   Uncommon.

AGE   Middle age; usually in the 40s.

ETIOLOGY, PATHOGENESIS, AND PREDISPOSING FACTORS   Neoplastic proliferation of helper/inducer T-cells invade the epidermis and upper dermis; progression leads to dissemination; some evidence indicates the etiology may involve a retrovirus.

SITES INVOLVED   Skin, epidermis, and dermis; one or several areas may be involved; with dissemination, Sézary syndrome involves blood, lymph nodes, and organs.

GROSS LESIONS   Early: red, scaly, eczematous patches, progressing to elevated plaques; late: red-brown cutaneous tumor nodules, which may ulcerate and become secondarily infected.

MICROSCOPIC LESIONS   Band of lymphocytes in the upper dermis; invasion of epidermis (epidermotropism); intraepidermal clusters of lymphocytes (Pautrier's microabscesses); cells have hyperconvoluted nuclei (Sézary cells).

COMPLICATIONS   Dissemination throughout blood, lymph nodes, and internal organs with organ system failure, infections, and cachexia.

SIGNS AND SYMPTOMS   Initially, scaly plaques resemble chronic dermatitis; later, plaques develop; pruritis is often intense; discolored tumor nodules develop in advanced cases; erythroderma characterizes Sézary syndrome.

CLINICAL DIAGNOSIS AND OTHER CLINICAL FEATURES   Several years elapse between initial skin lesions and confirmation of diagnosis; usually mistaken for chronic dermatitis or psoriasis; multiple skin biopsies are often required for diagnosis.

LABORATORY DIAGNOSIS   Histologic examination of skin biopsy; dermal infiltrate is usually polymorphous and nonspecific; atypical lymphocytes are found in Pautrier's microabscesses in the epidermis.

PROGNOSIS   Poor; median survival after diagnosis is less than 5 years; long-term remissions with therapy.

THERAPY   Topical chemotherapy; electron beam radiation therapy; photochemotherapy.

OTHER INFORMATION   Epidermotropism is a characteristic property of the neoplastic cells; as the tumor progresses, this property is lost, leading to tumor nodules and hematogenous and lymphatic dissemination.

Pemphigus

DESCRIPTION   A bullous skin disease produced by dyshesion (acantholysis) of epidermal cells, caused by autoantibodies to surface antigens of squamous cells; blisters form within the epidermis (suprabasal bullae).

DISEASE ENTITIES; SYNONYMS AND ACRONYMS   Pemphigus vulgaris, pemphigus vegetans, pemphigus foliaceous, pemphigus erythematosus.

INCIDENCE   Altogether rare; pemphigus vulgaris is the most common type.

AGE   Peak age range 30–50 years.

ETIOLOGY, PATHOGENESIS, AND PREDISPOSING FACTORS   Autoantibodies to a non–species-specific antigen on the surface of squamous cells causes dissolution of the intercellular attachments, possibly mediated by activation of plasmin protease.

SITES INVOLVED   Skin and mucosa; scalp, face, axilla, groin, trunk; pressure points; oral, esophageal, vaginal mucosa; oral lesions may precede skin lesions by months; bullae are intradermal.

GROSS LESIONS   Initially there are bullae filled with clear fluid; these break easily to leave erosions and superficial crusted ulcers that heal without significant scarring.

MICROSCOPIC LESIONS   Separation between epidermal cells (acantholysis); acantholytic cells are rounded and detached from other cells; dyshesion may extend into adnexa; mixed inflammatory infiltrate in upper dermis.

COMPLICATIONS   Denudation of large regions of skin can cause fluid and protein loss, electrolyte disturbances, and hypovolemic shock; secondary bacterial infections of denuded areas; hyperpigmentation with healing.

SIGNS AND SYMPTOMS   Large skin bullae on many skin sites, often extensive; erosions and superficial ulcers; mucosal lesions present as ulcers, often well in advance of the skin involvement.

CLINICAL DIAGNOSIS AND OTHER CLINICAL FEATURES   Recognition of bullous skin disease; categorization by skin biopsy; intact skin is easily dislodged by rubbing (Nikolsky's sign); often associated with another autoimmune disease or thymoma.

LABORATORY DIAGNOSIS   Histologic examination of skin biopsy; immunofluorescence shows IgG localization on the surface of epidermal cells, appearing as a net-like pattern; antibodies to intercellular substance in serum.

PROGNOSIS   Often fatal without therapy; controllable with steroids but side effects occur from therapy.

THERAPY   High-dose systemic steroids; methotrexate, azathioprine, gold; plasmapheresis.

OTHER INFORMATION   In bullous pemphigoid, bullae are subepidermal; immunofluorescence is linear along the basement membrane; autoantibody reacts with antigen in the lamina lucida below the basal cell layer.

Psoriasis

DESCRIPTION   A chronic skin disease that is often familial, characterized by reddened and scaly plaques occurring predominantly over dorsal and extensor surfaces.

DISEASE ENTITIES; SYNONYMS AND ACRONYMS   Pustular psoriasis; erythroderma; psoriatic arthritis.

INCIDENCE   Common; affects 1–2% of the population.

AGE   Any age; usually adults; average age at onset is in the late 20s.

ETIOLOGY, PATHOGENESIS, AND PREDISPOSING FACTORS   Exaggerated and persistent epidermal proliferation and PMN exudation in response to minor trauma; physical injury, infection, and sunlight induce lesions; genetic factors; severe cases occur in AIDS.

SITES INVOLVED   Most commonly involves skin over the dorsal extensor surfaces; elbows, knees, scalp, lumbosacral region, intergluteal cleft, glans penis; epidermis and upper dermis are involved.

GROSS LESIONS   Well-demarcated erythematous plaques covered by silver-white scales; usually 4–5 cm in diameter, sometimes much larger; erythroderma refers to whole body erythema; pustular psoriasis forms pustules.

MICROSCOPIC LESIONS   Epidermal thickening; parakeratosis; elongation of rete ridges; prominent venules in dermal papillae; PMN aggregates in upper epidermis (Monro's microabscesses); mononuclear infiltrates in dermis.

COMPLICATIONS   Pustular psoriasis can cause life-threatening disease with secondary infections and fluid loss; psoriatic arthritis is a deforming arthritis similar to rheumatoid arthritis.

SIGNS AND SYMPTOMS   Geographic scaly erythematous plaques over extensor surfaces: elbows, knees; scalp and trunk lesions; pitting of nails, discoloration, separation of nail plate (onycholysis); fever with pustular type.

CLINICAL DIAGNOSIS AND OTHER CLINICAL FEATURES   Recognition of typical lesions; punctate bleeding occurs when scales are scraped off (Auspitz sign); symmetric distribution of lesions; nail changes (pitting) is fairly specific.

LABORATORY DIAGNOSIS   Histologic examination of skin biopsy; certain other skin diseases may appear psoriasiform (seborrheic dermatitis, lichen simplex chronicus, and mycosis fungoides).

PROGNOSIS   Persistent chronic skin disease that can be successfully controlled in most cases.

THERAPY   Topical steroids, tar; psoralen and UV phototherapy (PUVA); methotrexate; etretinate; cyclosporine.

OTHER INFORMATION   Kobner response is the development of psoriasis at sites of injury. Variants of psoriasis: guttate, seborrheic, pustular, photosensitive, psoriatic erythroderma, Reiter's disease.

Squamous Cell Carcinoma

DESCRIPTION Primary malignant tumor of skin arising from keratinocytes, invading the dermis, and occasionally metastasizing to regional lymph nodes and distant sites.

DISEASE ENTITIES; SYNONYMS AND ACRONYMS Epidermoid carcinoma.

INCIDENCE Second most common skin cancer; more common in males.

AGE Most common in elderly.

ETIOLOGY, PATHOGENESIS, AND PREDISPOSING FACTORS UV radiation of sunlight (actinic radiation) causing DNA damage; chronic ulcers, draining osteomyelitis, burn scars; arsenic; ionizing radiation; industrial carcinogens; xeroderma pigmentosa.

SITES INVOLVED Skin, arising from squamous cells of epidermis, invading dermis; sun-exposed regions; face, especially scalp, ears, and lower lip; hands; areas of draining osteomyelitis, chronic ulcers, or burn sites.

GROSS LESIONS Premalignant and in situ lesions appear as keratotic, scaly, red plaques; invasive lesions are red, raised nodules that ulcerate and become necrotic centrally and have an indurated border.

MICROSCOPIC LESIONS Most are well differentiated squamous cell carcinomas with abundant keratinization in the form of horn pearls; others are poorly differentiated or anaplastic.

COMPLICATIONS Local invasion and destruction of underlying tissues; potential for metastasis is variable: 3% for cutaneous; 11% for mucocutaneous; 10–30% for those arising in ulcers, scars, or draining fistulas.

SIGNS AND SYMPTOMS Progressively enlarging and centrally ulcerating lesion that arises in sun-exposed site or chronic inflammatory process; lymph nodes draining the region may be enlarged.

CLINICAL DIAGNOSIS AND OTHER CLINICAL FEATURES Recognition of enlarging and ulcerative tumor; differentiated from basal cell carcinoma by its absence of pearly surface; rapidly growing tumors are usually keratoacanthoma; evaluation of lymph nodes.

LABORATORY DIAGNOSIS Histologic examination of excision or biopsy; tissue from central necrotic area may not be adequate for diagnosis; biopsy needs to be sufficiently deep to evaluate invasion.

PROGNOSIS Good, if excised early; overall, 5% metastasize and produce fatality.

THERAPY Complete excision, radiation therapy, Moh's microscopic controlled surgery.

OTHER INFORMATION Premalignant lesions are: actinic (solar) keratosis, leukoplakia, and Bowen's disease; keratoacanthoma is a rapidly growing tumor resembling squamous carcinoma that usually resolves spontaneously.

Urticaria

DESCRIPTION Pruritic skin wheals produced by localized dermal edema due to mast cell degranulation; in the variant angioedema, there is edema in the subcutaneous tissue as well as the dermis.

DISEASE ENTITIES; SYNONYMS AND ACRONYMS Hives; angioedema; hereditary angioneurotic edema or angioedema, HANE or HAE.

INCIDENCE Urticaria is common; affects at least 20% of the population at some time during their life.

AGE Acute urticaria: young males and females; chronic urticaria: women aged 30–50 years.

ETIOLOGY, PATHOGENESIS, AND PREDISPOSING FACTORS IgE-dependent reactions with allergens causing mast cell degranulation to release histamine, which increases vascular permeability; also IgE-independent reactions (drugs, physical contact, cold).

SITES INVOLVED Skin; dermis in urticaria, subcutaneous tissue and dermis in angioedema; lesions are most common at sites exposed to pressure; in anaphylaxis, generalized urticaria occurs with laryngeal edema.

GROSS LESIONS Raised papules and plaque-like wheals with a geographic border; linear or oval; up to many cm in diameter; reddish on light skin; in dermographism, wheals correspond to pressure strokes on the skin.

MICROSCOPIC LESIONS Acute lesions show wide separation of dermal collagen fibers, dilatation of lymphatics and venules; chronic lesions show an infiltrate of lymphocytes and eosinophils; vasculitis may be present.

COMPLICATIONS Urticaria may be part of systemic anaphylaxis, in which laryngeal edema, bronchospasm, and shock can be fatal; angioedema also may be complicated by laryngeal edema.

SIGNS AND SYMPTOMS Rapid appearance of numerous reddish pruritic wheals (hives) involving large areas of skin or localized to areas compressed by clothing; usually resolve within 24 hours but may persist for weeks.

CLINICAL DIAGNOSIS AND OTHER CLINICAL FEATURES Recognition of hives is easy; identification of cause requires consideration of allergies, clothing, pets, plants, unusual foods, laundry products, drugs, physical contact, fungal infections, stress.

LABORATORY DIAGNOSIS CBC with differential may show eosinophilia; elevations of IgE can be assessed with RAST test; cold agglutinins, cryofibrinogens, and cold agglutinins are associated with familial cold urticaria.

PROGNOSIS Good; lesions usually resolve completely; chronic urticaria is associated with fungal infections.

THERAPY Avoidance of cause; sympathomimetics (epinephrine), antihistamines, steroids; treatment of fungus.

OTHER INFORMATION HAE is due to autosomal dominant deficiency of activated C1 inhibitor, which results in intravascular activation of complement; acquired angioedema is often associated with lymphoid tumors.

Pathology Facts, by Richard C. Harruff, J.B. Lippincott Company, Philadelphia © 1994.

Chapter 23

Nervous System

Alzheimer's Disease

DESCRIPTION   A degenerative neurologic disease causing chronic dementia, characterized by cerebral atrophy, senile (neuritic) plaques, neurofibrillary tangles, granulovacuolar degeneration, and Hirano bodies.

DISEASE ENTITIES; SYNONYMS AND ACRONYMS   Presenile dementia; dementia of Alzheimer type.

INCIDENCE   The most common cause of dementia; affects up to 2 million people; causes 100,000 deaths per year.

AGE   Increasing incidence with age after 50 years; familial cases generally present earlier.

ETIOLOGY, PATHOGENESIS, AND PREDISPOSING FACTORS   Neuronal degeneration, cause unknown; research implicates abnormal metabolism of a precursor protein that leads to deposits of beta-amyloid in plaques and reduction in choline acetyltransferase.

SITES INVOLVED   Brain, cerebral cortex; temporal lobes, hippocampus, and amygdala; also frontal and parietal lobes; chromosome 21 carries genes for familial cases, beta-amyloid precursor protein, and Down's syndrome.

GROSS LESIONS   Cerebral cortex shows variable degrees of atrophy; sulci are widened and gyri narrowed; ventricles are dilated; brain often weighs less that 1000 g.

MICROSCOPIC LESIONS   Depletion of neurons; large neuritic plaques in cortex, neurofibrillary tangles in degenerating neurons; granulovacuolar degeneration of neurons; Hirano bodies are eosinophilic globs in dendrites.

COMPLICATIONS   Dementia; progressive neurologic deterioration; inability to care for self; disorientation, confusion; terminally there is wasting; bronchopneumonia usually causes death.

SIGNS AND SYMPTOMS   Initially there may be behavioral changes, depression, loss of sociability; intellectual function and judgment deteriorate; memory loss begins with recent knowledge, then past memories fade.

CLINICAL DIAGNOSIS AND OTHER CLINICAL FEATURES   Memory loss is a prominent sign; most patients are demented at presentation; differential includes cerebrovascular disease, Pick's disease, encephalitis, and Creutzfeldt-Jacob disease.

LABORATORY DIAGNOSIS   No specific antemortem test; postmortem confirmation of clinical diagnosis requires brain examination; plaques and neurofibrillary tangles are best demonstrated with silver or immunoperoxidase stains.

PROGNOSIS   Poor; progressive neurologic deterioration occurs over 3–8 years.

THERAPY   Supportive; usually long-term nursing home care; cholinergic drugs appear to have little benefit.

OTHER INFORMATION   Patients with Down's syndrome invariably develop Alzheimer type dementia after age 45. Amyloid (congophilic) angiopathy is highly associated with Alzheimer's disease.

Brain Abscess

DESCRIPTION Localized collection of purulence with suppurative necrosis of parenchyma; infective organisms are usually mixed and include anaerobes (especially Bacteroides) and aerobes (Staphylococcus, Streptococcus)

DISEASE ENTITIES; SYNONYMS AND ACRONYMS Necrotizing cerebritis; ventriculitis.

INCIDENCE Not common except in predisposed patients.

AGE Any age; peak in childhood and middle adulthood; less common in elderly and rare in infancy.

ETIOLOGY, PATHOGENESIS, AND PREDISPOSING FACTORS Hematogenous spread from another infection (bronchiectasis, endocarditis); contiguous spread from adjacent infection (chronic otitis media, mastoiditis, sinusitis); direct implantation from trauma.

SITES INVOLVED Brain, initially in subcortical white matter; progresses inwardly; temporal lobe abscesses are usually otogenous; parietal lobe abscesses, hematogenous; frontal lobe abscesses, from sinusitis.

GROSS LESIONS Cavity filled with thick liquefied pus, surrounded by a fibrous capsule of variable thickness; edema in brain around abscess; lesion often points or forms secondary abscesses in deeper white matter.

MICROSCOPIC LESIONS Central portion contains degenerated PMNs and cellular debris; capsule is composed of collagenous fibrous tissue with blood vessels and mixed inflammatory cells; acute cerebritis in early abscesses.

COMPLICATIONS Increased intracranial pressure from edema around abscess; transtentorial or cerebellar herniation; rupture of abscess into ventricles or subarachnoid space; seizures are a long-term complication.

SIGNS AND SYMPTOMS Headache, often localized to side of infection; progressive neurologic deficits that develop rapidly or over several weeks; vomiting, progressive loss of consciousness due to increased pressure.

CLINICAL DIAGNOSIS AND OTHER CLINICAL FEATURES Signs in a patient with chronic lung infection, congenital heart disease, endocarditis, or chronic ear or sinus infection; fever is often absent; CT, MRI, radionuclide scans, angiography.

LABORATORY DIAGNOSIS Examination of CSF shows lymphocytosis and normal glucose; PMNs indicate abscess has leaked into ventricle; culture and sensitivity of abscess fluid aspirated surgically.

PROGNOSIS Usually fatal if untreated; with modern therapy, mortality is less than 20%.

THERAPY Specific antibiotic therapy; surgical resection or aspiration drainage; anticonvulsants.

OTHER INFORMATION Patients with congenital heart disease with a left-to-right shunt are particularly predisposed because the normal filtering action of the pulmonary vasculature is lost.

Cerebral Aneurysm

DESCRIPTION Saccular dilatation of a cerebral artery due to congenital defect of media; their importance is the propensity to rupture and cause subarachnoid hemorrhage.

DISEASE ENTITIES; SYNONYMS AND ACRONYMS Congenital aneurysm, saccular aneurysm, berry aneurysm, medial defect aneurysm; subarachnoid hemorrhage.

INCIDENCE Fairly common; causes 6–8% of strokes; most common nontraumatic cause of subarachnoid hemorrhage.

AGE Middle age; 40–60 years; males predominate in younger cases; females predominate in older cases.

ETIOLOGY, PATHOGENESIS, AND PREDISPOSING FACTORS Congenital defect in medial smooth muscle at bifurcations of cerebral arteries; aneurysm progressively enlarges into adulthood until it ruptures, usually during an episode of elevated blood pressure.

SITES INVOLVED Cerebral arteries at bifurcations; 40% at internal carotid complex, usually at posterior communicating; 20–30% middle cerebral; 30% anterior communicating; 5% posterior communicating; often multiple.

GROSS LESIONS Thin-walled, sac-like outpouching of artery, usually less than 1 cm, at crotch where arteries branch; laminated thrombus and calcification may be present; subarachnoid hemorrhage occurs with rupture.

MICROSCOPIC LESIONS Medial smooth muscle and internal elastic lamina are absent from wall of aneurysm, which is composed of fibrous tissue and may contain thrombus; defect, hemorrhage, inflammation are seen with rupture.

COMPLICATIONS Fatal subarachnoid hemorrhage; vasospasm causing fatal cerebral ischemia; dissection of blood into parenchyma and ventricles; an enlarged aneurysm may produce cranial nerve palsies due to pressure.

SIGNS AND SYMPTOMS Sudden onset of intense headache, nausea, and vomiting, photophobia, confusion, collapse, and coma; focal neurologic signs are sometimes present; neck rigidity.

CLINICAL DIAGNOSIS AND OTHER CLINICAL FEATURES As many as 50% present days or weeks prior to final rupture with severe headache and signs of leak; cerebral angiography, CT, and MRI scans for localization; CSF is grossly bloody and under pressure.

LABORATORY DIAGNOSIS Microscopic examination of CSF confirms blood; xanthochromia differentiates subarachnoid hemorrhage from blood in traumatic tap.

PROGNOSIS Generally poor; at least 50% mortality with subarachnoid hemorrhage; severe disability in survivors.

THERAPY Surgical ligation or clipping of aneurysm; nimodipine reduces cerebral ischemia due to vasospasm.

OTHER INFORMATION Congenital aneurysms are associated with polycystic kidney disease and arteriovenous malformation; they may rupture during sexual activity, weight-lifting, or straining with a bowel movement.

Cerebral Cortical Contusion

DESCRIPTION   Traumatic brain injury characterized by disruption of small cortical blood vessels with bleeding into the cortical gray matter; laceration is a related lesion where the brain substance is torn.

DISEASE ENTITIES; SYNONYMS AND ACRONYMS   Cerebral contusion; coup contusion; contrecoup contusion; cerebral laceration.

INCIDENCE   Common consequence of head injury.

AGE   Any age.

ETIOLOGY, PATHOGENESIS, AND PREDISPOSING FACTORS   Head impact causes skull to deform and strike and bruise the brain surface; alternatively, head in motion and suddenly stopped causes brain to impact inner surface of skull.

SITES INVOLVED   Cerebral cortex, most commonly inferior frontal and temporal; coup lesions occur when a moving object strikes the fixed head; contrecoup contusions occur when the moving head strikes a fixed object.

GROSS LESIONS   Bluish-red discoloration on surface with associated subarachnoid hemorrhage; cut sections show linear streaks of cortical hemorrhage perpendicular to surface; old lesions are yellow craters.

MICROSCOPIC LESIONS   Streak-like and perivascular hemorrhages in cortex; subsequent cortical necrosis with liquefaction, infiltration of macrophages laden with lipid debris, hemosiderin, and astrocytic gliosis.

COMPLICATIONS   Bleeding into cortex and white matter with severe lesions; cerebral edema leading to increased intracranial pressure, herniations, and death; post-traumatic epilepsy.

SIGNS AND SYMPTOMS   Disorientation, confusion, poor motor responses, prolonged unconsciousness following head injury; signs of increased intracranial pressure with neurologic deficits.

CLINICAL DIAGNOSIS AND OTHER CLINICAL FEATURES   A likely injury with head impacts of all kinds, especially MVAs and falls and an unconscious patient; other injuries are usually present; CT scans with contrast and MRI scans show the contusion.

LABORATORY DIAGNOSIS   Histologic examination shows the features of cerebral cortical hemorrhage and necrosis.

PROGNOSIS   Depends on extent of injury and secondary brain swelling; usually good with limited injury.

THERAPY   Intravenous mannitol, mechanical hyperventilation, and dexamethasone to reduce intracranial pressure.

OTHER INFORMATION   Concussion causes loss of consciousness but no anatomic lesion; diffuse axonal injury refers to diffuse white matter degeneration that occurs with head impacts that do not produce cortical contusions.

Cerebral Infarction

DESCRIPTION   Infarction of cerebrum due to arterial occlusion by thrombus superimposed on atherosclerosis or by embolus from the heart or carotid artery; variants are lacunar infarct and transient ischemic attack.

DISEASE ENTITIES; SYNONYMS AND ACRONYMS   Ischemic stroke; cerebrovascular disease; cerebrovascular accident (CVA); transient ischemic attack (TIA); lacunae.

INCIDENCE   Strokes are third most common cause of death; ischemic strokes are the most common type of stroke.

AGE   Most common in older age groups, usually 60–70 years.

ETIOLOGY, PATHOGENESIS, AND PREDISPOSING FACTORS   Atherosclerosis with superimposed thrombosis is most common; embolism from cardiac mural thrombi, valve vegetations, or ruptured carotid plaques; minor causes: vasculitis, hematologic diseases.

SITES INVOLVED   Cerebral infarct: occlusion of internal carotid or circle of Willis and its branches, especially middle cerebral artery; brainstem infarct: basilar occlusion; lacunar infarcts: small parenchymal arteries.

GROSS LESIONS   Hemorrhagic or pale; liquefactive necrosis, often in region of middle cerebral artery; old infarcts are cystic cavities without fibrosis; lacunae are small holes around basal ganglia.

MICROSCOPIC LESIONS   Early: hypereosinophilic neurons with nuclear pyknosis, PMN response, disintegration of parenchyma; later: foamy macrophages filled with lipid; old: astrocytic gliosis around cystic cavity.

COMPLICATIONS   Disability, dementia, and death; motor, sensory, and autonomic neurologic defects depending on site and extent of infarct; edema that aggravates ischemia, worsens symptoms, and causes herniation.

SIGNS AND SYMPTOMS   Sudden onset of hemiplegia, hemianesthesia, aphasia, deviation of head and eyes, visual and cognitive defects, primitive reflexes, urinary incontinence, cranial nerve defects, dysphagia, dysphonia.

CLINICAL DIAGNOSIS AND OTHER CLINICAL FEATURES   Neurologic exam: head and eyes deviate to side of infarct; ipsilateral cranial nerve defects, contralateral extremity defects; aphasia with dominant hemisphere involvement; CT and MRI scans.

LABORATORY DIAGNOSIS   Brain-specific isoenzymes of lactic dehydrogenase and creatine kinase are elevated; microbiologic cultures are important during long-term care because of frequent respiratory and urinary infections.

PROGNOSIS   Depends on size, site and number of infarcts; 15–50% mortality, worse with embolic infarcts.

THERAPY   Supportive medical therapy; preventative: aspirin for TIAs; anticoagulation; carotid endarterectomy.

OTHER INFORMATION   TIAs are symptoms lasting a few minutes to less than 24 hours; about 50% of cerebral infarcts are preceded by TIAs.

Epidural Hematoma

DESCRIPTION Localized collection of blood between the skull and dura mater, resulting from skull fracture that lacerates a branch of the middle meningeal artery.

DISEASE ENTITIES; SYNONYMS AND ACRONYMS Extradural hematoma; epidural hemorrhage.

INCIDENCE Fairly common complication of head trauma.

AGE Any age; usually young adults due to higher incidence of trauma.

ETIOLOGY, PATHOGENESIS, AND PREDISPOSING FACTORS Skull fracture, usually in the temporoparietal region, lacerates a branch of the middle meningeal artery; arterial bleeding separates the dura from the inner skull to form hematoma.

SITES INVOLVED Space between skull and dura, temporoparietal region; normally the dura is firmly attached to the inner skull; arterial bleeding separates the dura to produce the space occupied by the blood.

GROSS LESIONS Disc-shaped mass of fresh blood, 30–50 mL, between skull and dura; mass indents cerebral cortex; secondary lesions: cingulate and uncal herniations, midbrain hemorrhages.

MICROSCOPIC LESIONS Minimal changes in cerebral cortex underlying hematoma; herniated structures may be necrotic; mesencephalon and upper pons show focal hemorrhages.

COMPLICATIONS Herniations: cingulate gyrus under falx, uncus through tentorium; midbrain compression; vascular stagnation; ischemia of the medullary reticular formation leading to death.

SIGNS AND SYMPTOMS Mental confusion and disorientation developing within a few minutes or hours after head injury; fixed and dilated pupil on same side as injury (oculomotor palsy); systolic hypertension, bradycardia.

CLINICAL DIAGNOSIS AND OTHER CLINICAL FEATURES Suspected in temporoparietal skull fracture; unconsciousness after injury may be temporary or absent; consciousness and mentation decline over several hours; CT and MRI scans are diagnostic.

LABORATORY DIAGNOSIS Material evacuated from the hematoma and sent to the histopathology laboratory shows only fresh blood clot.

PROGNOSIS Progresses to death in 6–10 hours if left untreated; timely treatment is life-saving.

THERAPY Emergency evacuation of hematoma by burr holes.

OTHER INFORMATION Classically, the patient loses consciousness immediately after injury and then regains it for a lucid interval of 4–8 hours as the blood enlarges the space between skull and dura.

Gliomas

DESCRIPTION   Primary brain tumors arising from the neuroectoderm, specifically the neuroglial elements, exhibiting varying degrees of anaplasia and biologic behavior.

DISEASE ENTITIES; SYNONYMS AND ACRONYMS   Astrocytoma; juvenile pilocytic astrocytoma; glioblastoma multiforme; oligodendroglioma; ependymoma.

INCIDENCE   Gliomas constitute about half of primary brain tumors; astrocytoma and glioblastoma are most common.

AGE   Mostly adults; juvenile pilocytic astrocytoma and brain stem glioma are more common in children.

ETIOLOGY, PATHOGENESIS, AND PREDISPOSING FACTORS   Neoplastic disease of unknown etiology; effects of tumor are produced by infiltration or destruction of tissue, blockage of CSF flow, displacement of brain, and production of cerebral edema.

SITES INVOLVED   Cerebrum, optic nerve, pons, cerebellum; juvenile pilocytic astrocytoma occurs in the cerebellum; ependymoma arises from 4th ventricle or central spinal cord; astrocytoma also occurs in spinal cord.

GROSS LESIONS   Astrocytoma: poorly defined, infiltrating; juvenile pilocytic: cystic; glioblastoma: hemorrhagic, necrotic; oligodendroglioma: well-circumscribed, calcospherites; ependymoma: circumscribed, papillary.

MICROSCOPIC LESIONS   Gliomas resemble their cell of origin; astrocytoma: fibrillary, protoplasmic, gemistocytic, pilocytic, or anaplastic cells; glioblastoma: anaplastic, foci of necrosis surrounded by palisading.

COMPLICATIONS   Expanding mass compresses and displaces brain, leading to functional loss and fatal herniations; hydrocephalus due to blockage of CSF; increased intracranial pressure; seizures.

SIGNS AND SYMPTOMS   Headache, worse in morning; nausea, vomiting with increased intracranial pressure; mental, behavioral changes; seizures; focal neurologic defects; dilated nonreactive pupil with uncal herniation.

CLINICAL DIAGNOSIS AND OTHER CLINICAL FEATURES   Recent onset of seizures or headaches are likely to indicate tumor; frontal lobe tumors cause behavioral changes; CT, MRI, and radionuclide scans; x-ray may show calcifications in oligodendroglioma.

LABORATORY DIAGNOSIS   Histologic examination of biopsy; well-differentiated, diffusely infiltrating astrocytoma may look deceptively normal; glioblastoma is markedly cellular, pleomorphic, anaplastic, and focally necrotic.

PROGNOSIS   Well-differentiated gliomas: 40–80% 5 year survival; glioblastoma: less than 1-year survival.

THERAPY   Surgical resection; radiotherapy; chemotherapy.

OTHER INFORMATION   Astrocytomas are graded according to differentiation; highest grades are anaplastic astrocytoma and glioblastoma multiforme; with time, astrocytomas progress to higher grades, often to glioblastoma.

Hypoxic Encephalopathy

DESCRIPTION Widespread damage of the brain due to generalized deficiency of oxygen delivered to the brain, resulting in necrosis with a pattern depending on vascular anatomy and neuronal vulnerability.

DISEASE ENTITIES; SYNONYMS AND ACRONYMS Ischemic or postanoxic encephalopathy, global ischemia; laminar necrosis; watershed, boundary zone infarct; brain death.

INCIDENCE Common, especially after severe shock or cardiopulmonary resuscitation following cardiac arrest.

AGE Any age.

ETIOLOGY, PATHOGENESIS, AND PREDISPOSING FACTORS Decreased blood flow to brain (cardiac arrest, hypotension, mechanical asphyxia); decreased oxygen in blood (anemia, CO poisoning, lung disease, decreased inspired oxygen); cytochrome toxin (CN).

SITES INVOLVED Brain, particularly neurons; Sommer's sector of hippocampus and cerebellar Purkinje cells are most sensitive; parasagittal cerebral cortex in boundary between middle and anterior cerebral arteries.

GROSS LESIONS Laminar necrosis: line of discoloration and disintegration in deep cerebral cortex; watershed infarcts: small infarcts along the sagittal sinus; old lesions show loss of cortex in involved areas.

MICROSCOPIC LESIONS Changes range from frank infarcts to ischemic injury of neurons only; ischemic neurons are hypereosinophilic with pyknotic nuclei (red neurons); gliosis develops with time.

COMPLICATIONS Major neurologic deficits involving motor and cognitive functions; persistent vegetative state; brain death.

SIGNS AND SYMPTOMS After cardiopulmonary resuscitation from cardiac arrest or from episode of severe shock, the patient remains comatose and exhibits loss of various cerebral functions and cranial reflexes.

CLINICAL DIAGNOSIS AND OTHER CLINICAL FEATURES Course is determined by the amount of damage; deficits in pupillary, corneal, and oculovestibular reflexes indicate a poor prognosis; brain scan and cerebral angiography establish brain death.

LABORATORY DIAGNOSIS No specific tests; carbon monoxide poisoning should always be remembered as a cause of neurologic symptoms; carboxyhemoglobin saturation in blood can be easily determined on many blood gas analyzers.

PROGNOSIS Often poor, especially if cranial reflex deficits persist more than 24 hours.

THERAPY Rapid reversal of hypoxic or hypotensive condition; supportive; dextrorphan to block excitotoxins.

OTHER INFORMATION Respirator brain is a condition where a patient is brain dead and has no cerebral blood flow but is maintained on a respirator; this promotes autolysis of the brain.

Increased Intracranial Pressure

DESCRIPTION   Elevation of the CSF pressure above 15 mm Hg, caused by intracranial mass, cerebral edema, or increased volume of CSF within the cranial cavity (hydrocephalus); resulting in herniations of the brain.

DISEASE ENTITIES; SYNONYMS AND ACRONYMS   Elevated ICP; cerebral edema, brain swelling; communicating hydrocephalus, noncommunicating (obstructive) hydrocephalus.

INCIDENCE   Common response to trauma, infection, hemorrhage, infarct, tumor, toxins, ischemia, anoxia.

AGE   Any age; hydrocephalus in infants causes head enlargement due to nonfused sutures.

ETIOLOGY, PATHOGENESIS, AND PREDISPOSING FACTORS   Cerebral edema: increased extracellular or intracellular fluid due to cerebral insult; hydrocephalus: blockage of flow of CSF (noncommunicating), interference with CSF absorption (communicating).

SITES INVOLVED   Brain; particularly white matter in cerebral edema; aqueduct of Sylvius, third ventricle, foramina of Munro or Magendie are possible sites of obstruction causing hydrocephalus.

GROSS LESIONS   Cerebral edema: brain is swollen, gyri flattened, sulci compressed; hydrocephalus: ventricular system proximal to obstruction enlarges; subarachnoid scarring is seen with communicating hydrocephalus.

MICROSCOPIC LESIONS   Vacuolation of cells and/or interstitial tissue; halos around nuclei; separation of myelin sheaths; cerebral edema may be diffuse or localized to vicinity of tumor, abscess, infarct, or contusion.

COMPLICATIONS   Herniations: cingulate gyrus under falx; uncus under tentorium; cerebellar tonsils in foramen magnum; compression of medulla; ischemia and brain death due to vascular compression; Duret's hemorrhages.

SIGNS AND SYMPTOMS   Headaches, nausea, projectile vomiting, confusion, coma; papilledema; dilated and fixed pupil indicates compression of third nerve by transtentorial herniation of uncus of temporal lobe.

CLINICAL DIAGNOSIS AND OTHER CLINICAL FEATURES   Lumbar puncture (contraindicated in case of papilledema) with manometer reading; intracranial pressure transducer; CT, MRI, angiography, brain scan; absent cerebral blood flow indicates brain death.

LABORATORY DIAGNOSIS   No specific tests; CSF analysis, including glucose, protein, white cell count with differential, and microbiologic culture may indicate cause of the elevated ICP.

PROGNOSIS   Often poor; when ICP exceeds cerebral arterial pressure, global ischemia results in brain death.

THERAPY   Mannitol, dexamethasone, hyperventilation; ventriculoperitoneal shunting for hydrocephalus.

OTHER INFORMATION   Hydrocephalus causes marked dilatation of ventricles and loss of brain mass, mostly white matter; hydrocephalus ex vacuo is ventricular dilatation due to atrophy.

Intracerebral Hemorrhage

DESCRIPTION   Spontaneous bleeding into the substance of the brain, usually in the deep structures, most often occurring as a complication of hypertension.

DISEASE ENTITIES; SYNONYMS AND ACRONYMS   Spontaneous cerebral hemorrhage; cerebral hematoma; hypertensive hemorrhage; hemorrhagic stroke.

INCIDENCE   Common, but less common than ischemic stroke; decreasing incidence due to control of hypertension.

AGE   More common in older age groups; 60–70 years.

ETIOLOGY, PATHOGENESIS, AND PREDISPOSING FACTORS   Hypertensive injury of small parenchymal arteries and arterioles, which rupture and bleed; amyloid angiopathy, arteriovenous malformation, hematologic diseases, vasculitis, hemorrhagic infarcts.

SITES INVOLVED   Brain: most commonly in the basal ganglia-thalamus-deep cortical white matter region; less often in pons; least often in cerebellum; secondary rupture into ventricles is common.

GROSS LESIONS   Mass of blood dissects through parenchyma in deep structures of brain; if lesion dissects into ventricles, clotted blood forms cast of ventricles and may appear at foramina of Magendie and Luschka.

MICROSCOPIC LESIONS   Hypertensive changes: hyaline arteriolosclerosis, lipohyalinosis, Charcot-Bouchard aneurysms; amyloid angiopathy stains with Congo red; fresh blood with inflammatory reaction; later, hemosiderin.

COMPLICATIONS   Disability, neurologic deficits, and death; expanding blood mass causes transtentorial herniations; intraventricular, pontine, and cerebellar hemorrhages result in compression of medulla.

SIGNS AND SYMPTOMS   Sudden onset that may evolve over several hours; severe headache, vomiting, loss of consciousness, hemiplegia, hemianesthesia, hemianopsia, ataxia, abnormalities in eye movements.

CLINICAL DIAGNOSIS AND OTHER CLINICAL FEATURES   It is often difficult to differentiate an infarct from a small intracerebral hemorrhage because the symptoms and neurologic findings overlap; CT and MRI scans usually provide the correct diagnosis.

LABORATORY DIAGNOSIS   No specific tests; postmortem brain examination differentiates the major etiologies: hypertensive arteriolosclerosis, amyloid angiopathy, and vascular malformation.

PROGNOSIS   Altogether poor; worse than for infarcts; as high as 80% mortality.

THERAPY   Supportive, occasionally surgical evacuation of hematoma; prevention by control of hypertension.

OTHER INFORMATION   Use of anticoagulants in thrombotic or embolic infarcts may produce secondary brain hemorrhage arising from the infarct.

Medulloblastoma

DESCRIPTION   A highly malignant primary brain tumor of children originating from primitive neuroectodermal cells of the cerebellum; despite its aggressive behavior, it is sensitive to radiation therapy.

DISEASE ENTITIES; SYNONYMS AND ACRONYMS   Desmoplastic medulloblastoma.

INCIDENCE   Constitutes less than 5% of all brain tumors but 20–25% of brain tumors in children.

AGE   Predominantly children under 10 years; a minority occur after 10 years.

ETIOLOGY, PATHOGENESIS, AND PREDISPOSING FACTORS   Neoplastic disease of unknown etiology; arises from undifferentiated neuroectodermal cells, possibly the fetal granular layer, which are capable of both glial and neuronal differentiation.

SITES INVOLVED   Brain; cerebellum, most often in the midline vermis; medulloblastomas in young adults are more likely to arise laterally; fourth ventricle is invaded and tumor cells seed throughout the CSF.

GROSS LESIONS   Light gray mass arising from the cerebellum, invading the cerebellar peduncles and fourth ventricle; often produces a diffuse coating on the leptomeningeal surfaces of brain and spinal cord.

MICROSCOPIC LESIONS   Sheets of crowded, small, oval hyperchromatic cells with scant cytoplasm; glial differentiation is indicated by spindle-shaped cell forms; neuronal differentiation by Homer-Wright pseudorosettes.

COMPLICATIONS   Dissemination throughout the CSF to produce multiple sites of tumor growth on the surface of brain or spinal cord; hydrocephalus due to obstruction of CSF flow in the fourth ventricle or aqueduct.

SIGNS AND SYMPTOMS   Headache, vomiting and ataxia in a child; papilledema.

CLINICAL DIAGNOSIS AND OTHER CLINICAL FEATURES   Signs of increased intracranial pressure in a child; tumor needs to be differentiated from glioma; CT, MRI, and radionuclide scans localize the lesion.

LABORATORY DIAGNOSIS   Histologic examination of tumor biopsy; densely cellular undifferentiated tumor is most likely medulloblastoma; finding of tumor cells in CSF examination indicates CSF dissemination.

PROGNOSIS   Rapidly fatal if untreated; 10-year survival of 50% with aggressive therapy.

THERAPY   Primarily surgical resection and radiation therapy; less importantly, chemotherapy.

OTHER INFORMATION   Astrocytoma, medulloblastoma, and ependymoma are, in order, the most common intracranial tumors in children, and the cerebellum is the most common site.

Meningioma

DESCRIPTION   Primary intracranial neoplasm arising from cells of the arachnoid granulations, characterized by slow growth, benign behavior, and expansile rather than infiltrative growth pattern.

DISEASE ENTITIES; SYNONYMS AND ACRONYMS   Syncytial, fibroblastic, and transitional meningioma; angioblastic meningioma; papillary, microcystic meningioma.

INCIDENCE   Constitute 20% of primary intracranial tumors; slightly more common in females.

AGE   Adult ages, usually middle ages.

ETIOLOGY, PATHOGENESIS, AND PREDISPOSING FACTORS   Neoplastic proliferation of arachnoidal cells; no defined etiology or predisposing conditions.

SITES INVOLVED   Surface of brain and expanding into brain, usually in the front half of the head; cerebral convexity, falx, sphenoid wing, olfactory groove, cerebellopontine angle, foramen magnum, spinal cord.

GROSS LESIONS   Well-circumscribed, rounded, firm, gritty mass that arises superficially and grows into the brain by expansion; indents and compresses brain but does not invade it.

MICROSCOPIC LESIONS   Several histologic variants (syncytial, fibroblastic, transitional); usually a whorling pattern of meningothelial cells with regular nuclei, indistinct cytoplasm, and psammoma bodies.

COMPLICATIONS   Compression and displacement of brain, leading to neurologic deficits and producing herniations; seizures; invasion of overlying bone complicates surgical resection.

SIGNS AND SYMPTOMS   Headaches, seizures; neurologic deficits involving motor, sensory, and visual functions; bitemporal hemianopsia; exophthalmos; cranial nerve defects; anosmia; spinal cord defects.

CLINICAL DIAGNOSIS AND OTHER CLINICAL FEATURES   Due to characteristic slow growth, symptoms develop over a long period; seizures are the most likely presentation; CT, MRI, radionuclide scans; bone invasion causes hyperostosis that is seen on x-ray.

LABORATORY DIAGNOSIS   Histologic examination of resected tumor or biopsy; the gross appearance is so characteristic that microscopic examination is largely for confirmation.

PROGNOSIS   Good, for those tumors that can be resected; slow recurrence for those partially removed.

THERAPY   Surgical resection; because it does not invade the brain, the tumor can often be completely removed.

OTHER INFORMATION   An occasional meningioma grows rapidly and invades the brain; these often show microscopic features similar to fibrosarcoma and are labeled malignant meningiomas.

Meningitis

DESCRIPTION   Inflammation of the pia, arachnoid, and subarachnoid space, often caused by bacterial infection; other causes are viral, tubercular, syphilitic, fungal infections and chemical irritation.

DISEASE ENTITIES; SYNONYMS AND ACRONYMS   Leptomeningitis; acute bacterial or pyogenic meningitis; viral, aseptic, lymphocytic meningitis; TB, fungal meningitis.

INCIDENCE   Fairly common; 25,000 new cases every year in US; most of these in children.

AGE   Infants: *E. coli, group B Strep.; children:* H. influenzae; *adults:* N. meningitidis, S. pneumoniae.

ETIOLOGY, PATHOGENESIS, AND PREDISPOSING FACTORS   Bacteria spread to meninges most commonly via blood, often from another infection (pneumonia, sinus, nasopharyngeal or middle ear infection); skull fractures, especially basilar, allow direct spread.

SITES INVOLVED   Surface of brain and spinal cord; pia, arachnoid and subarachnoid space; purulent exudate accumulates in sulci around vessels and concentrates in basal cisterns and Sylvian fissure.

GROSS LESIONS   Creamy pale yellow or greenish exudate covers surface of brain, within the leptomeningeal membranes, producing thickening and opacification of the leptomeninges.

MICROSCOPIC LESIONS   PMNs infiltrate pial and arachnoidal membranes and walls of blood vessels; exudate does not extend into surface of brain parenchyma; in nonbacterial meningitis, inflammatory cells are lymphocytes.

COMPLICATIONS   Seizures; cerebral edema with herniations; leptomeningeal fibrosis, hydrocephalus; sepsis, Waterhouse-Friderichsen syndrome; sagittal sinus thrombosis with parasagittal infarcts.

SIGNS AND SYMPTOMS   Headache, stiff neck, vomiting, fever developing over one to several days; declining consciousness progressing to coma; Kernig's and Brudzinski's signs; bulging fontanel in infants.

CLINICAL DIAGNOSIS AND OTHER CLINICAL FEATURES   Signs and symptoms are usually highly suspicious; lumbar puncture is required for confirmation; atypical presentations occur in infants and elderly patients; MRI and CT scans to exclude other lesions.

LABORATORY DIAGNOSIS   CSF analysis for cells, protein, and glucose; microbiologic culture; bacterial meningitis: PMNs, low glucose; viral: lymphocytes, normal glucose; TB or fungal: lymphocytes, low glucose.

PROGNOSIS   Fairly good with treatment, although 10–20% of patients have residual neurologic deficits.

THERAPY   Specific IV antibiotics; steroids; mannitol for cerebral edema; anticonvulsants for seizures.

OTHER INFORMATION   Lymphocytic infiltrates characterize viral and fungal meningitis; TB meningitis is granulomatous; India ink prep shows organism in cryptococcal meningitis, which affects immunosuppressed patients.

Multiple Sclerosis

DESCRIPTION A chronic demyelinating disease of unknown etiology, characterized by acute exacerbations and remissions of disease activity, producing progressive motor, sensory, and visual neurologic deficits.

DISEASE ENTITIES; SYNONYMS AND ACRONYMS MS; classical Charcot type of MS; Marburg variant (acute progressive MS); Devic's disease (neuromyelitis optica).

INCIDENCE Fairly common; 50–100 cases per 100,000 in temperate climates; much less common in tropics.

AGE Presents initially between ages 20–40 years and progresses thereafter over next 5–20 years.

ETIOLOGY, PATHOGENESIS, AND PREDISPOSING FACTORS Unproved hypotheses: viral infection, aberrant cellular immune reaction, genetic factors; more common with HLA-A3, B7, and DR2; plaques of demyelination interfere with axon conduction.

SITES INVOLVED White matter of cerebrum, brain stem, cerebellum, and spinal cord; plaques are distributed randomly but are more frequent in paraventricular regions; myelin is destroyed but the axons are preserved.

GROSS LESIONS Distinctive lesion is the plaque, which is a discrete, sharply bordered gray discoloration of the white matter, usually less than 2 cm in diameter; acute lesions are pink and edematous.

MICROSCOPIC LESIONS Loss of myelin in plaques, abruptly starting at plaque margin; axons are preserved; oligodendrocytes are sparse; rim of lymphocytes around edges of plaque; lipid-laden macrophages; astrocytic gliosis.

COMPLICATIONS Progression of neurologic deficits; motor defects leading to severe disability; visual disturbances and blindness; intellectual deterioration; urinary dysfunction with incontinence and infections.

SIGNS AND SYMPTOMS Episodes of a variety of motor, sensory, and visual disturbances that partially resolve but usually recur; visual system is particularly vulnerable (optic neuritis, ophthalmoplegia).

CLINICAL DIAGNOSIS AND OTHER CLINICAL FEATURES Diagnostic features include episodic attacks with remissions and evidence that CNS lesions affect several sites; evoked-potential abnormalities; CT and particularly MRI scans visualize plaques.

LABORATORY DIAGNOSIS Elevation of IgG/albumin ratio in CSF; oligoclonal bands of immunoglobulin in CSF but not serum; myelin basic protein (MBP) may be present in CSF during acute attacks.

PROGNOSIS Usually poor, leading to severe neurologic disability; time course is variable and unpredictable.

THERAPY Nonspecific supportive; avoidance of fatigue and stress; corticosteroids or ACTH for acute attacks.

OTHER INFORMATION Experimental allergic encephalomyelitis, a model of MS, is produced by injecting myelin basic protein; certain viral proteins have sequence homology with MBP, suggesting an autoimmune etiology for MS.

Nerve Sheath Tumors

DESCRIPTION   Primary tumors of nerves, arising from Schwann cells; most are benign and consist of schwannomas and neurofibromas; multiple neurofibromas are characteristic of von Recklinghausen's neurofibromatosis.

DISEASE ENTITIES; SYNONYMS AND ACRONYMS   Neurofibroma, plexiform neurofibroma; schwannoma, neurilemmoma.

INCIDENCE   Solitary neurofibromas are fairly common; neurofibromatosis is less common (35/100,000 population).

AGE   Adults; 40–50 years; neurofibromatosis presents much earlier.

ETIOLOGY, PATHOGENESIS, AND PREDISPOSING FACTORS   Most tumors are spontaneous neoplasms arising from nerve sheaths without known etiology; von Recklinghausen's disease is an autosomal dominant genetic disease.

SITES INVOLVED   Nerves, cranial and peripheral; spinal nerve roots; acoustic neuroma is a schwannoma of the 8th nerve; neurofibromas involve peripheral nerves and small cutaneous nerves; GI tract; retroperitoneum.

GROSS LESIONS   Schwannoma: encapsulated tumor attached to periphery of nerve; neurofibroma: diffuse enlargement of nerves (plexiform), soft skin nodules, nodules in the gastrointestinal tract, retroperitoneal mass.

MICROSCOPIC LESIONS   Schwannoma: spindle cells with a tightly interlaced pattern (Antoni A) and Verocay bodies, or a loose pattern (Antoni B); neurofibroma: loose pattern of spindle cells with intermixed nerve fibers.

COMPLICATIONS   Acoustic neuroma: compression of brain stem and cerebellum, herniations due to increased intracranial pressure; intraspinal tumors: spinal compression; others: sarcomatous transformation.

SIGNS AND SYMPTOMS   Acoustic neuroma: deafness, tinnitus; intraspinal tumor: radicular pain; distal nerves: enlargement, mass, sensory or motor dysfunction; cutaneous: soft dermal or subcutaneous nodule.

CLINICAL DIAGNOSIS AND OTHER CLINICAL FEATURES   Acoustic neuroma: CT, MRI scans, neurosurgical exploration; intraspinal: myelography, MRI, exploration; cutaneous lesions: neurofibroma is one possible diagnosis of skin nodule, confirmed by biopsy.

LABORATORY DIAGNOSIS   Histologic examination of lesion; microscopic pattern and location of tumor with respect to nerve distinguishes neurofibroma from schwannoma; mitotic count and nuclear pleomorphism indicate sarcoma.

PROGNOSIS   Depends on site and type; schwannomas are often resectable; neurofibromas may be unresectable.

THERAPY   Surgical resection.

OTHER INFORMATION   Features of von Recklinghausen's disease: bilateral acoustic neuromas, multiple cutaneous neurofibromas, plexiform neurofibromas, cafe-au-lait spots, Lisch nodules on iris, gliomas, meningiomas, etc.

Neural Tube Defects

DESCRIPTION Congenital failure of the embryonic neural tube to close, either caudally to produce variants of spina bifida, or rostrally to produce anencephaly; both may be present simultaneously.

DISEASE ENTITIES; SYNONYMS AND ACRONYMS Anencephaly, encephalocele, craniorachischisis; spina bifida, meningocele, meningomyelocele, myelocele, rachischisis.

INCIDENCE Common; anencephaly is the most common congenital defect of brain, occurring in 1/1000 live births.

AGE Dorsal fusion of the neural folds occurs between embryonic days 16 and 30; defect is seen at birth.

ETIOLOGY, PATHOGENESIS, AND PREDISPOSING FACTORS Failure of fusion at either end of neural tube; polygenetic and maternal factors; advanced maternal age, diabetes, nutritional and vitamin deficiencies; exposure to certain drugs or radiation.

SITES INVOLVED Anencephaly: brain and skull bones; spina bifida, meningocele, meningomyelocele: lumbosacral region skin, vertebral arches, spinal meninges, and caudal spinal cord.

GROSS LESIONS Anencephaly: small lump of neural tissue sits in large defect in skull; spina bifida and variants: varying defects of skin and vertebral arches with herniation of meninges and/or spinal cord.

MICROSCOPIC LESIONS Anencephaly: islands of immature glial and neural elements, vascular channels (cerebrovasculosa); spina bifida and variants: structures usually form normally despite defect.

COMPLICATIONS Anencephaly: incompatible with life; spina bifida: meningeal infection, hydrocephalus that presents after closure of the spinal defect, spinal nerve damage with urinary and orthopedic problems.

SIGNS AND SYMPTOMS Anencephaly and herniations of the spinal cord and meninges are obvious at birth; in spina bifida occulta, only the vertebral arches are defective and the condition is asymptomatic.

CLINICAL DIAGNOSIS AND OTHER CLINICAL FEATURES Presents no diagnostic challenge; spina bifida occulta may show a dimple or tuft of hair at lumbosacral region and is diagnosed by x-rays; in utero diagnosis by ultrasonography.

LABORATORY DIAGNOSIS Prenatal diagnosis by alphafetoprotein screening of maternal serum; measurement of alphafetoprotein in amniotic fluid; cytogenetic studies.

PROGNOSIS Nil for anencephaly; varying degrees of disability and shortened lifespan with spin bifida.

THERAPY Repair of spinal defect; ventriculoperitoneal shunt for hydrocephalus; urologic and orthopedic care.

OTHER INFORMATION Arnold-Chiari malformation, the downward displacement of the cerebellum and medulla through the foramen magnum, often accompanies meningomyelocele and is associated with hydrocephalus.

Parkinson's Disease

DESCRIPTION A degenerative disorder of the basal ganglia, particularly the dopaminergic neurons of the substantia nigra, characterized by muscular rigidity, disturbances of motor function, and resting tremor.

DISEASE ENTITIES; SYNONYMS AND ACRONYMS Idiopathic parkinsonism, paralysis agitans, postencephalitic parkinsonism.

INCIDENCE Fairly common; approximately 100 per 100,000 population.

AGE Initial symptoms start in late middle age and become progressively severe; peak onset 60–70 years.

ETIOLOGY, PATHOGENESIS, AND PREDISPOSING FACTORS Many cases occurred after the 1914–1918 influenza pandemic; a metabolite of MPTP causes parkinsonism in drug abusers; dopamine depletion in basal ganglia produces extrapyramidal dysfunction.

SITES INVOLVED Dopaminergic neurons are depleted in the substantia nigra and locus ceruleus; dopamine is depleted in the corpus striatum, which receives the projections of the substantia nigra neurons.

GROSS LESIONS Absence of brown/black pigment (melanin) from the substantia nigra, usually bilateral.

MICROSCOPIC LESIONS Pigmented neurons in substantia nigra are decreased; residual neurons contain Lewy bodies, which are eosinophilic cytoplasmic inclusions with halos, composed of dense aggregates of neurofilaments.

COMPLICATIONS Voluntary movements progressively deteriorate and muscular rigidity increases to the point of total disability culminating in death.

SIGNS AND SYMPTOMS Slowing in voluntary movement (bradykinesia), "cog-wheel" rigidity of limb muscles, facial immobility, rhythmic "pill-rolling" tremor at rest.

CLINICAL DIAGNOSIS AND OTHER CLINICAL FEATURES The complex of physical signs is fairly diagnostic; cerebrovascular disease and adverse drug reactions (e.g., phenothiazines) may produce similar findings.

LABORATORY DIAGNOSIS No specific tests; the diagnosis is a clinical one to be confirmed or rejected at autopsy.

PROGNOSIS Poor, but the time course of the progressive neurologic deterioration is prolonged.

THERAPY L-DOPA (levodopa); anticholinergics and antihistaminics; amantadine; bromocriptine.

OTHER INFORMATION Striatonigral degeneration, Shy-Drager syndrome, and supranuclear palsy present with parkinsonian disturbances; postencephalitic parkinsonism has neurofibrillary tangles rather than Lewy bodies.

Peripheral Neuropathies

DESCRIPTION   A group of diseases of the peripheral nerves that may affect all nerves (polyneuropathy) or just one (mononeuropathy) to cause motor, sensory, and autonomic dysfunction.

DISEASE ENTITIES; SYNONYMS AND ACRONYMS   Polyneuropathy, mononeuropathy multiplex; polyneuritis, Landry-Guillain-Barré syndrome; diabetic, alcoholic neuropathy.

INCIDENCE   Common; diabetic neuropathy is most common, followed by alcoholic neuropathy.

AGE   Usually adults; hereditary neuropathies present in childhood or teens.

ETIOLOGY, PATHOGENESIS, AND PREDISPOSING FACTORS   Metabolic (diabetes, uremia, hypothyroidism, porphyria); inflammatory or immune (Landry-Guillain-Barré); alcoholism; nutritional deficiencies; ischemia; toxic; amyloidosis; infections; hereditary.

SITES INVOLVED   Peripheral nerves; axons and/or myelin; primary involvement may involve the axon (axonopathic) or the myelin (demyelinating); neuropathy can also be due to motor neuron disease (neuronopathic).

GROSS LESIONS   Nerve lesions are not apparent, except in leprosy, which produces grossly visible enlargement of the peripheral nerves; severe motor neuropathy produces muscular atrophy.

MICROSCOPIC LESIONS   Metabolic, nutritional, and ischemic neuropathies show a mixture of segmental demyelination and axonal degeneration; inflammatory types show mononuclear infiltrates and segmental demyelination.

COMPLICATIONS   Distracting sensations in the extremities; motor weakness leading to disability; respiratory paralysis with pneumonia and/or respiratory failure in worst cases.

SIGNS AND SYMPTOMS   Distal muscle weakness; sensory loss with glove-stocking distribution; paresthesias, pains along distribution of nerves; autonomic dysfunction: constipation, postural hypotension, impotence.

CLINICAL DIAGNOSIS AND OTHER CLINICAL FEATURES   Etiology is often idiopathic; electromyography differentiates demyelination from axon degeneration; fasciculations indicate denervation; Guillain-Barré syndrome is preceded by viral illness.

LABORATORY DIAGNOSIS   In Guillain-Barré polyneuritis, CSF protein is markedly elevated and there are but a few lymphocytes in the CSF; there may be slight elevation of CSF protein in diabetic neuropathy.

PROGNOSIS   Usually good with control of underlying disease; Guillain-Barré has about a 5% mortality.

THERAPY   Control of diabetes, hypothyroidism, alcoholism; nutritional supplementation; ventilatory support.

OTHER INFORMATION   Hereditary motor sensory neuropathies: Charcot-Marie-Tooth: AD, affects lower leg; Dejerine-Sottas: AR, onset in early childhood; Refsum's disease: AR, multisystemic, accumulation of phytanic acid.

Subdural Hematoma

DESCRIPTION Traumatic lesion characterized by accumulation of blood between dura and arachnoid, caused by laceration of bridging veins; results in displacement of brain and cerebral herniations.

DISEASE ENTITIES; SYNONYMS AND ACRONYMS Acute subdural hematoma, subacute subdural hematoma, chronic subdural hematoma, subdural hygroma.

INCIDENCE A common consequence of head injury.

AGE Any age; elderly with cerebral atrophy are more susceptible to chronic subdural hematoma.

ETIOLOGY, PATHOGENESIS, AND PREDISPOSING FACTORS Head injury, especially when moving head strikes fixed object; shearing forces lacerate bridging veins that drain into dural sinuses; venous bleeding accumulates in the subdural space.

SITES INVOLVED Subdural space, often bilateral; hematoma becomes attached to the dura but not to the brain; outer membrane forms between the dura and hematoma; inner membrane forms on the surface of the hematoma.

GROSS LESIONS Acute: fresh nonadherent blood clot, cerebral cortex compressed, sulci remain wide; chronic: altered blood encased in thick adherent brown membranes, compressed and flattened cortex, sulci compressed.

MICROSCOPIC LESIONS Acute: fresh blood clot, organization occurs after several days; chronic: outer membrane composed of granulation and fibrous tissue with hemosiderin, inner membrane shows fibrous tissue only.

COMPLICATIONS Compression and displacement of brain with secondary herniations; acute hematoma causes brain swelling and increased intracranial pressure; chronic hematoma causes greater displacement of brain.

SIGNS AND SYMPTOMS Confusion, disorientation, obtundation, coma, weakness on contralateral side, headaches, seizures; onset may be gradual after injury: several hours, days, or even weeks in the case of chronic subdural.

CLINICAL DIAGNOSIS AND OTHER CLINICAL FEATURES Acute subdural hematoma is usually linked to obvious head injury (often MVA or fall on head); injury causing chronic subdural hematoma is often slight or forgotten; CT, MRI scans are diagnostic.

LABORATORY DIAGNOSIS Histologic examination of hematoma is used to estimate the age of the injury by the presence and appearance of the inner and outer membranes.

PROGNOSIS Depends on therapy; poor if untreated or if coma develops.

THERAPY Craniotomy with drainage of hematoma and resection of membranes if present.

OTHER INFORMATION Chronic subdural hematoma develops insidiously in elderly and chronic alcoholics, and often progressively enlarges due to rebleeding; symptoms may be mistaken for other causes of dementia.

Viral Encephalitis

DESCRIPTION   Infection of CNS by a neurotropic virus; currently herpes simplex virus (HSV), arboviruses, and human immunodeficiency virus (HIV) cause most cases; acute and slow viral infections are recognized.

DISEASE ENTITIES; SYNONYMS AND ACRONYMS   Herpes encephalitis; St. Louis, Eastern, and Western equine encephalitis; HIV encephalitis, AIDS encephalopathy.

INCIDENCE   Depends on etiology; arbovirus infections are epidemic; up to 50% of AIDS cases have encephalopathy.

AGE   Generally any age; neonate: HSV-2; older child, adult: HSV-1; polio was usually a childhood disease.

ETIOLOGY, PATHOGENESIS, AND PREDISPOSING FACTORS   Neonate acquires HSV infection by passage through infected birth canal; other HSV encephalitis are caused by reactivation of latent virus; arbovirus infections: mosquito transmission.

SITES INVOLVED   Brain; HSV infects neurons and glia, particularly in temporal lobes; HSV-1 lies dormant in the gasserian ganglion; arbovirus infections are usually diffuse cortical and sometimes meningeal infections.

GROSS LESIONS   Severe cases show diffuse brain swelling and regions of subarachnoid and parenchymal hemorrhage; with HSV encephalitis, there is hemorrhagic necrosis of the temporal lobes.

MICROSCOPIC LESIONS   Lymphocytic infiltrates in perivascular cuffs, focal necrosis, neuronophagia, glial nodules; nuclear or cytoplasmic inclusions are specific features; perivascular multinucleated giant cells in AIDS.

COMPLICATIONS   Irreversible neurologic damage; dementia, behavioral problems and personality change; residual seizures; cerebral edema with herniations, death; spinal paralysis (polio); parkinsonism (von Economo's).

SIGNS AND SYMPTOMS   Headache, fever, nausea, vomiting, seizures, fading consciousness, focal neurologic deficits including hemiparesis, visual disturbances, personality changes, ataxia, tremors.

CLINICAL DIAGNOSIS AND OTHER CLINICAL FEATURES   Suspected by the diffuse cerebral involvement and signs of infection; arbovirus infections are seasonal; HSV infections are related to genital or oral infections; EEG; CT, MRI scans; technetium scan.

LABORATORY DIAGNOSIS   Brain biopsy is most specific; histologic exam may show inclusion bodies; immunofluorescence; EM; viral culture; viral etiology is proved in only a third of cases.

PROGNOSIS   HSV: high mortality (70%), improved with therapy (30%); arbovirus: mortality ranges 2–20% or more.

THERAPY   Acyclovir for herpes encephalitis; supportive therapy for arbovirus and other encephalitis.

OTHER INFORMATION   Progressive multifocal leukoencephalopathy is an opportunistic viral (JC virus) encephalitis that produces demyelination by infecting and killing oligodendrocytes; infected cells show inclusions.

Bibliography

Pathology
Rubin E. and Farber J.L., Editors
J.B. Lippincott Company, 1988

Robbins Pathologic Basis of Disease
Fourth Edition
Cotran R.S., Kumar V., and Robbins S.L.
W.B. Saunders Company, 1989

Boyd's Textbook of Pathology
Ninth Edition
Ritchie A.C.
Lea and Febiger, 1990

Oxford Textbook of Pathology
McGee J.O. et. al., Editors
Oxford University Press, 1992

Greenfield's Neuropathology
Fifth Edition
Adams J.H. and Duchen L.W., Editors
Oxford University Press, 1992

Scientific American Medicine
Rubenstein E. and Federman D.D., Editors
Scientific American, 1978–1992

Harrison's Principles of Internal Medicine
Twelfth Edition
Wilson J.D. et. al., Editors
McGraw-Hill, 1991

Control of Communicable Diseases in Man
Fifteenth Edition
Benenson A.S., Editor
American Public Health Association, 1990

Index